PUBLIC HEALTH IN THE 21ST CENTURY

RESPONDING TO HIV/AIDS: NATIONAL STRATEGIES, PLANS AND PROGRAMS

PUBLIC HEALTH IN THE 21ST CENTURY

Additional books in this series can be found on Nova's website under the Series tab.

Additional E-books in this series can be found on Nova's website under the E-books tab.

HIV/AIDS - MEDICAL, SOCIAL AND PSYCHOLOGICAL ASPECTS

Additional books in this series can be found on Nova's website under the Series tab.

Additional E-books in this series can be found on Nova's website under the E-books tab.

PUBLIC HEALTH IN THE 21ST CENTURY

RESPONDING TO HIV/AIDS: NATIONAL STRATEGIES, PLANS AND PROGRAMS

LAWRENCE T. JENSEN
EDITOR

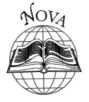

Nova Science Publishers, Inc.
New York

Copyright © 2011 by Nova Science Publishers, Inc.

All rights reserved. No part of this book may be reproduced, stored in a retrieval system or transmitted in any form or by any means: electronic, electrostatic, magnetic, tape, mechanical photocopying, recording or otherwise without the written permission of the Publisher.

For permission to use material from this book please contact us:
Telephone 631-231-7269; Fax 631-231-8175
Web Site: http://www.novapublishers.com

NOTICE TO THE READER

The Publisher has taken reasonable care in the preparation of this book, but makes no expressed or implied warranty of any kind and assumes no responsibility for any errors or omissions. No liability is assumed for incidental or consequential damages in connection with or arising out of information contained in this book. The Publisher shall not be liable for any special, consequential, or exemplary damages resulting, in whole or in part, from the readers' use of, or reliance upon, this material. Any parts of this book based on government reports are so indicated and copyright is claimed for those parts to the extent applicable to compilations of such works.

Independent verification should be sought for any data, advice or recommendations contained in this book. In addition, no responsibility is assumed by the publisher for any injury and/or damage to persons or property arising from any methods, products, instructions, ideas or otherwise contained in this publication.

This publication is designed to provide accurate and authoritative information with regard to the subject matter covered herein. It is sold with the clear understanding that the Publisher is not engaged in rendering legal or any other professional services. If legal or any other expert assistance is required, the services of a competent person should be sought. FROM A DECLARATION OF PARTICIPANTS JOINTLY ADOPTED BY A COMMITTEE OF THE AMERICAN BAR ASSOCIATION AND A COMMITTEE OF PUBLISHERS.

Additional color graphics may be available in the e-book version of this book.

Library of Congress Cataloging-in-Publication Data

Responding to HIV/AIDS : national strategies, plans, and programs / editor, Lawrence T. Jensen.
  p. ; cm.
Includes bibliographical references and index.
  ISBN 978-1-61324-618-4 (hardcover : alk. paper) 1. AIDS (Disease)--Government policy--United States. 2. HIV infections--Government policy--United States. I. Jensen, Lawrence T.
  [DNLM: 1. Acquired Immunodeficiency Syndrome--United States. 2. HIV Infections--United States. 3. Health Policy--United States. WC 503]
  RA643.83.R47 2011
  362.196'9792--dc23
                                                                        2011015637

Published by Nova Science Publishers, Inc. ✦ New York

CONTENTS

Preface		vii
Chapter 1	National HIV/AIDS Strategy for the United States *Office of the President of the United States*	1
Chapter 2	National HIV/AIDS Strategy: Federal Implementation Plan *Office of the President of the United States*	47
Chapter 3	Community Ideas for Improving the Response to the Domestic HIV Epidemic: A Report on a National Dialogue on HIV/AIDS *White House Office of National Aids Policy*	79
Chapter 4	The Ryan White HIV/AIDS Program *Judith A. Johnson*	141
Chapter 5	Housing for Persons Living with HIV/AIDS *Libby Perl*	161
Chapter 6	Federal and State Efforts to Identify Infected Individuals and Connect Them to Care *The United States Government Accountability Office*	183
Index		217

PREFACE

This book explores the strategies, plans and programs for responding to the HIV/AIDS epidemic in the United States. When one of our fellow citizens becomes infected with the human immunodeficiency virus (HIV) every 9-1/2 minutes, the epidemic affects all Americans. Without treatment, the virus slowly debilitates a person's immune system until they succumb to illness. The epidemic has claimed the lives of nearly 600,000 Americans and affects many more. We have the knowledge and tools needed to slow the spread of HIV infection and improve the health of people living with HIV. Despite this potential, however, the public's sense of urgency associated with combating the epidemic appears to be declining. Unless we take bold actions, we face a new era of rising infections, greater challenges in serving people living with HIV, and higher health care costs.

Chapter 1- When one of our fellow citizens becomes infected with the human immunodeficiency virus (HIV) every nine-and-a-half minutes, the epidemic affects all Americans. It has been nearly thirty years since the first cases of HIV garnered the world's attention. Without treatment, the virus slowly debilitates a person's immune system until they succumb to illness. The epidemic has claimed the lives of nearly 600,000 Americans and affects many more. Our Nation is at a crossroads. We have the knowledge and tools needed to slow the spread of HIV infection and improve the health of people living with HIV. Despite this potential, however, the public's sense of urgency associated with combating the epidemic appears to be declining. In 1995, 44 percent of the general public indicated that HIV/AIDS was the most urgent health problem facing the Nation, compared to only 6 percent in March 2009. While HIV transmission rates have been reduced substantially over time and people with HIV are living longer and more productive lives, approximately 56,000 people become infected each year and more Americans are living with HIV than ever before. Unless we take bold actions, we face a new era of rising infections, greater challenges in serving people living with HIV, and higher health care costs.

Chapter 2- President Obama committed to developing a National HIV/AIDS Strategy with three primary goals: 1) reducing the number of people who become infected with HIV, 2) increasing access to care and optimizing health outcomes for people living with HIV, and 3) reducing HIV-related health disparities. To accomplish these goals, we must undertake a more coordinated, vigorous national response to the HIV epidemic.

Chapter 3- At the beginning of his Administration, President Obama instructed the White House Office of National AIDS Policy (ONAP), a component of the Domestic Policy Council (DPC), to develop a National HIV/AIDS Strategy and re-focus our response to the HIV epidemic in the United States. The President directed that this strategy be driven by three primary goals:

Prevent new HIV infections.

Increase access to care and optimize health outcomes.

Reduce HIV-related health disparities.

Chapter 4- The Ryan White HIV/AIDS Program makes federal funds available to metropolitan areas and states to assist in health care costs and support services for individuals and families affected by the human immunodeficiency virus (HIV) or acquired immune deficiency syndrome (AIDS). The Ryan White program currently serves more than half a million low-income people with HIV/AIDS in the United States; 33% of those served are uninsured, and an additional 56% are underinsured. The program is administered by the Health Resources and Services Administration (HRSA) of the Department of Health and Human Services (HHS). Its statutory authority is Title XXVI of the Public Health Service (PHS) Act, originally enacted in 1990.

Chapter 5- Since the beginning of the acquired immunodeficiency syndrome (AIDS) epidemic in the early 1980s, many individuals living with the disease have had difficulty finding affordable, stable housing. As individuals become ill, they may find themselves unable to work, while at the same time facing health care expenses that leave few resources to pay for housing. In addition, many of those persons living with AIDS struggled to afford housing even before being diagnosed with the disease. The financial vulnerability associated with AIDS, as well as the human immunodeficiency virus (HIV) that causes AIDS, results in a greater likelihood of homelessness among persons living with the disease. At the same time, those who are homeless may be more likely to engage in activities through which they could acquire or transmit HIV. Further, recent research has indicated that those individuals living with HIV who live in stable housing have better health outcomes than those who are homeless or unstably housed, and that they spend fewer days in hospitals and emergency rooms.

Chapter 6- Of the estimated 1.1 million Americans living with HIV, not all are aware of their HIV-positive status. Timely testing of HIV-positive individuals is important to improve health outcomes and to slow the disease's transmission. It is also important that individuals have access to HIV care after being diagnosed, but not all diagnosed individuals are receiving such care.

The Centers for Disease Control and Prevention (CDC) provides grants to state and local health departments for HIV prevention and collects data on HIV. In 2006, CDC recommended routine HIV testing for all individuals ages 13- 64. The Health Resources and Services Administration (HRSA) provides grants to states and localities for HIV care and services.

In: Responding to HIV/AIDS
Editor: Lawrence T. Jensen

ISBN: 978-1-61324-618-4
© 2011 Nova Science Publishers, Inc.

Chapter 1

NATIONAL HIV/AIDS STRATEGY FOR THE UNITED STATES[*]

Office of the President of the United States

The White House
Washington, July 13, 2010

Thirty years ago, the first cases of human immunodeficiency virus (HIV) garnered the world's attention. Since then, over 575,000 Americans have lost their lives to AIDS and more than 56,000 people in the United States become infected with HIV each year. Currently, there are more than 1.1 million Americans living with HIV. Moreover, almost half of all Americans know someone living with HIV.

Our country is at a crossroads. Right now, we are experiencing a domestic epidemic that demands a renewed commitment, increased public attention, and leadership. Early in my Administration, I tasked the Office of National AIDS Policy with developing a National HIV/AIDS Strategy with three primary goals: 1) reducing the number of people who become infected with HIV; 2) increasing access to care and improving health outcomes for people living with HIV; and, 3) reducing HIV-related health disparities. To accomplish these goals, we must undertake a more coordinated national response to the epidemic. The Federal government can't do this alone, nor should it. Success will require the commitment of governments at all levels, businesses, faith communities, philanthropy, the scientific and medical communities, educational institutions, people living with HIV, and others.

Countless Americans have devoted their lives to fighting the HIV epidemic and thanks to their tireless work we've made real inroads. People living with HIV have transformed how we engage community members in setting policy, conducting research, and providing services. Researchers have produced a wealth of information about the disease, including a number of critical tools and interventions to diagnose, prevent, and treat HIV. Successful

---

[*] This is an edited, reformatted and augmented version of an Office of the President of the United States publication, dated July, 2010.

prevention efforts have averted more than 350,000 new infections in the United States. And health care and other services providers have taught us how to provide quality services in diverse settings and develop medical homes for people with HIV. This moment represents an opportunity for the Nation. Now is the time to build on and refocus our existing efforts to deliver better results for the American people.

I look forward to working with Congress, State, tribal, and local governments, and other stakeholders to support the implementation of a Strategy that is innovative, grounded in the best science, focuses on the areas of greatest need, and that provides a clear direction for moving forward together.

VISION FOR THE NATIONAL HIV/AIDS STRATEGY

"The United States will become a place where new HIV infections are rare and when they do occur, every person, regardless of age, gender, race/ethnicity, sexual orientation, gender identity or socio-economic circumstance, will have unfettered access to high quality, life-extending care, free from stigma and discrimination"

EXECUTIVE SUMMARY

When one of our fellow citizens becomes infected with the human immunodeficiency virus (HIV) every nine-and-a-half minutes, the epidemic affects all Americans. It has been nearly thirty years since the first cases of HIV garnered the world's attention. Without treatment, the virus slowly debilitates a person's immune system until they succumb to illness. The epidemic has claimed the lives of nearly 600,000 Americans and affects many more.[1] Our Nation is at a crossroads. We have the knowledge and tools needed to slow the spread of HIV infection and improve the health of people living with HIV. Despite this potential, however, the public's sense of urgency associated with combating the epidemic appears to be declining. In 1995, 44 percent of the general public indicated that HIV/AIDS was the most urgent health problem facing the Nation, compared to only 6 percent in March 2009.[2] While HIV transmission rates have been reduced substantially over time and people with HIV are living longer and more productive lives, approximately 56,000 people become infected each year and more Americans are living with HIV than ever before.[3,4] Unless we take bold actions, we face a new era of rising infections, greater challenges in serving people living with HIV, and higher health care costs.[5]

President Obama committed to developing a National HIV/AIDS Strategy with three primary goals: 1) reducing the number of people who become infected with HIV, 2) increasing access to care and optimizing health outcomes for people living with HIV, and 3) reducing HIV-related health disparities. To accomplish these goals, we must undertake a more coordinated national response to the HIV epidemic. The Strategy is intended to be a concise plan that will identify a set of priorities and strategic action steps tied to measurable outcomes. Accompanying the Strategy is a Federal Implementation Plan that outlines the specific steps to be taken by various Federal agencies to support the high-level priorities outlined in the Strategy. This is an ambitious plan that will challenge us to meet all of the goals that we set. The job, however, does not fall to the Federal Government alone, nor should it. Success will require the commitment of all parts of society, including State, tribal and local governments, businesses, faith communities, philanthropy, the scientific and medical communities, educational institutions, people living with HIV, and others. The vision for the National HIV/AIDS Strategy is simple:

The United States will become a place where new HIV infections are rare and when they do occur, every person, regardless of age, gender, race/ethnicity, sexual orientation, gender identity or socioeconomic circumstance, will have unfettered access to high quality, life-extending care, free from stigma and discrimination.

REDUCING NEW HIV INFECTIONS

More must be done to ensure that new prevention methods are identified and that prevention resources are more strategically concentrated in specific communities at high risk for HIV infection. Almost half of all Americans know someone living with HIV (43 percent in 2009).[6] Our national commitment to ending the HIV epidemic, however, cannot be tied only to our own perception of how closely HIV affects us personally. Just as we mobilize the country to support cancer prevention and research whether or not we believe that we are at high risk of cancer, or just as we support investments in public education whether or not we have children, success at fighting HIV calls on all Americans to help us sustain a longterm effort against HIV. While anyone can become infected with HIV, some Americans are at greater risk than others. This includes gay and bisexual men of all races and ethnicities, Black men and women, Latinos and Latinas, people struggling with addiction, including injection drug users, and people in geographic hot spots, including the United States South and Northeast, as well as Puerto Rico and the U.S. Virgin Islands. By focusing our efforts in communities where HIV is concentrated, we can have the biggest impact in lowering all communities' collective risk of acquiring HIV.

We must also move away from thinking that one approach to HIV prevention will work, whether it is condoms, pills, or information. Instead, we need to develop, evaluate, and implement effective prevention strategies and combinations of approaches including efforts such as expanded HIV testing (since people who know their status are less likely to transmit HIV), education and support to encourage people to reduce risky behaviors, the strategic use of medications and biomedical interventions (which have allowed us, for example, to nearly eliminate HIV transmission to newborns), the development of vaccines and microbicides, and the expansion of evidence-based mental health and substance abuse prevention and treatment programs. It is essential that all Americans have access to a shared base of factual information about HIV. The Strategy also provides an opportunity for working together to advance a public health approach to sexual health that includes HIV prevention as one component. To successfully reduce the number of new HIV infections, there must be a concerted effort by the public and private sectors, including government at all levels, individuals, and communities, to:

- Intensify HIV prevention efforts in communities where HIV is most heavily concentrated.
- Expand targeted efforts to prevent HIV infection using a combination of effective, evidence-based approaches.
- Educate all Americans about the threat of HIV and how to prevent it.

INCREASING ACCESS TO CARE AND IMPROVING HEALTH OUTCOMES FOR PEOPLE LIVING WITH HIV

As a result of our ongoing investments in research and years of clinical experience, people living with HIV can enjoy long and healthy lives. To make this a reality for everyone, it is important to get people with HIV into care early after infection to protect their health and reduce their potential of transmitting the virus to others. For these reasons, it is important that all people living with HIV are well supported in a regular system of care. The Affordable Care Act, which will greatly expand access to insurance coverage for people living with HIV, will provide a platform for improvements in health care coverage and quality. High risk pools are available immediately. High risk pools will be established in every state to provide coverage to uninsured people with chronic conditions. In 2014, Medicaid will be expanded to all lower income individuals (below 133% of the Federal poverty level, or about $15,000 for a single individual in 2010) under age 65. Uninsured people with incomes up to 400% of the Federal poverty level (about $43,000 for a single individual in 2010) will have access to Federal tax credits and the opportunity to purchase private insurance coverage through competitive insurance exchanges. New consumer protections will better protect people with private insurance coverage by ending discrimination based on health status and pre-existing conditions. Gaps in essential care and services for people living with HIV will continue to need to be addressed along with the unique biological, psychological, and social effects of living with HIV. Therefore, the Ryan White HIV/AIDS Program and other Federal and State HIV-focused programs will continue to be necessary after the law is implemented. Additionally, improving health outcomes requires continued investments in research to develop safer, cheaper, and more effective treatments. Both public and private sector entities must take the following steps to improve service delivery for people living with HIV:

- Establish a seamless system to immediately link people to continuous and coordinated quality care when they are diagnosed with HIV.
- Take deliberate steps to increase the number and diversity of available providers of clinical care and related services for people living with HIV.
- Support people living with HIV with co-occurring health conditions and those who have challenges meeting their basic needs, such as housing.

REDUCING HIV-RELATED HEALTH DISPARITIES

The stigma associated with HIV remains extremely high and fear of discrimination causes some Americans to avoid learning their HIV status, disclosing their status, or accessing medical care.[7] Data indicate that HIV disproportionately affects the most vulnerable in our society—those Americans who have less access to prevention and treatment services and, as a result, often have poorer health outcomes. Further, in some heavily affected communities, HIV may not be viewed as a primary concern, such as in communities experiencing problems with crime, unemployment, lack of housing, and other pressing issues. Therefore, to successfully address HIV, we need more and better community-level approaches that integrate HIV prevention and care with more comprehensive responses to social service needs. Key steps for the public and private sector to take to reduce HIV-related health disparities are:

- Reduce HIV-related mortality in communities at high risk for HIV infection.
- Adopt community-level approaches to reduce HIV infection in high-risk communities.
- Reduce stigma and discrimination against people living with HIV.

ACHIEVING A MORE COORDINATED NATIONAL RESPONSE TO THE HIV EPIDEMIC IN THE UNITED STATES

The Nation can succeed at meeting the President's goals. It will require the Federal Government and State, tribal and local governments, however, to do some things differently. Foremost is the need for an unprecedented commitment to collaboration, efficiency, and innovation. We also must be prepared to adjust course as needed. This Strategy is intended to complement other related efforts across the Administration. For example, *the President's Emergency Plan for AIDS Relief (PEPFAR)* has taught us valuable lessons about fighting HIV and scaling up efforts around the world that can be applied to the domestic epidemic. The President's National Drug Control Strategy serves as a blueprint for reducing drug use and its consequences, and the Federal Strategic Plan to Prevent and End Homelessness focuses efforts to reduce homelessness and increase housing security. The White House Office of National AIDS Policy (ONAP) will work collaboratively with the Office of National Drug Control Policy and other White House offices, as well as relevant agencies to further the goals of the Strategy. The Strategy is intended to promote greater investment in HIV/AIDS, but this is not a budget document. Nonetheless, it will inform the Federal budget development process within the context of the fiscal goals that the President has articulated. The United States currently provides more than $19 billion in annual funding for domestic HIV prevention, care, and research, and there are constraints on the magnitude of any potential new investments in the Federal budget. The Strategy should be used to refocus our existing efforts and deliver better results to the American people within current funding levels, as well as to highlight the need for additional investments. Our national progress will require sustaining broader public commitment to HIV, and this calls for more regular communications to ensure transparency about whether we are meeting national goals. Key steps are to:

- Increase the coordination of HIV programs across the Federal government and between federal agencies and state, territorial, tribal, and local governments.
- Develop improved mechanisms to monitor and report on progress toward achieving national goals.

This Strategy provides a basic framework for moving forward. With government at all levels doing its part, a committed private sector, and leadership from people living with HIV and affected communities, the United States can dramatically reduce HIV transmission and better support people living with HIV and their families.

INTRODUCTION

It has been nearly thirty years since the first cases of human immunodeficiency virus (HIV) garnered the world's attention. Without treatment, the virus slowly debilitates a person's immune system until they succumb to illness. The epidemic has claimed the lives of nearly 600,000 Americans and affects many more.[8] Our Nation is at a crossroads: the urgency associated with combating the epidemic appears to be declining as people with HIV live longer and more productive lives. In 1995, 44 percent of the general public indicated that HIV/AIDS was the most urgent health problem facing the Nation, compared to only six percent in March 2009.[9] Approximately 56,000 people become infected each year, and more than 1.1 million Americans are living with HIV.[10,11], Unless we take bold actions, however, we anticipate a new era of rising infections and even greater challenges in serving people living with HIV.[12]

President Obama committed to developing a National HIV/AIDS Strategy with three primary goals:

- Reducing the number of people who become infected with HIV;
- Increasing access to care and optimizing health outcomes for people living with HIV; and,
- Reducing HIV-related health disparities.

To accomplish these goals, we must achieve a more coordinated national response to the HIV epidemic.

Where Things Stand: HIV in the United States

Although the United States has accomplished many successes in fighting HIV, much more needs to be done to curb the epidemic. Research has produced a wealth of information about HIV disease, including a number of critical tools and interventions to diagnose, prevent, and treat HIV infection. HIV transmission rates have been dramatically reduced in the United States and people with HIV are living healthier and more productive lives than ever before. Nevertheless, much more needs to be done. With more than one million Americans living with HIV, there are more people in need of testing, prevention, and treatment services than at any point in history, and ongoing research efforts are needed to find a cure for HIV/AIDS and continue to develop improved prevention tools and effective treatments. The Strategy cannot succeed without continued and sustained progress in biomedical and behavioral research.

The challenges we face are sobering:

- Approximately one in five people living with HIV are unaware of their status, placing them at greater risk for spreading the virus to others.[13]
- Roughly three-fourths of HIV/AIDS cases in the United States are among men, the majority of whom are gay and bisexual men.[14,15]
- One-fourth of Americans living with HIV are women, and the disease disproportionately impacts women of color. The HIV diagnosis rate for Black

women is more than 19 times the rate for White women.[16,17]
- Racial and ethnic minorities are disproportionately represented in the HIV epidemic and die sooner than Whites.[18,19]
- The South and Northeast, along with Puerto Rico and the U.S. Virgin Islands, are disproportionately impacted by HIV.[20]
- One quarter of new HIV infections occur among adolescents and young adults (ages 13 to 29).[21]
- Twenty-four percent of people living with HIV are 50 or older, and 15 percent of new HIV/AIDS cases occur among people in this age group.[22]

Development of the National HIV/AIDS Strategy

Since taking office, the Obama Administration has worked to engage the public to evaluate what we are doing right and identify new approaches that will strengthen our response to the domestic epidemic. The White House Office of National AIDS Policy (ONAP), a component of the Domestic Policy Council, has been tasked with leading the effort to develop a national strategy. Throughout the process, ONAP has taken steps to engage as many Americans as possible to hear their ideas for making progress in the fight against HIV. ONAP's outreach included hosting 14 HIV/AIDS Community Discussions with thousands of people across the United States, reviewing suggestions from the public via the White House website, conducting a series of expert meetings on several HIV-specific topics, and working with Federal and community partners who organized their own meetings to support the development of a national strategy. A report summarizing public recommendations for the strategy, entitled Community Ideas for Improving the Response to the Domestic HIV Epidemic, was published in April 2010.[23]

To develop the Strategy, ONAP convened a panel of Federal officials from across government to assist in reviewing the public recommendations, assessing the scientific evidence for or against various recommendations, and making their own recommendations for the Strategy. ONAP also has contracted with the Institute of Medicine to examine several key policy issues.

This document provides a roadmap to move the Nation forward in responding to the domestic HIV epidemic. It is not intended to be a comprehensive list of all activities needed to address HIV/AIDS in the United States, but is intended to be a concise plan that identifies a set of priorities and strategic action steps tied to measurable outcomes. The National HIV/AIDS Strategy outlines top-line priorities. Additional details on the specific actions that the Federal Government will take to implement its part of the Strategy are included in a Federal Implementation Plan. This is an ambitious plan that will challenge us to meet all of the goals that we set. Both the National HIV/AIDS Strategy and the Federal Implementation Plan may be accessed at www.WhiteHouse.gov/ONAP.

The job of implementing the National HIV/AIDS Strategy, however, does not fall to the Federal Government alone, nor should it. Success will require the commitment of all parts of society, including State, tribal and local governments, businesses, faith communities, philanthropy, the scientific and medical communities, educational institutions, people living with HIV, and others.

REDUCING NEW HIV INFECTIONS

Plan to Lower New HIV Infections at-a-Glance

There have been many successes in preventing HIV, but more must be done. In order to reduce HIV incidence, we must:

- Intensify HIV prevention efforts in communities where HIV is most heavily concentrated.
- Expand targeted efforts to prevent HIV infection using a combination of effective, evidence-based approaches.
- Educate all Americans about the threat of HIV and how to prevent it.

Anticipated Results

By 2015

- Lower the annual number of new infections by 25 percent;

To achieve this incidence goal, it will require our Nation to:

- Reduce the HIV transmission rate, which is a measure of annual transmissions in relation to the number of people living with HIV, by 30 percent; and,
- Increase from 79 percent to 90 percent the percentage of people living with HIV who know their serostatus.

The Opportunity

Within a few short years in the 1980s, HIV went from an unknown condition to an epidemic that was infecting more than 130,000 people annually.[24] The United States succeeded in mounting a response that involved affected communities, businesses, the public sector, foundations, pharmaceutical companies, scientific, medical, and public health professionals, faith communities, and others. These collective efforts were important for helping to reduce HIV infection rates. By 2000, the number of Americans becoming infected each year had fallen to an estimated 56,300.[25] Activities that contributed to our success in reducing HIV infections include:

- HIV testing: HIV testing has enabled individuals with HIV to become aware of their health status and to take appropriate precautions to preserve their health. Moreover, studies show that individuals diagnosed with HIV take steps to reduce the likelihood of transmitting HIV to others.
- Effective screening of the blood supply: Early in the epidemic, people contracted HIV through blood transfusions, but because of government research and the

implementation of effective blood screening procedures, HIV transmission through blood transfusion is very rare.[26,27]

- Screening and treating expectant mothers during pregnancy: Government-sponsored research in the 1990s demonstrated that taking antiretroviral medication prevents HIV transmission from mother to child during pregnancy and delivery. Cases declined from an estimated 1,650 a year in 1991 to fewer than 200 per year by 2004.[28]
- Minimizing infections from injection drug use: Comprehensive, evidence-based drug prevention and treatment strategies have contributed to reducing HIV infections. In 1993, injection drug users comprised [31] percent of AIDS cases nationally compared to 17 percent by 2007.[29] Studies show that comprehensive prevention and drug treatment programs, including needle exchange, have dramatically cut the number of new HIV infections among people who inject drugs by 80 percent since the mid-1990s.[30, 31, 32]
- Advances in HIV therapies: HIV medications can extend the length and quality of life for infected individuals, and lower the amount of the virus circulating in a person's body, thereby reducing their risk of transmitting HIV to others.[33]

Because of these and other prevention efforts, the annual number of new infections has not risen despite a growing number of people living with HIV, and thus, a larger pool of people capable of transmitting HIV to others (Figure 1). Unless we mount more intensive prevention efforts and keep innovating to develop more and better prevention methods, the number of new HIV infections will likely rise.[34]

The following are challenges that must be overcome:

- Too many people living with HIV are unaware of their status: An estimated 21 percent of people with HIV in the United States do not know their status.[35] Studies show that people who do not know that they are HIV-positive are more likely to engage in risk behaviors associated with HIV transmission.[36] Some of these individuals are already accessing health care services, but opportunities to diagnose them are being missed.[37]
- Access to HIV prevention is too limited: HIV prevention services have never been sufficient to reach all people at risk for HIV. Since Federal resources are limited and many States have reduced HIV prevention budgets in response to the economic downturn, we need to do a better job of evaluating and allocating existing resources based on their demonstrated health impact.
- Insufficient access to care: HIV medications not only improve the health of the individual, they also reduce their infectiousness, reducing their risk of transmitting HIV to others. An estimated one-third of people living with HIV in the United States are not in care.[38] Large numbers of uninsured and underinsured people with HIV mean that not everyone has sufficient access to HIV therapy.
- Diminished public attention: Media and public attention to the HIV epidemic has waned. The Kaiser Family Foundation found that in 2009, only 45 percent of respondents in a poll of the general public said that they had heard "some" or "a lot" about the problems of AIDS in the United States in the last year, compared to 70

percent of respondents in 2004.39 Because HIV is treatable, many people now think that it is no longer a public health emergency.

HIV infection is preventable. Allowing the number of new infections to rise or remain the same imposes costs on the country because the lifetime cost of treating HIV is estimated to be approximately $355,000 per person.40 If we do not substantially reduce HIV incidence in the United States, the numbers of people living with HIV and the cost of their care will continue to grow. We need to get better results from existing resources, and promote new investments from Federal, State, tribal, and local governments, as well as philanthropy, businesses, and community resources to achieve the goals that we set.

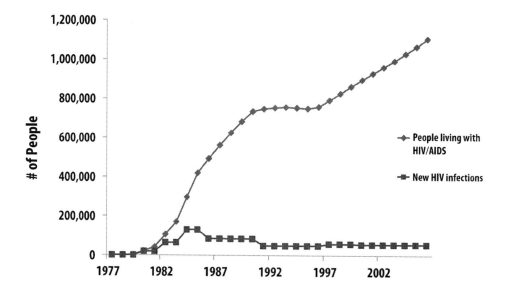

Sources: Hall et al, JAMA, 2008; and MMWR, October 3, 2008.

Figure 1. Estimates of Annual HIV Infections and People Living with HIV/AIDS (1977-2006).

Steps to be Taken

There are three critical steps that we must take to reduce HIV infections:

1. Intensify HIV prevention efforts in communities where HIV is most heavily concentrated.
2. Expand targeted efforts to prevent HIV infection using a combination of effective, evidence-based approaches.
3. Educate all Americans about the threat of HIV and how to prevent it.

Anticipated Results

By working together, we hope to meet the following benchmarks by 2015:[41]

- Lower the annual number of new infections by 25 percent (from 56,300 to 42,225);
- Reduce the HIV transmission rate, which is a measure of annual transmissions in relation to the number of people living with HIV, by 30 percent (from 5 persons infected each year per 100 people with HIV to 3.5 persons infected each year per 100 people with HIV); and,
- Increase from 79 percent to 90 percent the percentage of people living with HIV who know their serostatus (from 948,000 to 1,080,000 people).

Recommended Actions

Step 1. Intensify HIV Prevention Efforts in the Communities where HIV is Most Heavily Concentrated

In the beginning of the HIV epidemic, there was widespread fear that the epidemic would spread to the general population. The public heard about growing infection rates and that HIV had spread to all parts of the country. While this is true, nearly three decades later, the U.S. epidemic has not run the course that was previously feared. In contrast to HIV epidemics in sub-Saharan Africa and parts of Asia where nearly all sexually active adults are at high risk of becoming infected, HIV cases in the United States are concentrated in specific locations and populations.[42] More must be done to ensure that prevention resources are more strategically concentrated in specific communities at high risk for HIV infection.

Almost half of all Americans know someone living with HIV (43 percent in 2009), but our national commitment to ending the HIV epidemic cannot be tied only to perceptions of how closely HIV affects us personally.[43] All Americans have a stake in preventing HIV transmission and need to remain invested in sustaining our collective efforts to reduce HIV transmission. By intensifying our efforts in communities where HIV is concentrated, however, we can have the biggest impact that will lower all communities' collective risk of acquiring HIV infection. Just as we mobilize the country to support cancer prevention and research whether or not we believe that we are at high risk of cancer and we support public education whether or not we have children, fighting HIV requires widespread public support to sustain a long-term effort. *Not every person or group has an equal chance of becoming infected with HIV* Yet, for many years, too much of our Nation's response has been conducted as though everyone is equally at risk for HIV infection.

Stopping HIV transmission requires that we focus more intently on the groups and communities where the most cases of new infections are occurring (Figure 2). These numbers alone, however, do not give a complete picture of which populations are at greatest relative risk.

Figure 3 shows how the number of new infections in the high-risk groups listed in Figure 2 compares to the total size of each population. Estimating the size of some high-risk populations is challenging and group sizes may be imprecise. Nevertheless, it is clear that some communities are heavily disproportionately impacted compared to others. While we must focus most heavily on those groups with the largest numbers of new infections (Figure 2), the estimated relative risk of infection helps us to better understand disparities among these populations and how to prioritize efforts between and within groups (Figure 3). Further, some groups may be at very high risk of infection in relation to their group size, but they contribute relatively few cases to national totals of new infections.

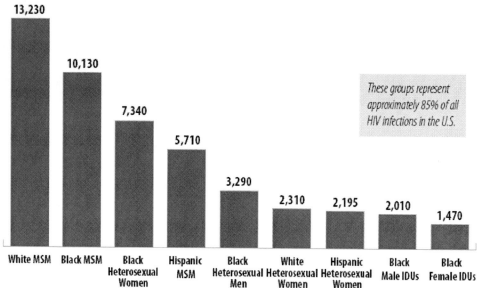

Sources: MMWR, October 3, 2008 and MMWR, June 5, 2009 with the addition of incidence data for Puerto Rico based on an analysis by Holtgrave, D., Johns Hopkins Bloomberg School of Public Health. For this analysis, all Puerto Rico cases were classified as Hispanic. Chart based upon CDC, HIV Prevention in the United States at a Critical Crossroads, 2009. MSM = men who have sex with men (gay and bisexual men) and IDUs = injection drug users.

Figure 2. Numbers of Annual HIV Infections by High-Risk Groups (2006).

For example, Figure 3 shows that Black male and female injection drug users are at the greatest risk for new HIV infection relative to their population size, but, as indicated in Figure 2, they represent a small fraction of new infections each year among the highest risk groups. Some other groups not shown here may be at high risk of infection in relation to their population size, but they contribute fewer cases to national totals of new infections (e.g. Latino[44] injection drug users).

At a time of limited resources, we must re-orient our efforts by giving much more attention and resources to the following populations at highest risk of HIV infection:

- *Gay and bisexual men*: According to the Centers for Disease Control and Prevention, gay men comprise approximately 2 percent of the U.S. population, but 53 percent of new infections.[45] Among gay men, White gay men constitute the greatest number of new infections, but Black and Latino gay men are at disproportionate risk for infection;[46]
- *Black men and women:* Black men and women represent only 13 percent of the population, but account for 46% of people living with HIV.[47] Among Blacks, gay and bisexual men are at greatest risk for HIV infection followed by women, and

heterosexual men.[48] One study of five major cities found that nearly 50 percent of all Black gay and bisexual men were HIV-positive.[49] Sixty-four percent of all women living with HIV/AIDS are Black.[50]

- *Latinos and Latinas:* According to the CDC, the rate of new AIDS diagnoses among Latino men is three times that of White men, and the rate among Latinas is five times that of White women.[51] Gay and bisexual men represent the greatest proportion of HIV cases among Latinos followed by heterosexual Latinas.[52]

- *Substance abusers:* People who inject drugs are a relatively small share of the U.S. population, but they are disproportionately represented in the HIV epidemic. It is estimated that there are about 1 million injection drug users (IDUs), but injection drug use accounts for approximately 16 percent of new HIV infections in the United States.[53,54] Although Figure 2 reflects new HIV cases among injection drug users, use of non-injection drugs such as methamphetamine, amyl nitrites and other drugs are also associated with sexual transmission of HIV infection and should be targeted with prevention efforts.[55,56,57]

Many individuals in these groups may not engage in greater risk behaviors than others, but they still can be more likely to become infected with HIV. Research has shown that the higher risk for these groups is associated with the sheer number of HIV-positive persons in the communities where they live. As a result, any instance of risk behavior carries a far greater likelihood of infection than other communities with fewer cases of HIV.

Thus, unprotected sex even once for individuals in some communities carries a greater risk of HIV infection than for individuals in other communities.[58,59] The Northeast and the South, as well as Puerto Rico and the U.S. Virgin Islands, are more impacted by HIV than other parts of the country.[60,61]

Women and men have different biological, psychological, and cultural factors that increase their vulnerability to infection and disease progression. Additional research is needed into the unique factors that place women at risk for HIV infection. Since most infections among women occur through heterosexual sex, their risk is predicated on the risk behaviors of their male partners. This raises complex policy and research questions, as negotiating safer sexual practices can be especially challenging for women who may be vulnerable to physical violence, or who may be emotionally or economically dependent on men.[62] Given the extreme disparities in infection rates among Black women and Latinas when compared to White women, it is also important to consider the unique factors that place them at higher risk for infection. One such issue, although certainly not the only one, relates to a higher proportion of injection drug use by their male partners than in other communities.[63] Another issue involves trying to assess the effect of incarceration on these communities and the impact it has on HIV transmission.

Although the available data suggests that relatively few infections occur in prison settings, there is evidence that some people with HIV who had received medical care while incarcerated have difficulty accessing HIV medications upon release—affecting their health and potentially increasing the likelihood that they will transmit HIV.[64,65,66] High rates of incarceration within certain communities can also be destabilizing. When large numbers of men are incarcerated, the gender imbalance in the communities they leave behind can fuel HIV transmissions by increasing the likelihood that the remaining men will have multiple,

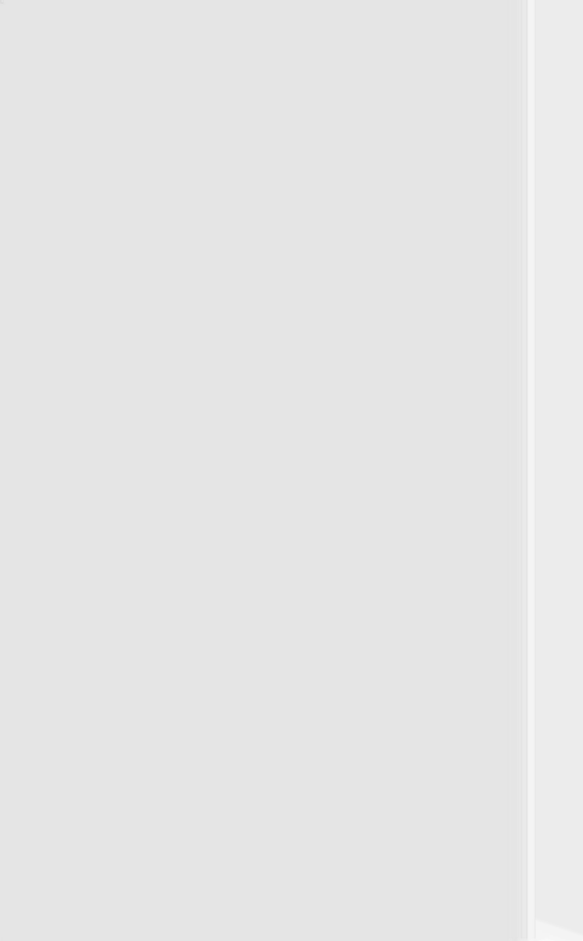

In addition, when the size of the population is taken into account, American Indians and Alaska Natives (AI/AN) have ranked third behind Blacks and Latinos in rates of HIV/AIDS diagnoses.[69] Although we must focus our national efforts in those communities with the highest numbers of new infections, targeted surveillance efforts must continue to be supported in localities with concentrations of AAPI and Native American communities.

It is clear that African Americans overall and gay and bisexual men (irrespective of race or ethnicity) continue to bear the brunt of HIV infections in the United States. In recent years, policy makers, community leaders and others have begun to mobilize responses to HIV among African Americans. Black Americans represent 13 percent of the U.S. population, but 46 percent of the estimated 1.1 million people living with HIV in the United States are Black.[70] AIDS cases among African Americans surpassed AIDS cases among Whites in 1994 and have steadily increased.[71] Blacks comprise the greatest proportion of HIV/AIDS cases across many transmission categories, including among women, heterosexual men, injection drug users, and infants. HIV/AIDS case rates among Black women are almost twenty times higher than among White women.[72] What is sometimes less recognized is the extent to which the HIV epidemic among African Americans remains concentrated among Black gay men, who comprise the single largest group of African Americans living with HIV.[73] Fighting HIV among African Americans is not mutually exclusive with fighting HIV among gay and bisexual men. Efforts to reduce HIV among Blacks must confront the epidemic among Black gay and bisexual men as forcefully as existing efforts to confront the epidemic among other groups. These overlapping communities both need intensive efforts to stem HIV infection.

Gay and bisexual men have comprised the largest proportion of the HIV epidemic in the United States since the first cases were reported in the 1980s, and that has not changed. They still comprise the greatest proportion of infections nationally. Although not reflected in Figures 2 or 3 because of small numbers, gay and bisexual men also represent the greatest proportion of HIV cases in the AAPI community and in AI/AN communities.[74,75] Given the starkness and the enduring nature of the disparate impact on gay and bisexual men, it is important to significantly reprioritize resources and attention on this community. *The United States cannot reduce the number of HIV infections nationally without better addressing HIV among gay and bisexual men.* Our national commitment to this population has not always reached a level of HIV prevention funding reflective of their risk.[76] Even though gay and bisexual men comprise only two percent of the U.S. population (4 percent of men):

- Gay and bisexual men of all races are the only group in the United States where the estimated number of new HIV infections is rising annually.[77]
- They are 44 to 86 times more likely to become infected with HIV than other men, and 40 to 77 times more likely to become infected than women.[78]
- Approximately one-half of the 1.1 million persons living with HIV in the United States are gay and bisexual men, and they account for the majority (53 percent) of new HIV infections each year.[79]
- High rates of HIV among gay men are found not only in large urban areas. More than half of all AIDS cases diagnosed in the United States are among gay and bisexual men irrespective of town or city size.[80]

As with gay and bisexual men, transgender individuals are also at high risk for HIV infection. Some studies have found that as many as 30 percent of transgender individuals are HIV-positive.[81] Yet, historically, efforts targeting this specific population have been minimal.

The burden of addressing the HIV epidemic among gay and bisexual men and transgender individuals does not rest with the government alone. Early in the epidemic, the lesbian, gay, bisexual and transgender (LGBT) community developed its own education campaigns and institutions to reduce HIV infection in the wake of inaction by government and other institutions. Continuing these efforts is important to our success. Despite our earlier achievements, CDC reports that HIV diagnoses among young gay men (ages 13-24) of all races and ethnicities rose between 2001 and 2006.[82]

Recommended Actions

To refocus our HIV prevention efforts, the following actions are needed:

1.1. Allocate public funding to geographic areas consistent with the epidemic: Governments at all levels should ensure that HIV prevention funding is allocated consistent with the latest epidemiological data and is targeted to the highest prevalence populations and communities.
1.2. Target high-risk populations: Federal agencies should develop new mechanisms for ensuring that grant funding to State and local health departments and community-based organizations is based on the epidemiological profile within the jurisdiction.

   1.2.1. Prevent HIV among gay and bisexual men and transgender individuals: Congress and State legislatures should consider the implementation of laws that promote public health practice and underscore the existing best evidence in HIV prevention for sexual minorities.
   1.2.2. Prevent HIV among Black Americans: To lower risks for all Americans, prevention efforts should acknowledge the heavy burden of HIV among Black Americans and target resources appropriately.
   1.2.3. Prevent HIV among Latino Americans: HIV prevention efforts that target Latino communities must be culturally appropriate and available to acculturated and non-acculturated Latino populations.
   1.2.4. Prevent HIV among substance users: Substance use is associated with a greater likelihood of acquiring HIV infection. HIV screening and other comprehensive HIV prevention services should be coupled with substance treatment programs.

1.3. Address HIV prevention in Asian American and Pacific Islander and American Indian and Alaska Native populations: Federal and State agencies should consider efforts to support surveillance activities to better characterize HIV among smaller populations such as AAPIs and AI/ANs.
1.4. .Enhance program accountability: New tools are needed to hold recipients of public funds accountable for achieving results.

Step 2. Expand Targeted Efforts to Prevent HIV Infection Using a Combination of Effective, Evidence-Based Approaches

One of the hardest lessons of the HIV/AIDS epidemic is that there is no single 'magic bullet' that will stem the tide of new HIV infections. In the past, some have focused on one method of HIV prevention in favor of others. The public discourse has over-simplified the policy issues and has led some people to believe that a single solution, whether it is education, condom use, or biomedical innovations, held the key to reducing HIV infections. Our prevention efforts have been hampered by not deploying adequate overlapping, combination approaches to HIV prevention.[83,84] Further, we have not consistently utilized the most effective, cost-efficient tools to prevent HIV or tools that will have a sustainable impact over the long term.[85] Evaluating and employing multiple scientifically proven methods will have a greater impact to keep people from becoming infected. Additional research can also help identify new prevention strategies and the most effective combination approaches to prevent new HIV infections.

Prevention for people who are HIV-positive is critical to reducing new HIV infections. To prevent HIV, we should strive to ensure that all people living with HIV know their HIV status and are linked to and maintained in high-quality care that includes timely offering of, and promotes adherence to, HIV antiretroviral therapy, consistent with current clinical practice standards.[86] In addition, all people who are diagnosed with HIV should receive (1) services to assist with notifying recent sex and drug-use partners of the need to get tested for HIV; (2) access to behavioral and biomedical interventions that have been shown to sustainably reduce the probability of transmitting HIV to others and reduce acquisition of other sexually transmitted diseases; and (3) be screened for, and linked to, other medical and social services (as needed, including drug treatment, family planning, housing, and mental health services) that support individuals in reducing their transmission risk.

Moreover, all HIV-negative people at high-risk for HIV infection, especially those in sexual relationships with HIV-positive individuals or those with multiple sex partners, should be tested for HIV and STDs at least once a year. They should also have access to behavioral and biomedical interventions with longterm and sustainable outcomes that reduce the probability of HIV acquisition and also receive other medical and social services (as needed) that reduce the risk of acquiring HIV.

The following are scientifically proven biomedical and behavioral approaches that reduce the probability of HIV transmission:

- Abstinence from sex or drug use: Abstaining from sexual activity and substance use reduces the risk of HIV infection. In cases where this may not be possible, limiting the number of partners and taking other steps can lower the risk of acquiring HIV.
- HIV testing: There is evidence that people who test HIV-positive take steps to keep others from being exposed to the virus.[87] People who are unaware of their HIV status for an extended period of time may also enter care too late to have the maximum benefit from therapy, and they may unintentionally expose others to HIV.[88]
- Condom availability: Condom use is the most effective method to reduce risk of HIV infection during sexual activity. Correct and consistent use of male condoms is estimated to reduce the risk of HIV transmission by 80 percent.[89]

- Access to sterile needles and syringes: Among injection drug users, sharing needles and other drug paraphernalia increases the risk of HIV infection. Several studies have found that providing sterilized equipment to injection drug users substantially reduces risk of HIV infection, increases the probability that they will initiate drug treatment, and does not increase drug use.[90,91]
- HIV treatment: In addition to benefiting their own health, studies show that HIV-positive individuals who are adhering to effective antiretroviral therapy are less likely to transmit the virus compared to HIV-positive individuals who are not on medication.[92] There are also specific HIV medications that a person can take immediately after being exposed to HIV that can reduce the risk of HIV infection, called post exposure prophylaxis (PEP).[93] Antiretroviral therapy for pregnant women with HIV also dramatically reduces the risk of HIV transmission during pregnancy and childbirth.[94]

Some other biomedical and behavioral interventions have not been consistently associated with reducing HIV transmission, but may still contribute to our prevention efforts. For example, having an untreated sexually transmitted infection (STI) such as herpes, gonorrhea or syphilis substantially increases a person's chance of acquiring HIV, but research has not yet shown that treating STIs lowers HIV infection at a population level.[95, 96] Nevertheless, all people screened for STIs should also be screened for HIV infection because these infections are driven by the same risk behaviors.[97] Similarly, there are scientifically proven behavioral interventions that reduce HIV risk behaviors such as sexual risk behavior or drug use.[98] Even though these interventions have not been proven to reduce HIV infections, they promote responsible sexual behaviors that may lower a person's risk for becoming infected with HIV and some have been associated with reducing STIs.[99, 100, 101] Not all of the interventions, however, are equally effective over the long-term and not all of them are readily scalable, meaning that they can be effectively and affordably disseminated to large groups of people.[102] Given limited resources and substantial needs in communities heavily impacted by HIV, behavioral interventions that can effectively reach large groups of individuals should be prioritized. Additionally, more operational research is needed to determine which behavioral interventions are scalable and produce robust and sustainable outcomes.

The quality of information that we have to understand the epidemic we face and how it is changing depends on having an effective HIV surveillance system. The National HIV Surveillance System is the primary source of data used to monitor the epidemic in the United States HIV surveillance data are used extensively to target and evaluate HIV prevention and care programs. Therefore, completeness and timeliness of the data are critical. Surveillance of HIV disease necessitates a complex system of reporting from providers, laboratories, and State and local health departments to coordinate accurate, complete and timely reporting. While the system has performed well, there are few tools to accurately detect people who are newly infected with HIV. This is critical because people who are newly infected with HIV are more infectious than those individuals who have been living with HIV for an extended period of time.[103] Aside from tools to diagnose acute HIV infection, not all HIV surveillance sites track the same key measures in the same way (e.g., viral load, CD4).

Current approaches to preventing HIV must be coupled with research on new and innovative prevention methods that can have a long-term impact. Vaccines and microbicides are two biomedical approaches that are of promising, but safe and effective vaccines and microbicides are not yet available and investments in research to produce safe and effective vaccines and microbicides must continue. In addition, an important area to study is the feasibility and effectiveness of using treatment to prevent new infections. Such strategies include: 1) pre-exposure prophylaxis (PrEP), the use of antiretroviral therapy by high-risk uninfected populations, such as by HIV-negative individuals in committed relationships with HIV-positive individuals; and 2) potential prevention strategies known as 'test and treat' or 'test, treat and link to care' to determine whether a community-wide HIV testing program with an offer of immediate treatment can decrease the overall rate of new HIV infections in that community. Studies are currently underway to test the feasibility of PrEP and 'test and treat' in the United States and multiple sites around the world. Even if these prevention strategies are successful, additional research will be needed to assess the cost effectiveness of these approaches and their adaptability outside of carefully controlled research studies. There will also be a need to couple these approaches with behavioral interventions to ensure that any positive outcomes from PrEP, 'test and treat' or other innovative interventions are not erased by changes in risk behaviors.

There is an opportunity to get better results from our investments in HIV prevention by piloting, evaluating, and expanding access to effective combinations of prevention services.

Recommended Actions

To expand effective approaches to HIV prevention, the following actions are needed:

2.1. Design and evaluate innovative prevention strategies and combination approaches for preventing HIV in high-risk communities: Government agencies should fund and evaluate demonstration projects to test which combinations of effective interventions are cost-efficient, produce sustainable outcomes, and have the greatest impact in preventing HIV in specific communities.
2.2. Support and strengthen HIV screening and surveillance activities: There is a need to support existing surveillance methods to identify populations at greatest risk that need to be targeted for HIV prevention services.
2.3. Expand access to effective prevention services: Federal funds should support and State and local governments should be encouraged to expand access to effective HIV prevention services with the greatest potential for population-level impact for high-risk populations.
2.4. Expand prevention with HIV-positive individuals: Although most people diagnosed with HIV do not transmit the virus to others, there are effective approaches that support people living with HIV in avoiding transmitting HIV to others.

Step 3. Educate All Americans about the Threat of HIV and How to Prevent it

If a central tenet of the National HIV/AIDS Strategy is that we need to focus our public investments to achieve a maximal response, it is predicated on all Americans having access to a common baseline of information about the current HIV epidemic. This includes knowing how HIV is transmitted and prevented, and knowing which behaviors place individuals at greatest risk for infection. In some communities, many people no longer consider HIV a priority or something that could affect them personally. While we recognize that HIV is concentrated in certain communities, we need to provide all Americans with clear information about how to avoid HIV infection.

Broader HIV education is needed across the age span. Twenty-four percent of people living with HIV are over age 50, and 15 percent of new HIV cases occur in this age group.[104] HIV awareness and education should be universally integrated into all educational environments and health and wellness initiatives. Information about HIV is important to include in any wellness context promoting healthy behaviors, including sexual health. We must also ensure that all health and wellness practitioners (peer counselors, intake specialists, doctors, nurses, and other health professionals) are also educated about HIV, especially in programs for underserved communities. We should ensure that this education reaches populations that may be overlooked, including people with other disabilities. The focus of the education and awareness effort is to improve individual understanding of HIV infection, HIV-related risk factors and risk reduction, and HIV-related stigma and discrimination.

It is also important to educate Americans about how HIV is not transmitted. A significant proportion of the American public harbors misconceptions about how HIV is transmitted. The Kaiser Family Foundation released the results of a survey in 2009, where between one in five or one in ten Americans believed that HIV could be transmitted through sharing a drinking glass, touching a toilet seat, or swimming in a pool with someone who is HIV-positive. Misperceptions varied by demographics and were more common among the elderly, but as many as a third of young people (ages 18-29) held one of these misperceptions. Strikingly, the percentage of the American public that holds these misperceptions has not changed since 1987.[105]

Finally, educating young people about HIV before they begin engaging in behaviors that place them at risk for HIV infection should be a priority. Appropriately, it is a parent's job to instill values and to provide the moral and ethical foundation for their children, but schools have an important role in providing access to current and accurate information about the biological and scientific aspects of health education. It is important to provide access to a baseline of health education information that is grounded in the benefits of abstinence and delaying or limiting sexual activity, while ensuring that youth who make the decision to be sexually active have the information they need to take steps to protect themselves.

Recommended Actions

To better educate the American people about HIV/AIDS, the following is needed:

3.1. Utilize evidence-based social marketing and education campaigns: Outreach and engagement through traditional media (radio, television, and print) and networked media (such as online health sites, search providers, social media, and mobile applications) must be increased to educate and engage the public about how HIV is transmitted and to reduce misperceptions about HIV transmission. Efforts will be made to utilize and build upon World AIDS Day (December 1st) and National HIV Testing Day (June 27th), as well as other key dates and ongoing activities throughout the year.

3.2. Promote age-appropriate HIV and STI prevention education for all Americans: Too many Americans do not have the basic facts about HIV and other sexually transmitted infections. Sustained and reinforcing education is needed to effectively encourage people across the age span to take steps to reduce their risk for infection.

INCREASING ACCESS TO CARE AND IMPROVING HEALTH OUTCOMES FOR PEOPLE LIVING WITH HIV

Plan to Increase Access to Care and Improve Health Outcomes at-a-Glance

To increase access to care and improve health outcomes, we must work to:

- Establish a seamless system to immediately link people to continuous and coordinated quality care when they are diagnosed with HIV.
- Take deliberate steps to increase the number and diversity of available providers of clinical care and related services for people living with HIV.
- Support people living with HIV with co-occurring health conditions and those who have challenges meeting their basic needs, such as housing.

Anticipated Results

By 2015

- Increase the proportion of newly diagnosed patients linked to clinical care within three months of their HIV diagnosis from 65 percent to 85 percent.
- Increase the proportion of Ryan White HIV/AIDS Program clients who are in continuous care (at least 2 visits for routine HIV medical care in 12 months at least 3 months apart) from 73 percent to 80 percent.
- Increase the percentage of Ryan White HIV/AIDS Program clients with permanent housing from 82 percent to 86 percent. (This serves as a measurable proxy of our efforts to expand access to HUD and other housing supports to all needy people living with HIV.)

The Opportunity

While there is not yet a cure for HIV infection, there are a growing number of treatments that can extend life expectancy for those who have access to them. Research remains essential to finding a cure for HIV and to developing safer, more effective therapies and regimens to treat HIV and its associated complications. Access to treatment can be difficult, however, due to the high cost of care which makes insurance coverage a necessity. On average, HIV therapy costs approximately $25,000 per year, and medications are only one portion of a person's total health care needs.[106] Other factors can also prevent people from entering into care and staying on a course of treatment.

Despite our significant public investments in health care services through Medicaid, Medicare, and the Ryan White HIV/AIDS Program, too many people living with HIV do not have access to the medical care that they need. Further, difficult economic times have caused a number of States to reduce or eliminate funding for HIV programs. Waiting lists and other limitations on lifesaving HIV medications are increasing concerns that threaten our progress at getting people with HIV into care.

The Affordable Care Act, which will greatly expand access to insurance coverage for people living with HIV, will provide a platform for improvements in health care coverage and quality.[107] High risk pools are available immediately. High risk pools will be established in every state to provide coverage to uninsured people with chronic conditions. In 2014, Medicaid will be expanded to all lower income individuals (below 133% of the Federal poverty level, or about $15,000 for a single individual in 2010) under age 65. Uninsured people with incomes up to 400% of the Federal poverty level (about $43,000 for a single individual in 2010) will have access to Federal tax credits and have the opportunity to purchase private insurance coverage through competitive insurance exchanges. New consumer protections will better protect people with private insurance coverage by ending discrimination based on health status and pre-existing conditions. Gaps in essential care and services for people living with HIV will continue to need to be addressed along with the unique biological, psychological, and social effects of living with HIV. As the new law takes effect, it also will be important to ensure that people living with HIV and HIV health care providers are included in the various initiatives that seek to improve the quality of care and integration of services.

The Ryan White HIV/AIDS Program is entering its twentieth year and exists to provide services to the uninsured and to fill in gaps left by private and public insurance coverage. While the program has done impressive work, the level of need has always exceeded available funding. There are ongoing debates about how to fairly allocate limited resources among needy groups or which services to prioritize. Expanded access to insurance coverage will not take care of all needs, but implementation of health insurance reform presents the Nation with an opportunity to re-think what will be needed from the Ryan White HIV/AIDS Program in order to bring people with HIV into care and retain them in care once more people have insurance coverage. Therefore, the Ryan White HIV/AIDS Program and other Federal and State HIV-focused programs will continue to be necessary after the law is implemented to address gaps in essential services for people living with HIV.

People with HIV also have other significant challenges. Many people living with HIV have other co-occurring conditions, such as heart disease, depression or other mental health problems, or drug or alcohol addiction.[108] In addition, poverty, unemployment, domestic violence, homelessness, hunger, lack of access to transportation, and other issues can prevent people from accessing health care. There are also differences in health care access and treatment outcomes by race/ethnicity, gender, and geography. HIV-positive African Americans and Latinos are more likely to die sooner after an AIDS diagnosis compared to HIV-positive Whites; HIV-positive women are less likely to access therapy compared to HIV-positive men; and access to care and supportive services is particularly difficult for HIV-positive persons in rural areas, as well as other underserved communities.[109,110] While research has already brought us a long way, continued research is needed to develop safer, less expensive, and more effective treatments and drug regimens, as well as to evaluate new approaches to meeting HIV treatment needs while also responding to co-occurring conditions or other barriers to care.

To address these issues, we need to expand our approaches to connecting people to services and keeping them in care.

Steps to be Taken

We must pursue a concerted national effort to get and keep people living with HIV in care. The following steps are critical to achieving success:

1. Establish a seamless system to immediately link people to continuous and coordinated quality care when they are diagnosed with HIV.
2. Take deliberate steps to increase the number and diversity of available providers of clinical care and related services for people living with HIV.
3. Support people living with HIV with co-occurring health conditions and those who have challenges meeting their basic needs, such as housing.

Anticipated Results

By 2015

- Increase the proportion of newly diagnosed patients linked to clinical care within three months of their HIV diagnosis from 65 percent to 85 percent (from 26,824 to 35,079 people).
- Increase the proportion of Ryan White HIV/AIDS Program clients who are in continuous care (at least 2 visits for routine HIV medical care in 12 months at least 3 months apart) from 73 percent to 80 percent (or 237,924 people in continuous care to 260,739 people in continuous care).
- Increase the percentage of Ryan White HIV/AIDS Program clients with permanent housing from 82 percent to 86 percent (from 434,000 to 455,800 people). This serves as a measurable proxy of our efforts to expand access to HUD and other housing supports to all needy people living with HIV.

Recommended Actions

Step 1. Establish a Seamless System to Immediately Link People to Continuous and Coordinated Quality Care when They Learn they are Infected with HIV

Since effective antiretroviral therapies became available in the mid-1990s, questions about when to initiate therapy and how to minimize side effects and complications of long-term medication therapy have been debated. The Federal Government's treatment guidelines, which are the standard of care, have evolved over time and are regularly updated to reflect the most current research findings.[111] While decisions about when to start treatment must remain voluntary and require an individual to be ready to start a long-term regimen, growing evidence suggests that early initiation of treatment leads to improved outcomes.[112] To achieve this clinical goal requires that people are identified soon after their infection and systems are put in place to link them to care. This is particularly important given that over 230,000 people living with HIV do not know they are HIV positive, and therefore are not receiving regular medical care to manage the disease.[113]

Since 2006, CDC has recommended routine HIV screening for adults and adolescents ages 13-64 in health care settings. Testing, however, is only one of several critical services needed to get people into care. People who receive a diagnosis of HIV infection need to be connected to appropriate clinical care, prevention, and supportive services. It is essential to provide linkage coordination when and where HIV screening services are provided to help overcome barriers to obtaining care.

One approach to improving linkage to care is co-location of testing and care services. Another approach is using nontraditional sites to provide HIV screening and referral services. A recent study sponsored by the Substance Abuse and Mental Health Services Administration (SAMHSA) indicated that fewer than half of all substance abuse treatment facilities surveyed nationwide reported that they conduct on-site infectious disease screening.[114] Facilities that provided hospital inpatient treatment were more likely than facilities providing only outpatient or nonhospital residential treatment to offer screening for HIV, sexually transmitted diseases (STDs), hepatitis B, hepatitis C, or tuberculosis. Encouraging these types of facilities and nontraditional sites like community centers, mental health centers, or faith institutions to get trained and offer HIV screening and referrals could help build service provider capacity and connect people to the care and treatment they need to address HIV and other co-occurring conditions. This is also one element of a strategy to better meet the HIV prevention and care needs of people living in rural or under-resourced areas. It also provides an opportunity for providers to begin to take a more holistic approach to health, rather than focusing only on HIV. Some of the same behaviors that help to prevent HIV infection also will help to prevent STDs and hepatitis B and C.

Being linked to care is not enough. It is estimated that as many as 30 percent of people diagnosed with HIV are not accessing care. There is a need to re-engage people diagnosed with HIV who have never been in care or who have subsequently fallen out of care. There is also a need for ongoing support to maintain the necessary high levels of adherence to antiretroviral treatment. Government, academic, and pharmaceutical industry research has brought us simpler, more easily tolerated therapies than the initial generation of effective antiretroviral therapies. Safer, more potent, and more durable treatments are still needed. Additionally, we need to better understand how to manage the clinical complications and consequences of HIV infection and long-term use of antiretroviral drugs—including issues related to accelerated heart disease, kidney disease, cancers, and premature aging.[115,116] More work is also needed to understand differences in treatment response between women and men and among racial and ethnic minorities. Public and private insurers and health care providers must also take steps to ensure that all HIV care providers have the knowledge and training to provide quality HIV care consistent with the latest treatment guidelines.

Recommended Actions

To put this key action step into practice, the following are needed:

1.1. Facilitate linkages to care: HIV resources should be targeted to include support for linkage coordinators in a range of settings where at risk populations receive health and social services.
1.2. Promote collaboration among providers: All levels of government should increase collaboration between HIV medical care providers and agencies providing HIV counseling and testing services, mental health treatment, substance abuse treatment, housing and supportive services to link people with HIV to care.
1.3. Maintain people living with HIV in care: Clinical care providers should ensure that all eligible HIV-positive persons have access to antiretroviral therapy. Those who start therapy need to be maintained on a medication regimen, as recommended by the HHS treatment guidelines.

Step 2. Take Deliberate Steps to Increase the Number and Diversity of Available Providers of Clinical Care and Related Services for People Living with HIV

To improve health outcomes, we need to adopt policies that will produce a workforce that is large enough to care for all people living with HIV, is diverse, has the appropriate training and technical expertise to provide high-quality care consistent with the latest treatment guidelines, and has the capacity, through shared experiences or training, to provide care in a non-stigmatizing manner and create relationships of trust with their patients. Specialized HIV care should also incorporate prevention. Efforts to expand the HIV workforce of highly skilled professionals should target the areas where the need is greatest.

For too long, our nation has suffered from a severe shortage of primary care health professionals. The Affordable Care Act provides for significant new policies and resources to begin to address these issues. In addition, the provider workforce of physicians, nurses, and other health professionals that specialize in HIV care is aging, and new recruits are needed to address the workforce shortage. According to the Association of American Medical Colleges, nearly one fourth (24.7 percent) of the active physician workforce in the United States was age 60 or older in 2008.[117] Within a medical specialty like infectious disease, the problem of limited physician supply is more pronounced. The Affordable Care Act and its investments in the National Health Service Corps will help to alleviate primary care workforce shortages in underserved areas, but it is also necessary to encourage more health care providers, including nonphysician providers, to obtain specialized HIV training and include people living with HIV in their practices. Surveys by HIV provider associations indicate that the pending shortage of HIV providers and the increases in HIV patient loads during recent years require an urgent response in order to maintain a robust HIV care system in the United States.[118] Specialized training, task shifting and use of interdisciplinary health teams all can help alleviate HIV workforce shortages. Providers should also consider including peer-based programming, such as peer treatment educators, to reduce workforce burden and to help retain HIV-positive people, especially among hard-to-reach populations, in care.

Enhanced program integration is another approach that can be useful in expanding the workforce of professionals providing HIV services. For example, by integrating HIV screening along with reproductive health care, it is possible to effectively address concurrent sexually transmitted infections (STIs), which increase risk for HIV transmission. Providing better integrated, coordinated care will help ensure individuals receive services to prevent and treat opportunistic infections and have their other chronic health needs met, ultimately leading to improved health outcomes and better quality of life.

Strategies available to increase the number of HIV providers include health professions training grants, the National Health Service Corps Scholarship and Loan Repayment Programs, financial incentives to compensate providers for HIV care management, and program coordination so that providers who are not HIV specialists are adequately equipped to provide prevention services to high-risk populations and link patients who test positive to HIV clinical care providers. For example, substance abuse treatment providers may not be HIV specialists, but their patient population may be engaging in behaviors that put them at risk for HIV infection. Therefore, substance abuse and mental health treatment providers are potential providers of HIV prevention services. Oral health care plays an important role because HIV disease can cause certain symptoms identifiable only through dental exams. Dental care providers who are educated about HIV can be referral sources to other services that people living with HIV may need. Similarly, gynecologists and family planning services can be a source of HIV prevention services for women who may or may not be engaging in high-risk behaviors, but who might not actively seek services from an HIV or sexually transmitted disease clinic. Over 70 percent of women ages 15-44 received at least one family planning or medical care service from a medical care provider in the last 12 months.[119] Increasing the number of HIV providers, as well as increasing knowledge among all health professionals about HIV risks and prevention is a critical need. This involves a wide range of health professionals in all health care settings including physicians, registered nurses, nurse practitioners, physician assistants, social workers, pharmacists, and dentists.

Health care services that are respectful of and responsive to the health beliefs, practices and cultural and linguistic needs of diverse patients can help bring about positive health outcomes.[120] Many people living with HIV come from communities that have been historically poorly served by the mainstream health care system. For example, among some African Americans, there is mistrust of the medical establishment, and it may lead some to question clinical recommendations that are widely accepted by others.[121] Heterosexual providers may not be comfortable asking about sexual history when taking a patient's history and this may limit appropriate care.[122] Transgender individuals are particularly challenged in finding providers who respect them and with whom they can have honest discussions about hormone use and other practices, and this results in lower satisfaction with their care providers, less trust, and poorer health outcomes.[123] Findings from an AHRQ-funded study indicated that poor health literacy among people with living with HIV negatively impacts their adherence to antiretroviral medications and their health outcomes.[124] In addition to having HIV expertise, care providers should be culturally competent and able to clearly and effectively communicate to help their patients understand the benefits of following treatment plans.

Recommended Actions

To put this key action step into practice, the following are needed:

2.1. Increase the number of available providers of HIV care: Federal agencies should develop strategies encouraging more clinicians including primary care providers, reproductive health care providers and sexually transmitted disease experts, mental health providers, substance abuse treatment professionals to provide HIV services.

2.2. Strengthen the current provider workforce to improve quality of HIV care and health outcomes for people living with HIV: Federal agencies should engage clinical providers and professional medical societies on the importance of routine, voluntary HIV screening and quality HIV care in clinical settings consistent with CDC guidelines.

Step 3. Support People Living with HIV with Co-Occurring Health Conditions and those Who Have Challenges Meeting Their Basic Needs, Such as Housing

To support the provision of quality care for people living with HIV, it is important to reduce barriers that impede access to services. The concept of a medical home is a model for the provision of coordinated, person-centered care for individuals with chronic or prolonged illnesses requiring regular medical monitoring, care management, and treatment. The Ryan White HIV/AIDS Program has supported the development of medical homes for people living with HIV and has experience to share, which can be valuable to other providers including community health centers and private physicians in their provision of HIV care.[125]

Chronic diseases like heart disease, cancer, and diabetes are leading causes of death and disability in the United States. Many people with HIV have these and other chronic conditions, such as hepatitis, diabetes, and mental illness. Co-infection with other sexually transmitted infections like herpes, syphilis and gonorrhea is also common. It is estimated that up to 50 percent of people with HIV have a mental illness such as depression, and 13 percent have both mental illness and substance abuse issues.[126] Co-infection with HIV and Hepatitis C occurs in 50-90 percent of HIV-infected injection drug users.[127] As people age, the likelihood of having multiple chronic illnesses increases, even among people who do not have HIV. HIV disease itself, as well as long-term use of HIV therapies may also contribute to common chronic conditions, such as heart disease and kidney disease.[128] Additional research is needed to better understand, prevent, and treat these co-infections and complications of HIV disease.

Optimal clinical care should include a range of integrated clinical and preventive services to reduce HIV-related morbidity and mortality. Patient-centered care–defined by the Institute of Medicine as health care that establishes a partnership among practitioners, patients, and their families (when appropriate) to ensure that decisions respect patients' wants, needs, and preferences–should be the standard. In addition to ensuring that clinical care services are well coordinated, non-medical services and assistance to meet basic needs are important supports for achieving good clinical outcomes. Access to medical treatment should be supplemented with ongoing case management services to facilitate continuity of care. Supportive services such as transportation, legal assistance, nutrition services, mental health services, substance use treatment, and child care are essential for certain populations facing difficulties with everyday needs.

Access to housing is an important precursor to getting many people into a stable treatment regimen. Individuals living with HIV who lack stable housing are more likely to delay HIV care, have poorer access to regular care, are less likely to receive optimal antiretroviral therapy, and are less likely to adhere to therapy. A large-scale study from 2007 comparing the health of homeless and stably housed people living with HIV found that housing status was more significant than individual characteristics as a predictor of health care access and outcomes.[129] A long-term study of people living with HIV in New York City found that over a 12-year period, receipt of housing assistance was one of the strongest predictors of accessing HIV primary care, maintaining continuous care, receiving care that meets clinical practice standards, and entry into HIV care.[130] Receipt of housing assistance had a direct impact on improved medical care, regardless of demographics, drug use, health and mental health status, or receipt of other services. Opening Doors: Federal Strategic Plan to Prevent and End Homelessness focuses efforts to reduce homelessness and increase housing security. Planning efforts will be undertaken in collaboration with community partners to address the housing needs of vulnerable Americans who are in homeless situations or present risks of homelessness.

People with competing demands and challenges meeting their basic needs for housing, food, and child care often have problems staying in care. Access to legal services can be important to help people resolve issues with discrimination, access to public benefits including health care, and resolving problems with employment and other issues that can create serious barriers to staying in care. Support from social workers and/or case managers can help with identifying resources, and peer networks among people living with HIV may also be valuable for information sharing and other support. Programs that provide family-centered care can be especially important for women living with HIV. Further, both women and men with HIV can be at risk for intimate partner violence, which can impede adherence and stability in care. As HIV service providers develop ways to improve delivery of care for these and other specific populations, including youth, people in or transitioning from correctional settings, and people living in remote or rural areas, it will be important to disseminate information about effective models to enable other providers to better serve those groups and overcome common barriers to care.

Recommended Actions

To put this key action step into practice, the following are needed:

3.1. Enhance client assessment tools and measurement of health outcomes: Federal and State agencies should support case management and clinical services that contribute to improving health outcomes for people living with HIV and work toward increasing access to non-medical supportive services (e.g., housing, food, transportation) as critical elements of an effective HIV care system.

3.2. Address policies to promote access to housing and supportive services for people living with HIV: Federal agencies should consider additional efforts to support housing assistance and other services that enable people living with HIV to obtain and adhere to HIV treatment.

REDUCING HIV-RELATED DISPARITIES AND HEALTH INEQUITIES

Plan to Reduce HIV-Related

Disparities and Health Inequities at-a-Glance

Disparities in HIV prevention and care persist among racial/ethnic minorities, as well as among sexual minorities. While working to improve access to prevention and care services for all Americans, the following steps will help to reduce inequities across groups:

- Reduce HIV-related mortality in communities at high risk for HIV infection.
- Adopt community-level approaches to reduce HIV infection in high-risk communities.
- Reduce stigma and discrimination against people living with HIV.

Anticipated Results

By 2015

- Increase the proportion of HIV diagnosed gay and bisexual men with undetectable viral load by 20 percent.
- Increase the proportion of HIV diagnosed Blacks with undetectable viral load by 20 percent.
- Increase the proportion of HIV diagnosed Latinos with undetectable viral load by 20 percent.

The Opportunity

The transmission of HIV has long been concentrated in groups that have been marginalized or underserved.[131] For persons living with HIV, this issue often transcends discrete measures such as incidence, morbidity and mortality rates, but speaks to a confluence of factors that lead to poorer health overall. In some communities, a major challenge is overcoming a sense of fatalism where people believe that they are destined to become infected with HIV. In other communities, although the threat of HIV is real, it is only one of many issues individuals face on a daily basis and may rank lower than more immediate needs such as shelter, food, or safety. In still other communities, people may want to prioritize HIV prevention and care, but services are not easily accessible to them. A national response to the HIV epidemic needs to be mindful of the size, diversity and richness of our country, as well as the needs of the most affected communities.

HIV exists within a health care system where different groups have varying access to services—and achieve varying health outcomes. The Affordable Care Act represents the broadest Federal effort, to date, to address health inequities.

The law says that a group is a health disparity population when:

> "there is a significant disparity in the overall rate of disease incidence, prevalence, morbidity, mortality, or survival rates in the population as compared to the health status of the general population." In addition, it may be determined, "that such term includes populations for which there is a significant disparity in the quality, outcomes, cost, or use of healthcare services or access to or satisfaction with such services as compared to the general population."

By greatly expanding access to health care for all, taking specific steps to support treatment adherence for people living with HIV, conducting research on the causes of differences in health outcomes, and refocusing our prevention efforts on combination strategies targeted to the highest risk communities, we will create the conditions where serious progress can be made in reducing HIV-related health disparities. What is missing are community-level approaches to altering the conditions in which HIV is transmitted and addressing the factors that influence disparate health outcomes among people living with HIV, including lessening stigma and discrimination.

Steps to Be Taken

A concerted national effort to increase the capacity of whole communities to prevent HIV and support community members living with HIV is needed. The following steps are critical to achieving success:

1. Reduce HIV-related mortality in communities at high risk for HIV infection.
2. Adopt community-level approaches to reduce HIV infection in high-risk communities.
3. Reduce stigma and discrimination against people living with HIV.

Anticipated Results

By 2015

- Increase the proportion of HIV diagnosed gay and bisexual men with undetectable viral load by 20 percent.
- Increase the proportion of HIV diagnosed Blacks with undetectable viral load by 20 percent.
- Increase the proportion of HIV diagnosed Latinos with undetectable viral load by 20 percent.

Recommended Actions

Step 1. Reduce HIV-Related Mortality in Communities at High Risk for HIV Infection

Significant racial disparities in HIV infection exist in the United States (Figure 4). According to CDC, the overall rate of HIV diagnosis for Blacks was roughly eight times the rate for Whites in 2006. The HIV diagnosis rate for all Black males (119.1 per 100,000 population) remains the highest of any racial/ethnic group and is more than seven times that for White males, twice the rate for Latino males, and twice the rate for Black females.[132] Additionally, the diagnosis rate for Latino males was approximately three times that for White males. The HIV diagnosis rate in 2006 for Black females and Latinas was more than 19 times and 5 times (respectively) the rate for White females. Disparities in HIV infection also exist between gay and bisexual men and heterosexual populations. Recently, the CDC announced that gay and bisexual men in the United States are 44 to 86 times more likely to become infected with HIV than heterosexual men, and 40 to 77 times more likely to become infected than women.[133]

Unfortunately, these disparities in HIV infection also translate into disparities in premature death. Even though HIV-related mortality has been declining since the availability of effective medications, Black and Latino Americans are more likely than White Americans to die earlier from AIDS.[134] Racial disparities in HIV-related deaths also exist among gay men, where Black and Latino gay men are more likely to die from AIDS compared to White men, and among women with Black women and Latinas at greater risk for death compared to White women.[135,136] Gay and bisexual men comprise the majority of people with HIV who have died in the United States.[137]

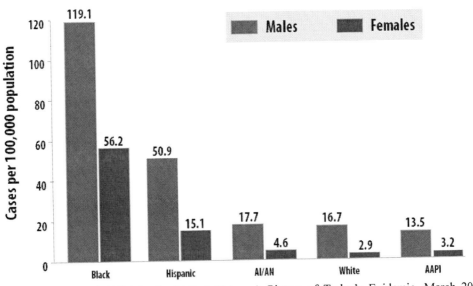

Source: CDC, HIV and AIDS in the United States: A Picture of Today's Epidemic, March 2008.
AI/AN = American Indian or Alaska Native and AAPI = Asian and Pacific Islander.

Figure 4. HIV Diagnoses by Race/Ethnicity.

Decisions about when to start therapies for HIV are personal. There is accumulating scientific evidence, however, that early initiation of antiretroviral therapy improves health outcomes among people living with HIV.[138,139] To achieve these results, it is necessary for people on therapy to be adherent to their medication regimen. Antiretroviral therapy reduces the amount of virus in the bloodstream and improves the health of people living with HIV, in addition to reducing the transmissibility of HIV.

A key indicator for health and transmissibility is viral load, which is a way of measuring the amount of virus in a person's body. A high viral load (5,000 to 10,000 copies per milliliter of blood) means that a person's HIV disease is progressing and that they are more infectious. A low viral load (40 to 500 copies per milliliter of blood) indicates that a person's HIV disease progression is not as rapid.[140] Besides disease progression, people with high viral loads are more likely to transmit HIV to uninfected partners than people with low viral loads.[141] If we are able to increase the number of people with HIV in heavily affected communities who have a low viral load, it may reduce disparities in HIV infection rates and mortality in these groups.

Recommended Actions

1.1. Ensure that high-risk groups have access to regular viral load and CD4 tests: All persons living with HIV should have access to tests that track their health, but more must be done to make sure that these tests are available to African Americans, Latinos, and gay and bisexual men.

Step 2. Adopt Community-Level Approaches to Reduce HIV Infection in High-Risk Communities

In order to reduce disparities among groups, we need effective approaches to reduce the risk of HIV transmission not only at the individual level but at the community level. In some heavily impacted communities, preventing HIV one individual at a time will not meaningfully impact the overall epidemic. As mentioned earlier, individuals in some communities are at higher risk for HIV infection even if they personally engage in comparable or lower risk behavior than individuals in other communities.[142, 143] To address this greater vulnerability to HIV infection, it is necessary to reduce the high proportion of individuals in these communities who are living with HIV. The viral load of a person living with HIV is associated with transmissibility. Moreover, the scientific evidence shows that the average viral load among all diagnosed HIV-positive individuals in a given community who are in care is strongly associated with the number of new infections that occur in that community.[144, 145] Thus, neighborhoods with a high community viral load are also places where uninfected individuals are at greater risk for acquiring HIV than neighborhoods or other localities with a comparatively lower viral load. Innovative solutions such as reducing community viral load may help reduce the number of new HIV infections in specific communities that may, in turn, reduce disparities in HIV infection.[146] Recently, NIH has launched a pilot study in Washington, D.C., and is working with CDC to launch a companion study in the Bronx, New York, to test this approach.[147]

HIV is often only one of many conditions that plague communities at greater risk for HIV infection. In many cases, it is not possible to effectively address HIV transmission or care without also addressing sexually transmitted diseases, substance use, poverty, homelessness and other issues.[148,149] For example, a recent study found that hunger was associated with poor viral suppression among homeless and marginally housed HIV-positive adults taking antiretroviral therapy.[150] Because of these many co-occurring issues, it is important to employ a holistic approach to HIV prevention and care that extends beyond risk behaviors of the individual and address not only mental health, but contextual factors such as sexual and drug use networks, joblessness or homelessness and others that increase risk for infection or suboptimal access or response to care. Although there have been some successful efforts in this regard, such as interventions that examine the link between homelessness and HIV risk behavior, there are too few proven models associated with reducing HIV incidence or increasing access to care that have had a community-level impact.

Recommended Actions

To achieve a community-level impact at lowering HIV infections, the following actions are needed:

2.1. Establish pilot programs that utilize community models: In order to reduce disparities between various groups affected by the epidemic, testing community-level approaches is needed to identify effective interventions that reduce the risk of infection in high prevalence communities.

2.2. Measure and utilize community viral load: Ensure that all high prevalence localities are able to collect data necessary to calculate community viral load, measure the viral load in specific communities, and reduce viral load in those communities where HIV incidence is high.

2.3. Promote a more holistic approach to health: Promote a more holistic approach to health that addresses not only HIV prevention among African Americans, Latinos, gay and bisexual men, women, and substance users, but also the prevention of HIV related co-morbidities, such as STDs and hepatitis B and C.

Step 3. Reduce Stigma and Discrimination Against People Living with HIV

In the earliest days of the HIV epidemic, fear, ignorance, and denial led to harsh, ugly treatment of people living with the disease, and some Americans even called for forced quarantine of all people living with HIV.[151] Although such extreme measures never occurred, the stigma and discrimination faced by people living with HIV was often extremely high. Even today, some people living with HIV still face discrimination in many areas of life including employment, housing, provision of health care services, and access to public accommodations. This undermines efforts to encourage all people to learn their HIV status, and it makes it harder for people to disclose their HIV status to their medical providers, their sex partners, and even clergy and others from whom they may seek understanding and support.

Time and again, an essential element of what has caused social attitudes to change has been when the public sees and interacts with people who are openly living with HIV. For decades, community organizations have operated speakers bureaus where people with HIV go into schools, businesses, and churches to talk about living with HIV. In the 1990s, both major political parties had memorable keynote speakers at their presidential nominating conventions that were living with HIV.[152] We know that many people feel shame and embarrassment when they learn their HIV status. And, there is too much social stigma that seeks to assign blame to people who acquire HIV. Encouraging more individuals to disclose their HIV status directly lessens the stigma associated with HIV. As we promote disclosure, however, we must also ensure that we are protecting people who are openly living with HIV. This calls for a continued commitment to civil rights enforcement.

This year marks the twentieth anniversary of the Americans with Disabilities Act, the landmark civil rights law that has proven so vital to the protection of people with disabilities including HIV. To be free of discrimination on the basis of HIV status is both a human and a civil right. Vigorous enforcement of the Americans with Disabilities Act, the Fair Housing Act, the Rehabilitation Act, and other civil rights laws is vital to establishing an environment where people will feel safe in getting tested and seeking treatment. Recently, the Obama Administration completed the process begun in the Bush Administration to eliminate the HIV entry ban that restricted noncitizens living with HIV from entering the United States. These and other policy actions have been positive steps forward in lessening the stigma associated with living with HIV.

Working to end the stigma and discrimination experienced by people living with HIV is a critical component of curtailing the epidemic. The success of public health policy depends upon the cooperation of the affected populations. People at high risk for HIV cannot be expected to, nor will they seek testing or treatment services if they fear that it would result in adverse consequences of discrimination. HIV stigma has been shown to be a barrier to HIV testing and people living with HIV who experience more stigma have poorer physical and mental health and are more likely to miss doses of their medication.[153]

An important step we can take is to ensure that laws and policies support our current understanding of best public health practices for preventing and treating HIV. At least 32 states have HIV-specific laws that criminalize behavior by people living with HIV.[154] Some criminalize behavior like spitting and biting by people with HIV, and were initially enacted at a time when there was less knowledge about HIV's transmissibility. Since it is now clear that spitting and biting do not pose significant risks for HIV transmission, many believe that it is unfair to single out people with HIV for engaging in these behaviors and should be dealt with in a consistent manner without consideration of HIV status. Some laws criminalize consensual sexual activity between adults on the basis that one of the individuals is a person with HIV who failed to disclose their status to their partner. CDC data and other studies, however, tell us that intentional HIV transmission is atypical and uncommon.[155] A recent research study also found that HIV-specific laws do not influence the behavior of people living with HIV in those states where these laws exist.[156] While we understand the intent behind such laws, they may not have the desired effect and they may make people less willing to disclose their status by making people feel at even greater risk of discrimination. In some cases, it may be appropriate for legislators to reconsider whether existing laws continue to further the public interest and public health. In many instances, the continued existence and enforcement of these types of laws run counter to scientific evidence about routes of HIV transmission and may undermine the public health goals of promoting HIV screening and treatment.[157,158]

Recommended Actions

To reduce stigma and discrimination experienced by people living with HIV, the following are needed:

3.1. Engage communities to affirm support for people living with HIV: Faith communities, businesses, schools, community-based organizations, social gathering sites, and all types of media outlets should take responsibility for affirming nonjudgmental support for people living with HIV and high-risk communities.
3.2. Promote public leadership of people living with HIV: Governments and other institutions (including HIV prevention community planning groups and Ryan White planning councils and consortia) should work with people with AIDS coalitions, HIV services organizations, and other institutions to actively promote public leadership by people living with HIV.
3.3. Promote public health approaches to HIV prevention and care: State legislatures should consider reviewing HIV-specific criminal statutes to ensure that they are consistent with current knowledge of HIV transmission and support public health approaches to preventing and treating HIV.
3.4. Strengthen enforcement of civil rights laws: The Department of Justice and Federal agencies must enhance cooperation to facilitate enforcement of Federal antidiscrimination laws.

ACHIEVING A MORE COORDINATED NATIONAL RESPONSE TO THE HIV EPIDEMIC

Plan to Achieve a More Coordinated National Response to the HIV Epidemic in the United States at-a-Glance

In Order for the National HIV/AIDS
Strategy to be successful, emphasis must be placed on coordination of activities among agencies and across all levels of government.

- Increase the coordination of HIV programs across the Federal Government and between Federal agencies and State, territorial, local, and tribal governments.
- Develop improved mechanisms to monitor and report on progress toward achieving national goals.

The Opportunity

The United States does many things right in how it responds to HIV. Persistent advocacy, research accomplishments, and observable successes in preventing HIV and providing health care and social supports to people with HIV have left us with a legacy of global leadership. We have also learned important lessons about how to engage affected communities and how to mobilize broad sectors of society to care about a condition that is highly stigmatized, associated with sexuality, drug use, and other issues that magnify our cultural divides. The United States investment in responding to the domestic HIV epidemic has risen to more than $19 billion per year.[159] This number alone says nothing about whether it is sufficient to meet existing needs or if these resources are used most effectively–and we believe that evaluation of existing funds along with increased investments in certain key areas are warranted. Nonetheless, it is clear that the Nation has devoted significant financial resources to mount a serious and sustained response to ending the HIV epidemic. What has been missing and what is needed at this time is an enhanced focus on coordinating our efforts across Federal agencies, across all levels of government, with external partners, and throughout the health care system. Further, with dispersed responsibility for responding to HIV, there is a need for a clearer understanding of roles and increased accountability. Since our ultimate success at ending the HIV epidemic depends on the American people understanding the urgency of the challenge and remaining supportive of the important investments we are making in research, care, and prevention, a greater priority should be placed on communicating to the public the challenges we face and the progress we are making.

The many Federal agencies that operate critical HIV programs operate under their own statutory authority as established by Congress. It is not possible or desirable to merge all HIV programs under one roof. At the same time, improved coordination is possible and we can improve the Federal response by insisting that agencies work in closer collaboration with each other.

In our Federal system, the role of the Federal Government is not to direct all activities by all entities. Indeed, in our diverse country, the most effective responses are often those that originate at the State or local level, or even at the level of individual neighborhoods. In this environment, Federal leadership is critical in identifying overarching national priorities, as well as supporting research to evaluate which activities are most effective and then ensuring that Federal resources are deployed to maximal effect. Many Federal HIV prevention and care programs operate largely by providing resources to State, local and tribal governments to provide services within Federal rules and guidelines. While flexibility is critical to respond to varied needs, our three decades of experience of fighting HIV has given the Nation a greater sense of what is effective. Therefore, it is appropriate for the Federal Government to focus the use of its resources on tools that have been shown to work effectively in addressing the Administration's National HIV/AIDS Strategy goals and to prioritize the utilization of epidemiological data in the policy-making process.

Much can be achieved by prioritizing enhanced collaboration and accountability.

Steps to be Taken

The following steps are critical to achieving a more coordinated response to HIV:

1) 1 Increase the coordination of HIV programs across the Federal government and between federal agencies and state, territorial, tribal, and local governments.
2) 2 Develop improved mechanisms to monitor and report on progress toward achieving national goals.

Recommended Actions

Step 1. Increase the Coordination of HIV Programs across the Federal Government and between Federal Agencies and State, Territorial, Tribal, and Local Governments

Funding for HIV services is spread across multiple departments, including Health and Human Services (HHS), Housing and Urban Development (HUD), Justice, Veterans Affairs (VA), and Defense (Figure 5). Within HHS, in particular, responsibility for HIV programs is spread across multiple agencies including the Centers for Medicare & Medicaid Services (CMS), the Health Resources and Services Administration (HRSA), CDC, the Indian Health Service (IHS), the Food and Drug Administration, the Office of HIV/AIDS Policy, the Office of Minority Health, and others. Responsibility for HIV research is primarily carried by NIH, but CDC, VA, Department of Defense, and USAID also support research initiatives. This dispersion of responsibility is appropriate, as each agency has its own expertise, and different agencies operate different programs with varying purposes and with unique histories. Spreading the response to HIV across the Federal Government has helped our response to HIV. At the same time, it imposes costs and challenges us in getting the greatest results.

Roughly half of Federal funding for domestic HIV services flows through Medicaid and Medicare, two programs that are administered by the Centers for Medicare & Medicaid Services (CMS) (Figure 5).

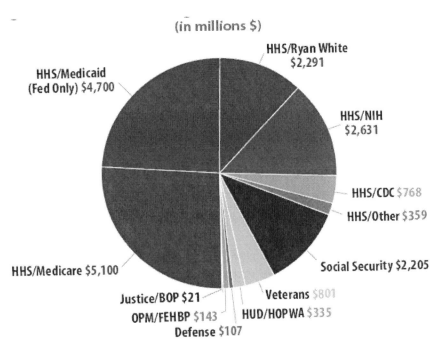

Source: FY 2010 Appropriations. HHS other includes (in millions $) SAMHSA ($178), FDA ($109), Office of the Secretary ($64), Indian Health Service ($5), and AHRQ ($3).

Figure 5. Federal Funding for Domestic HIV/AIDS, FY 2010.

These programs provide essential guarantees of access to lifesaving medical care for all eligible beneficiaries, but the structure of the programs makes it difficult to adapt to HIV policy goals. Most services must be provided to all beneficiaries, and this limits the ability to target prevention and care services to high-risk populations. Moreover, data limitations make it hard to monitor people living with HIV as a distinct group. Other programs are more flexible, but competing rules, data collection requirements, and purposes create administrative burdens for the government, grantees and other external partners.

Laws governing HIV programs have changed over time, but have not all evolved in a way that places resources where they are most needed. For instance, some localities receive more funding for HIV prevention and care services than others despite having fewer persons living with HIV/AIDS. A recent analysis found that States with a low number of existing HIV/AIDS cases received the highest HIV prevention funding per case from CDC. The five States with 50 percent of the persons living with AIDS receive only 43 percent of CDC prevention funds for the Health Department Prevention, Expanded Testing Initiative, and Core Surveillance cooperative agreements, whereas the twenty jurisdictions that account for the last two percent of AIDS cases received nearly seven percent of the budget for these cooperative agreements.[160] If we are to target our efforts to more effectively address the epidemic, then resources to prevent HIV infection should be proportionate to disease burden. To achieve this, HIV prevention funding should be based upon more current HIV surveillance data rather than historical AIDS data. CDC is moving toward this goal and will be able to provide HIV in addition to AIDS data from all localities by the 2012 HIV surveillance report.

Another issue with Federal HIV funding programs is that few are designed to encourage efficient coordination across programs. As a result, HIV services providers often receive funding from multiple sources with different grant application processes and funding schedules, and varied reporting requirements. These issues are not unique at the Federal level, and overlapping and competing programs also hinder efforts at the State and local levels.

We need to integrate services and reduce redundancy, encourage collaboration across different levels of government and with nongovernment partners, and ensure accountability for achieving positive results. In this regard, the President's Emergency Plan for AIDS Relief (PEPFAR) has taught us valuable lessons about fighting HIV and scaling up efforts around the world that can be applied to the domestic epidemic.

Recommended Actions

To increase coordination across programs, the following are needed:

1.1. Ensure coordinated program administration: The Federal Government should increase focus on coordinated planning for HIV programs and services agencies.
1.2. Promote equitable resource allocation: The Federal Government should review the methods used to distribute Federal funds and take steps to ensure that resources go to the States and localities with the greatest need.
1.3. Streamline and standardize data collection: The Federal Government should take short and longer-term efforts to simplify grant administration activities, including work to standardize data collection, consolidating grant announcements, and grantee reporting requirements for Federal HIV programs.

Step 2. Develop Improved Mechanisms to Monitor and Report on Progress toward Achieving National Goals

The HIV epidemic in America requires a bold public health response. Annual AIDS deaths have declined, but the number of new infections has been static and the number of people living with HIV is growing. We need to be able to critically evaluate our current efforts to gauge the extent to which an impact is being made. Moreover, because of budget shortfalls at the state level, it is increasingly important that existing State and local efforts are concentrated and aligned with the Strategy goals. We need to measure the results of our efforts to reduce incidence and improve health outcomes to chart our progress in fighting HIV and AIDS nationally, and refine our response to this public health problem over time. This requires a monitoring system that evaluates the implementation of the Strategy, its progress, and the impact of the Strategy efforts. A system of regular public reporting will help to sustain public attention and support.

Recommended Actions

To monitor and communicate our progress, the following are needed:

2.1. Provide rigorous evaluation of current programs and redirect resources to the most effective programs: Prioritize programs that are 1) scientifically proven to reduce HIV infection, increase access to care, or reduce HIV-related disparities, 2) able to demonstrate sustained and long lasting (>1 year) outcomes toward achieving any of these goals, 3) scalable to produce desired outcomes at the community level, and 4) cost efficient.
2.2. Provide regular public reporting: Progress in reaching Strategy goals will be reported by the Federal Government through an annual report at the end of each year.
2.3. Encourage States to provide regular progress reports: The Federal Government will encourage States to provide annual reports to ONAP and HHS OS on progress made implementing their comprehensive HIV/AIDS plans. ONAP will incorporate the State reports into the national progress report at the end of each year.

CONCLUSION

HIV is a complex epidemic that creates many challenges and calls on all of us to take steps to protect ourselves, the communities where we live, and our Nation as a whole. There are many actions that should be taken, and there are many things that the United States has done well that offer lessons for future action. The development of a National HIV/AIDS Strategy is important because it is an effort to reflect on what is and is not working in order to increase the outcomes that we receive for our public and private investments. The Strategy is intended to refocus our existing efforts and deliver better results to the American people within current funding levels, as well as make the case for new investments. It is also a new attempt to set clear priorities and provide leadership for all public and private stakeholders to align their efforts toward a common purpose.

A perspective that arises out of the inclusive process used to develop this strategy leads us to recommend the following steps:

1. Resources will always be tight, and we will have to make tough choices about the most effective use of funds. Therefore, all resource allocation decisions for programs should be grounded in the latest epidemiological data about who is being most affected and other data that tell us which are the most urgent unmet needs to be addressed.
2. People living with HIV have unique experience that should be valued and relied upon as a critical source of input in setting policy.
3. Communities themselves are often the best equipped to make difficult trade-offs, and priority setting and resource allocation is best done as close to ground as possible.
4. Continued investment in research is needed. This includes biomedical research to develop new prevention strategies, safer, better therapies, and eventually a cure. There is also a need for additional health services research, operations research, and behavioral research and biomedical prevention research that have a population-level impact.
5. A commitment to innovation is needed to keep pace with an evolving epidemic, a scarcity of resources, and to support communities for which HIV is just one of many major challenges.

The steps outlined in this document merely provide a path forward. Because they are the result of broad-based engagement with Federal and community partners, we believe that they contain an informed wisdom from multiple perspectives and experiences. If they are to have any impact, individuals and groups all over the country will need to follow the path described and produce a more coordinated, collective response to HIV.

With government at all levels doing its part, a committed private sector, and leadership from people living with HIV and affected communities, the United States can dramatically reduce HIV transmission and better support people living with HIV and their families.

End Notes

[1] CDC. HIV/AIDS Surveillance Report. 2007; 19: 7. Available at http://www.cdc.gov/hiv/topics /surveillance /resources/reports/2007report/pdf/2007SurveillanceReport.pdf.

[2] Kaiser Family Foundation. 2009 Survey of Americans on HIV/AIDS: Summary of Findings on the Domestic Epidemic. April 2009.

[3] CDC. Estimates of new HIV infections in the United States. August 2008. Available at http://www. kff.org /kaiserpolls/upload/7889.pdf.

[4] CDC. HIV Prevalence Estimates—United States, 2006. MMWR 2008;57(39):1073-76.

[5] If the HIV transmission rate remained constant at 5.0 persons infected each year per 100 people living with HIV, within a decade, the number of new infections would increase to more than 75,000 per year and the number of people living with HIV would grow to more than 1,500,000 (JAIDS, in press).

[6] Kaiser Family Foundation. 2009 Survey of Americans on HIV/AIDS: Summary of Findings on the Domestic Epidemic. April 2009. Available at http://www.kff.org/kaiserpolls/upload/7889.pdf.

[7] Mahajan AP, Sayles JN, Patel VA, et al. Stigma in the HIV/AIDS epidemic: A review of the literature and recommendations for the way forward. AIDS 2008;22(Suppl 2):S67-S69.

[8] CDC. HIV/AIDS Surveillance Report. 2007; 19: 7. Available at http://www.cdc.gov/hiv/topics/surveillance /resources/reports/2007report/pdf/2007SurveillanceReport.pdf.

[9] Kaiser Family Foundation. 2009 Survey of Americans on HIV/AIDS: Summary of Findings on the Domestic Epidemic. April 2009. Available at http://www.kff.org/kaiserpolls/upload/7889.pdf.

[10] Hall HI, Song R, Rhodes P, et al. Estimation of HIV incidence in the United States. JAMA 2008;300(5):520-529.

[11.] CDC. HIV Prevalence Estimates—United States, 2006. MMWR 2008;57(39):1073-76.

[12] If the HIV transmission rate remained constant at 5.0 persons infected each year per 100 people living with HIV, within a decade, the number of new infections would increase to more than 75,000 per year, and the number of people living with HIV would grow to more than 1,500,000 (JAIDS, in press).

[13] CDC. Estimates of new HIV infections in the United States. August 2008. Available at www.cdc.gov/hiv/topics/surveillance/resources/factsheets/pdf/incidence.pdf.

[14] CDC. HIV/AIDS Surveillance Report. 2007; 19: 7. Available at http://www.cdc.gov/hiv/topics/surveillance/resources/reports/2007report/pdf/2007SurveillanceReport.pdf.

[15] Throughout this document we use the terms "gay and bisexual men" and "gay men" interchangeably, and we intend these terms to be inclusive of all men who have sex with men (MSM), even those who do not identify as gay or bisexual.

[16] Throughout this document we use the terms "Black" and "African American" interchangeably, and we intend these terms to be inclusive of all individuals from the African Diaspora who identify as Black and/or African American.

[17] CDC. HIV and AIDS in the United States: *A Picture of Today's Epidemic.* 2007. Available at http://www.cdc.gov/hiv/topics/surveillance/united_states.htm.

[18] CDC. HIV/AIDS Surveillance Report. 2007; 19: 7. Available at http://www.cdc.gov/hiv/topics/surveillance/resources/reports/2007report/pdf/2007SurveillanceReport.pdf.

[19] Losina E, Schackman BR, Sadownik SN, et al. Racial and Sex Disparities in Life Expectancy Losses among HIV-Infected Persons in the United States. *Clin. Infect. Dis.* 2009;49(10):1570-8.

[20] CDC. HIV/AIDS Surveillance Report. 2007; 19: 7. Available at http://www.cdc.gov/hiv/topics/surveillance/resources/reports/2007report/pdf/2007SurveillanceReport.pdf.

[21] CDC. Estimates of new HIV infections in the United States. August 2008. Available at www.cdc.gov/hiv/topics/surveillance/resources/factsheets/pdf/incidence.pdf.

[22] CDC. HIV and AIDS among persons aged 50 and over. 2008. Available at www.cdc.gov/hiv/topics/over50/resources/factsheets/pdf/over50.pdf. Accessed February 18, 2010.

[23] See www.WhiteHouse.gov/ONAP.

[24] Hall HI, Song R, Rhodes P, et al. Estimation of HIV incidence in the United States. *JAMA* 2008;300(5):520-529.

[25] Hall HI, Song R, Rhodes P, et al. Estimation of HIV incidence in the United States. *JAMA* 2008;300(5):520-529.

[26] CDC. HIV and AIDS-United States, 1981-2000. MMWR 2001 50(21);430-4.

[27] Phelps R, Robbins K, Liberti T, et al. Window-period human immunodeficiency virus transmission to two recipients by an adolescent blood donor. *Transfusion.* 2004;44:929-933.

[28] CDC. HIV/AIDS Fact Sheet: Pregnancy and Childbirth. 2007. Available at http://www.cdc.gov/hiv/topics/perinatal/overview_partner.htm.

[29] CDC. HIV/AIDS Surveillance in Injection Drug Users (through 2007). Available at http://www.cdc.gov/hiv/idu/resources/slides/index.htm.

[30] Des Jarlais DC, Perlis T, Kamyar A, et al. HIV Incidence Among Injection Drug Users in New York City, 1990 to 2002: Use of Serologic Test Algorithm to Assess Expansion of HIV Prevention Services. *Am. J. Public Health.* 2005;95:1439-1444.

[31] Strathdee SA, Patrick DM, Currie SL, et al. Needle exchange is not enough: lessons from the Vancouver injecting drug use study. *AIDS.* 1997;11:F59-65.

[32] CDC. HIV infection among injection-drug users—34 States, 2004-2007. MMWR. 2009;58:1291-1295.

[33] Donnell D, Baeten JM, Kiarie J, et al. Heterosexual HIV-1 transmission after initiation of antiretroviral therapy: a prospective cohort analysis. *Lancet.* 2010.

[34] If the HIV transmission rate remained constant at 5.0 persons infected each year per 100 people living with HIV, within a decade, the number of new infections would increase to more than 75,000 per year and the number of people living with HIV would grow to more than 1,500,000 (JAIDS, in press).

[35] CDC. HIV prevalence estimates—United States, 2006. MMWR. 2008; 57: 1073-1076.

[36] Marks G, Crepaz N, Janssen RS. Estimating sexual transmission of HIV from persons aware and unaware that they are infected with the virus in the USA. AIDS 2006; 26;10:1447-50.

[37] Jenkins TC, Gardener EM, Thrun MW, et al., Risk-Based Human Immunodeficiency Virus (HIV) Testing Fails to Detect the Majority of HIV-Infected Persons in Medical Care Settings. Sex Transm Dis. 2006; 33:329-333.

[38] HRSA. HIV/AIDS Bureau. Outreach: Engaging People in HIV Care. August 2006. Available at http:// hab.

hrsa.gov/tools/HIVoutreach.

[39] Kaiser Family Foundation. 2009 Survey of Americans on HIV/AIDS: Summary of Findings on the Domestic Epidemic. April 2009. Available at http://www.kff.org/kaiserpolls/upload/7889.pdf.

[40] Schackman BR, Gebo KA, Walensky RP, et al. The lifetime cost of current human immunodeficiency virus care in the United States. Med Care 2006;44(11):990-97.

[41] For more information about how these and other targets in the National HIV/AIDS Strategy were derived, see the National HIV/ AIDS Strategy: Federal Implementation Plan at www.WhiteHouse.gov/ONAP. All numbers are based on current estimates.

[42] El-Sadr W, Mayer KH, Hodder SL. AIDS in America—Forgotten but not Gone. New Engl J Med. 2010.

[43] Kaiser Family Foundation. 2009 Survey of Americans on HIV/AIDS: Summary of Findings on the Domestic Epidemic. April 2009. Available at http://www.kff.org/kaiserpolls/upload/7889.pdf.

[44] Throughout this document we use the terms "Latino" and "Hispanic" interchangeably. "Hispanic' is used in the Figures to match data sources.

[45] CDC Press release. CDC analysis provides new look at disproportionate impact of HIV and syphilis among U.S. gay and bisexual men. March 19, 2010. Available at http://www.cdc.gov/nchhstp/ newsroom/ msmpressrelease.html This press release includes data from the CDC that is based on the most comprehensive analysis to date of nationally representative surveys. The estimate of 2% is based on a range of 1.4-2.7% in the overall U.S. population age 13 and older who have engaged in same sex behavior in the last five years. (Data source: DW Purcell, C Johnson, A Lansky, et al. Calculating HIV and Syphilis Rates for Risk Groups: Estimating the National Population Size of Men Who Have Sex with Men 2010 National STD Prevention Conference; Atlanta, GA Latebreaker #22896 Presented March 10, 2010).

[46] CDC. HIV Prevention in the United States at a Critical Crossroads. 2009. Available at http://www.cdc.gov/hiv/resources/reports/pdf/hiv_prev_us.pdf.

[47] CDC Fact Sheet. HIV/AIDS among African Americans. August 2009. Available at http://www.cdc.gov/hiv/topics/aa/resources/factsheets/aa.htm.

[48] CDC. HIV Prevention in the United States at a Critical Crossroads. 2009. Available at http://www.cdc.gov/hiv/resources/reports/pdf/hiv_prev_us.pdf.

[49] CDC. HIV Prevalence, Unrecognized Infection, and HIV Testing Among Men Who Have Sex with Men - Five U.S. Cities, June 2004-April 2005. MMWR Weekly 54(24);597-601.

[50] CDC Fact Sheet. HIV/AIDS Among Women, August 2008. Available at http://www.cdc.gov/hiv/topics /women /resources/factsheets/pdf/women.pdf.

[51] CDC Fact Sheet. HIV/AIDS among Hispanics/Latinos. 2009. Available at http://www.cdc.gov/hiv /hispanics/ resources/factsheets/hispanic.htm.

[52] CDC. HIV Prevention in the United States at a Critical Crossroads. 2009. Available at http://www.cdc.gov/hiv/resources/reports/pdf/hiv_prev_us.pdf.

[53] Brady JE, Friedman SR, Cooper HLF, et al. Risk-based prevalence of infection drug users in the U.S. and in large U.S. metropolitan areas from 1992-2002. J. Urban Health.2008;85:323-351.

[54] Hall HI, Song R, Rhodes P, et al. Estimation of HIV incidence in the United States. JAMA 2008;300(5):520-529.

[55] Strathdee SA, Sherman SG. The role of sexual transmission of HIV infection among injection and non-injection drug users. J. Urban Health. 2003; 80:iii7-14.

[56] Molitor F, Truax SR, Ruiz JD, Sun RK. Association of methamphetamine use during sex with risky sexual behaviors and HIV infection among non-injection drug users. West. J. Med. 1998;168(2):93-97.

[57] Buchbinder SP, Vittinghoff E, Heagerty P, et al. Sexual Risk, Nitrite Inhalant Use, and Lack of Circumcision associated with HIV Seroconversion in Men who have Sex with Men in the United States. J. Acquir. Immune Def. Syn. 2005;39(1):82-89.

[58] Millett GA, Flores SA, Peterson J, Bakeman R. Explaining disparities in HIV infection among Black and White men who have sex with men: A meta-analysis of HIV risk behaviors. AIDS 2007;21(15): 2083-2091.

[59] Hallfors DD, Iritani BJ, Miller WC, Bauer DJ. Sexual and Drug Behavior Patterns and HIV/STD Racial Disparities: The Need for New Directions. Am. J. Public Health. 2007;97(1):125-132.

[60] CDC. HIV/AIDS Surveillance in Urban and Nonurban Areas (through 2007) Slide Set. 2009. Available at http://www.cdc.gov/hiv/topics/surveillance/resources/slides/urban-nonurban/index.htm

[61] HHS Fact Sheet: HIV/AIDS in the Caribbean. Available at http://www.kff.org/hivaids/upload/7505-06.pdf

[62] Amaro H, Raj A. One the margin: Power and women's HIV risk reduction strategies. Sex Roles. 2000;42:723-749.

[63] CDC. HIV/AIDS Surveillance in Injection Drug Users (through 2007) Slide set. Available at http://www.cdc.gov/hiv/idu/resources/slides/index.htm

[64] CDC. HIV Transmission among Male Inmates in a State Prison System—Georgia, 1992-2005. 2006. Available at

http://www.cdc.gov/mmwr/preview/mmwrhtml/mm5515a1.htm. Accessed June 14, 2010.

[65] Federal Bureau Of Prisons. HIV Seroconversion Study. Presented at International Emerging Infectious Diseases Conference. March 19-22, Atlanta, GA. 2006.

[66] Baillargeon J, Giordano TP, Rich JD, et al. Accessing antiretroviral therapy following release from prison. *JAMA* 2009;301(8):848-857.

[67] Adimora AA, Schoenbach VJ, Doherty IA. HIV and African Americans in the Southern United States: Sexual Networks and Social Context. *Sex Transm. Dis.* 2006; 33(7):S39-S45.

[68] CDC Fact Sheet. HIV/AIDS among Asians and Pacific Islanders. August 2008. Available at http://www.cdc.gov/hiv/resources/factsheets/API.htm

[69] CDC Fact Sheet. HIV/AIDS among American Indians and Alaska Natives. August 2008. Available at http://www.cdc.gov/hiv/resources/factsheets/aian.htm

[70] CDC Fact Sheet. HIV/AIDS among African-Americans. August 2009. Available at http://www.cdc.gov/hiv/topics/aa/resources/factsheets/aa.htm

[71] CDC. HIV/AIDS Surveillance by Race/Ethnicity (through 2007) Slide set. April 2009. Available at http://www.cdc.gov/hiv/topics/surveillance/resources/slides/race-ethnicity/index.htm

[72] CDC. HIV/AIDS Surveillance Report. 2007; 19:7. Available at http://www.cdc.gov/hiv/topics/surveillance/resources/reports/2007report/pdf/2007SurveillanceReport.pdf

[73] CDC. HIV Prevention in the United States at a Critical Crossroads. 2009. Available at http://www.cdc.gov/hiv/resources/reports/pdf/hiv_prev_us.pdf

[74] CDC. HIV/AIDS among Asians and Pacific Islanders. August 2008. Available at http://www.cdc.gov/hiv/resources/factsheets/API.htm

[75] CDC. HIV/AIDS among American Indians and Alaska Natives. August 2008. Available at http://www.cdc.gov/hiv/resources/factsheets/aian.htm

[76] NASTAD and Kaiser Family Foundation. The National HIV Prevention Inventory: The State of HIV Prevention Across the U.S. July 2009. Available at http://www.kff.org/hivaids/upload/7932.pdf.

[77] CDC. CDC Fact Sheet: HIV and AIDS among Gay and Bisexual Men. June 2010. Available at http://www.cdc.gov/nchhstp/newsroom/docs/FastFacts-MSM-FINAL508COMP.pdf.

[78] DW Purcell, C Johnson, A Lansky, et al. Calculating HIV and Syphilis Rates for Risk Groups: Estimating the National Population Size of Men Who Have Sex with Men 2010 National STD Prevention Conference; Atlanta, GA Latebreaker #22896 Presented March 10, 2010.

[79] CDC. CDC Fact Sheet: HIV and AIDS among Gay and Bisexual Men. June 2010. Available at http://www.cdc.gov/nchhstp/newsroom/docs/FastFacts-MSM-FINAL508COMP.pdf.

[80] CDC. HIV/AIDS Surveillance in Urban and Nonurban Areas (through 2007). Available at http://www.cdc.gov/hiv/topics/surveillance/resources/slides/urban-nonurban/index.htm.

[81] Operario D, Soma T, Underhill K. Sex work and HIV Status among Transgender Women: Systematic Review and Meta-Analysis. *J. Acquir .Immune Def. Syndr.* 2008;48(1)97-103.

[82] CDC. Trends in HIV/AIDS Diagnoses among men who have sex with men—33 states, 2001-2006. MMWR June 2008;57(25):681- 686.

[83] Auerbach JD, Coates TJ. HIV Prevention Research: Accomplishment and Challenges for the Third decade of AIDS. Am J Public Health. 2000;90:1029-1032.

[84] UNAIDS. UNAIDS promotes combination HIV prevention towards universal access goals. March 2009. Available at http://www.unaids.org/en/KnowledgeCentre/Resources/PressCentre/PressReleases/2009/20090318_ComprehensivePrevention.asp.

[85] Piot P, Bartos M, Larson H, Zewdie D, Mane P Coming to terms with complexity: a call to action for HIV prevention. *Lancet.*2008 (9641);372:845-859.

[86] The National Institutes of Health (NIH) publishes and updates the Department of Health and Human Services clinical practice guidelines for the use of antiretroviral therapy for people living with HIV. The most recent versions of the guidelines for specific populations may be found at http://www.aidsinfo.nih.gov/Guidelines/.

[87] Marks G, Crepaz Nicole, Janssen, RS. Estimating sexual transmission of HIV from persons aware and unaware that they are infected with the virus in the USA. AIDS.2006;20(10): 1447-1450.

[88] Bisset L, Cone RW, Huber W, et al. Highly active antiretroviral therapy during early HIV infection reverses T-cell activation and maturation abnormalities. AIDS 1998;12(16):2115-23.

[89] Weller S, Davis, K. Condom effectiveness in reducing heterosexual HIV transmission (Cochrane Review). In: The Cochrane Library, Issue 4, 2003. Chichester, UK: John Wiley & Sons, Ltd.

[90] Latkin, C, Davey, M, and Hua, W. Needle Exchange Program Utilization and Entry into Drug User Treatment: Is There a Long-Term Connection in Baltimore, Maryland? Subst Use Misuse, 41(14):1991-2001.

[91] Vlahov D, Junge B. The role of needle exchange programs in HIV prevention. *Public Health Rep.* 1998;113

(Suppl 1):75-80.

[92] Donnell D, Baeten JM, Kiarie J, et al. Heterosexual HIV-1 transmission after initiation of antiretroviral therapy: a prospective cohort analysis. *Lancet.* 2010.

[93] Smith DK, Grohskopf LA, Black RJ, et al. Antiretroviral postexposure prophylaxis after sexual, injection-drug use, or other nonoccupational exposure to HIV in the United States. MMWR. 2005; 54:1-20.

[94] HHS. Recommendations for Use of Antiretroviral Drugs in Pregnant HIV-1 Infected Women for Maternal Health and Interventions to Reduce Perinatal HIV Transmission in the United States. May 24, 2010.

[95] Celum C, Wald A, Hughes J, et al. Effect of acyclovir on HIV-1 acquisition in herpes simplex virus 2 seropositive women and men who have sex with men. *Lancet.* 2008;371:2109-19.

[96] Gray RH, Wawer MJ. Reassessing the hypothesis on STI control for Prevention. *Lancet.* 2008; 371(9630): 2064-2065.

[97] National Alliance of State and Territorial AIDS Directors, National Coalition of STD Directors. STD/HIV prevention integration; 2002Available from: URL: http://www.ncsddc.org/docs/STDHIVIssuePaperFinal.pdf

[98] CDC. 2009 compendium of evidence-based HIV prevention interventions. Available from URL: http://www.cdc.gov/hiv/topics/research/prs/evidence-based-interventions.htm.

[99] Coates T, Richter L, Caceres C. Behavioural strategies to reduce HIV transmission: how to make them better. *Lancet.* 2008;372(9639):669-684.

[100] Koblin B, Chesney M, Coates TJ, for the EXPLORE Study Team. Effects of a behavioural intervention to reduce acquisition of HIV infection among men who have sex with men: the EXPLORE randomised controlled study. *Lancet.* 2004; 364: 41–50.

[101] Crepaz N, Horn AK, Rama SM, et al. The efficacy of behavioral interventions in reducing HIV risk sex behaviors and incident sexually transmitted disease in black and Hispanic sexually transmitted disease clinic patients in the United States: a meta-analytic review. *Sex Transm. Dis.* 2007;34(6):319-32.

[102] Coates T, Richter L, Caceres C. Behavioural strategies to reduce HIV transmission: how to make them better. *Lancet.* 2008;372(9639):669-684.

[103] Pilcher CD, Tien HC, Eron JJ, et al. Brief but efficient: Acute HIV infection and the sexual transmission of HIV. *J. Infect. Dis.* 2004; 189(10):1785-1792.

[104] CDC. HIV/AIDS among Persons Aged 50 and Older. February 2008. Available at http://www.cdc.gov/hiv/topics/over50/resources/factsheets/over50.htm.

[105] Kaiser Family Foundation. 2009 Survey of Americans on HIV/AIDS: Summary of Findings on the Domestic Epidemic. Available at http://www.kff.org/kaiserpolls/upload/7889.pdf.

[106] Schackman BR, Gebo KA, Walensky RP, et al. The lifetime cost of current human immunodeficiency virus care in the United States. *Med. Care* 2006; 44(11):990-7.

[107] The Patient Protection and Affordable Care Act (Affordable Care Act), P.L. 111-148 includes numerous provisions that will expand access to insurance coverage for people living with HIV. See, for example, Title II which includes expands Medicaid eligibility and Title I which includes various insurance market reforms.

[108] Moore, R.M., Gebo, K.A., Lucas, G.M., Keruly, J.C. Rate of Co-morbidities Not Related to HIV infection or AIDS among HIV-Infected Patients, by CD4 Count and HAART Use Status. *Clin. Infect. Dis.* 2008; 47(8):1102-1104.

[109] Hall IH, McDavid K, Ling Q, Sloggett A. Determinants of Progression to AIDS or Death After HIV Diagnosis, United States, 1996 to 2001. *Ann. Epidemiol.* 2006;16(11): 824-33.

[110] Heckman TG, Somlai AM, Peters J, Walker J, Otto-Sajal CA, Galdabni CA, Kelly JA. Barriers to care among persons living with HIV/AIDS in urban and rural areas. *AIDS Care* 1998;10(3):365-75.

[111] The National Institutes of Health (NIH) publishes and updates the Department of Health and Human Services clinical practice guidelines for the use of antiretroviral therapy for people living with HIV. The most recent versions of the guidelines for specific populations may be found at http://www.aidsinfo.nih.gov/Guidelines/.

[112] Kitahata MM, Gange SJ, Abraham AG, et al. Effect of early versus deferred antiretroviral therapy for HIV on survival. *New Engl. iMed.* 2009; 360(18):1815-1826.

[113] CDC. HIV prevalence estimates—United States, 2006.MMWR. 2008; 57: 1073-1076.

[114] SAMHSA. National Survey of Substance Abuse Treatment Services. The N-SSATS Report. February 25, 2010.

[115] Aberg JA, Kaplan JE, Libman H, et al. Primary care guidelines for the management of persons infected with human immunodeficiency virus: 2009 update by the HIV Medicine Association of the Infectious Diseases Society of America. *Clin. Infect. Dis.* 2009;49(5):651-81.

[116] DHHS Panel on Antiretroviral Guidelines for Adults and Adolescents. Guidelines for the use of antiretroviral agents in HIV-1-infected adults and adolescents. Department of Health and Human Services. December 1, 2009; 1-161. Available at http://www.aidsinfo.nih.gov/ContentFiles/AdultandAdolescentGL.pdf.

[117] Association of American Medical Colleges. 2009 State Physician Workforce Data Book. November 2009.

[118] AAHIVM and HIVMA Medical Workforce Working Group. Averting a Crisis in HIV Care: A Joint Statement of the American Academy of HIV Medicine (AAHIVM) and the HIV Medicine Association (HIVMA) on the HIV Medical Workforce. June 2009.

[119] CDC. National Survey of Family Growth. Available at http://www.cdc.gov/nchs/nsfg/abc_list.htm.

[120] AHRQ. 2009 National Healthcare Quality Report. March 2010.

[121] Cargill VA, Stone VE. HIV/AIDS: a minority health issue. Med Clin North Am 200;89(4):895-912.

[122] Solursh DS, Ernst JL, Lewis RW et al. The human sexuality education of physicians in North American Schools. *Int. J. Imp. Res.* 2003;15(Suppl 5):S41-5.

[123] Williamson C.. Providing care to transgender persons: a clinical approach to primary care, hormones, and HIV management. *J. Assoc. Nurses AIDS Care* 2010;21(3):221-229.

[124] Kalichman SC, Ramachandran B, Catz S. Adherence to combination antiretroviral therapies in HIV patients of low health literacy. *J. Gen. Intern. Med.* 1999;14(5):267-73

[125] Saag MS. Ryan White: An Unintentional Home Builder. AIDS Reader 2009; 19:166-168.

[126] Bing EG, Burnman MA, Longshore D, et al. Psychiatric disorders and drug use among human immunodeficiency virus-infected adults in the United States. Arch Gen Psych 2001 58(8):721-728.

[127] CDC Fact Sheet. Coinfection with HIV and Hepatitis C Virus. November 2005. Available at http://www.cdc.gov/hiv/resources/factsheets/coinfection.htm.

[128] El-Sadr WM, Lundgren JD, Neaton JD, et a. Strategies for Management of Antiretroviral Therapy (SMART) Study Group. CD4+ count-guided interruption of antiretroviral treatment. *N. Engl. J. Med.* 2001,355(22):2283-2296.

[129] Kidder DP, Wolitski RJ, Campsmith,ML, Nakamura, GV. Health status, health care use, medication use, and medication adherence in homeless and housed people living with HIV/AIDS. *Am. J. Public Health.* 2007; 97(12):2238-2245.

[130] Aidala, AA, Lee, G, Abramson, DM, Messeri, P, Siegler, A. Housing need, housing assistance, and connection to medical care. *AIDS Behav.* 2007;11(Supp 2): S101-S115.

[131] El-Sadr W, Mayer KH, Hodder SL. AIDS in America—Forgotten but not Gone. New Engl. J. Med. 2010.

[132] CDC. HIV and AIDS in the United States: A Picture of Today's Epidemic. 2008. Available at http://www.cdc.gov/hiv/topics/surveillance/united_states.htm.

[133] DW Purcell, C Johnson, A Lansky, et al. Calculating HIV and Syphilis Rates for Risk Groups: Estimating the National Population Size of Men Who Have Sex with Men 2010 National STD Prevention Conference; Atlanta, GA Latebreaker #22896 Presented March 10, 2010.

[134] Losina E, Schackman BR, Sadownik SN, et al. Racial and Sex Disparities in Life Expectancy Losses among HIV-Infected Persons in the United States. *Clin. Infect. Dis.* 2009;49(10):1570-8.

[135] Hall HI, Byers RH, Ling Q, Espinoza L. Racial/Ethnic and Age Disparities in HIV Prevalence and Disease Progression Among Men Who Have Sex With Men in the United States. *Am. J. Public Health.* 2007;97(6):1060-66.

[136] Losina E, Schackman BR, Sadownik SN, et al. Racial and Sex Disparities in Life Expectancy Losses among HIV-Infected Persons in the United States. *Clin. Infect. Dis.* 2009;49(10):1570-8.

[137] CDC. HIV in the United States: An overview. June 2010. Available at http://www.cdc.gov /hiv/ topics /surveillance/resources/factsheets/us_overview.htm.

[138] Quinn TC, Wawer MJ, Sewankambo N, et al. Viral Load and Heterosexual Transmission of Human Immunodeficiency Virus Type 1. *New Engl. J. Med.* 2000;342(13):921-29.

[139] Donnell D, Baeten JM, Kiarie J, et al. Heterosexual HIV-1 transmission after initiation of antiretroviral therapy: a prospective cohort analysis. *Lancet* 2010;375(9731):2092-8.

[140] Sterling TR, Vlahov D, Astemborski J, et al. Initial Plasma HIV-1 RNA levels and progression to AIDS in women and men. *New Engl. J. Med.* 2001; 344(10):720-725.

[141] Donnell D, Baeten JM, Kiarie J, et al. Heterosexual HIV-1 transmission after initiation of antiretroviral therapy: a prospective cohort analysis. *Lancet* 2010;375(9731):2092-8.

[142] Millett GA, Flores SA, Peterson J, Bakeman R. Explaining disparities in HIV infection among Black and White men who have sex with men: A meta-analysis of HIV risk behaviors. *AIDS* 2007;21(15): 2083-2091.

[143] Hallfors DD, Iritani BJ, Miller WC, Bauer DJ. Sexual and Drug Behavior Patterns and HIV/STD Racial Disparities: The Need for New Directions. *Am. J. Public Health.* 2007;97(1):125-132.

[144] Das M, Chu PL, Santos G-M, Scheer S, Vittinghoff E, et al. 2010 Decreases in Community Viral Load Are Accompanied by Reductions in New HIV Infections in San Francisco. PLoS ONE 5(6): e11068. doi:10.1371/journal.pone.0011068.

[145] Wood E, Kerr T, Marshall BDL, et al. Longitudinal community plasma HIV-1 RNA concentrations and incidence of HIV-1 among injecting drug users: prospective cohort study. BMJ. 2009;338:b1649.

[146] Montaner J et al. Association of expanded HAART coverage with a decrease in new HIV diagnoses, particularly among injection drug users in British Columbia, Canada. 17th Conference on Retroviruses and Opportunistic Infections, San Francisco, abstract 88LB, 2010.

[147] NIH Press Release: NIH and D.C. Department of Health Team up to Combat District's HIV/AIDS Epidemic, January 12, 2010. Available at http://www.nih.gov/news/health/jan2010/niaid-12.htm.

[148] Holtgrave DR, Crosby RA. Social capital, poverty, and income inequality as predictors of gonorrhoea, syphilis, chlamydia and AIDS case rates in the United States. *Sex Transm. Infect.* 2003;79(1):62-64.

[149] Stall R, Mills TC, Williamson J, et al. Association of Co-Occurring Psychosocial Health Problems and Increased Vulnerability to HIV/AIDS Among Urban Men Who Have Sex With Men. Am) *Public Health.* 2003;93(6):939-942.

[150] Weiser SD, Frongillo EA, Ragland K, Hogg RS, Riley ED, Bangsberg DR. Food insecurity is associated with incomplete HIV RNA suppression among homeless and marginally housed HIV-infected individuals in San Francisco.) *Gen. Internal. Med.* 2009; 24(1):14-20.

[151] National Library of Medicine. Profiles in Science: Visual Culture and Health - HIV/AIDS. 2003.

[152] In 1992, Bob Hattoy addressed the Democratic National Convention and Mary Fischer addressed the Republican National Convention, and both openly acknowledged living with HIV.

[153] Valdiserri, RO. HIV/AIDS stigma: an impediment to public health. Am J Public Health 2002;92(3):341-342.

[154] Kaiser Family Foundation. Criminal statutes on HIV transmission. 2008. Available at http://www. Statehealth facts.org/comparetable.jsp?ind=569&cat=11.

[155] CDC. HIV Prevention in the United States at a Critical Crossroads. 2009. Available at http://www.cdc.gov/hiv/resources/reports/pdf/hiv_prev_us.pdf.

[156] Horvath KJ, Weinmeyer R, Rosser S. An examination of attitudes among US men who have sex with men and the impact of state law. AIDS Care. 2010 (in press).

[157] Burris S, Cameron E. The case against criminalization of HIV transmission. *JAMA.* 2008;300(5): 578-581.

[158] UNAIDS. Criminal law, public health and HIV transmission: A policy options paper. June 2002. Available at http://data.unaids.org/publications/IRC-pub02/jc733-criminallaw_en.pdf.

[159] FY 2010 Appropriations.

[160] CDC analysis. Please refer to www.cdc.gov/hiv for the budget information and http://www.cdc.gov/hiv/topics/surveillance/resources/reports/ for surveillance data.

In: Responding to HIV/AIDS
Editor: Lawrence T. Jensen

ISBN: 978-1-61324-618-4
© 2011 Nova Science Publishers, Inc.

Chapter 2

NATIONAL HIV/AIDS STRATEGY: FEDERAL IMPLEMENTATION PLAN*

Office of the President of the United States

LIST OF ACRONYMS

AAPI	Asian American and Pacific Islander
ADAP	AIDS Drug Assistance Program
AETC	AIDS Education and Training Center
AHRQ	Agency for Healthcare Research and Quality, http://www.ahrq.gov/
AI/AN	American Indian/Alaska Native
AIDS	Acquired Immune deficiency Syndrome
ASH	Assistant Secretary for Health, Department of Health and Human Services
BOP	Bureau of Prisons, Department of Justice, http://www.bop.gov/
CBO	Community-based organization(s)
CDC	Centers for Disease Control and Prevention, http://www.cdc.gov/
CMS	Centers for Medicare and Medicaid Services, http://www.cms.gov/
DOJ	Department of Justice, http://www.justice.gov/
DOL	Department of Labor, http://www.dol.gov/
FDA	Food and Drug Administration, http://www.fda.gov/
HAART	Highly-Active Antiretroviral Therapy
HIV	Human Immunodeficiency Virus
HHS	Department of Health and Human Services, http://www.hhs.gov/
HOPWA	Housing Opportunities for Persons with AIDS, http://www.hud.gov/offices/cpd/aidshousing/programs/
HRSA	Health Resources and Services Administration, http://www.hrsa.gov/
HUD	Department of Housing and Urban Development, http://portal.hud.gov/ portal/page/portal/HUD

---

* This is an edited, reformatted and augmented version of an Office of the President of the United States publication, dated July, 2010.

IDU	Injection Drug Use/User
HIS	Indian Health Service, http://wwww.ihs.gov
LGBT	Lesbian, Gay, Bisexual, and Transgender
NIH	National Institutes of Health, http://www.nih.gov/
OGAC	Office of the Global AIDS Coordinator, Department of State, http://www.state.gov/ogac/
OMB	Office of Management and Budget, http://www.whitehouse.gov/omb/
OMH	Office of Minority Health, http://minorityhealth.hhs.gov
ONAP	Office of National AIDS Policy, http://www.whitehouse.gov /administration /eop/onap/
PACHA	Presidential Advisory Council on HIV/AIDS, http://www.whitehouse.gov/administration/eop/onap/pacha
SAMHSA	Substance Abuse and Mental Health Services Administration, http://samhsa.gov/
SSA	Social Security Administration, http://www.ssa.gov/
STD	Sexually Transmitted Disease
STI	Sexually Transmitted Infection
VA	Department of Veterans Affairs, http://www.va.gov/

INTRODUCTION

President Obama committed to developing a National HIV/AIDS Strategy with three primary goals: 1) reducing the number of people who become infected with HIV, 2) increasing access to care and optimizing health outcomes for people living with HIV, and 3) reducing HIV-related health disparities. To accomplish these goals, we must undertake a more coordinated, vigorous national response to the HIV epidemic.

The President also promised that the Strategy would rely on sound science and include measurable goals, timelines, and accountability mechanisms. This document is a companion to the National HIV/ AIDS Strategy for the United States. It presents the Administration's plan for measuring progress toward meeting the Strategy's goals, and includes immediate and short-term Federal actions (those that can be achieved in calendar years 2010 and 2011) that will move the Nation toward improving its response to HIV/AIDS.[1] Where appropriate, we have highlighted some longer-term actions, but our immediate emphasis has been on identifying initial steps for moving forward. In 2011, ONAP will consult with Federal agencies to develop specific actions for 2012, and the plan will be updated annually, thereafter. This is a living document—we will evaluate our progress and modify it as necessary as we achieve certain milestones or experience unanticipated setbacks. Additionally, as the Federal agencies do their work to implement the Strategy, we anticipate that new activities will also be developed.

The job of implementing the National HIV/AIDS Strategy, however, does not fall to the Federal Government alone, nor should it. The success of the Strategy will require States, tribal and local governments, communities, and other partners to work together to better coordinate their responses to HIV/AIDS at the State and local levels. Therefore, we hope that the strategy will serve as a catalyst for all levels of government and other stakeholders to develop their own implementation plans for achieving the goals of the National HIV/AIDS Strategy.

The vision for the National HIV/AIDS Strategy is simple:

> The United States will become a place where new HIV infections are rare and when they do occur, every person, regardless of age, gender, race/ethnicity, sexual orientation, gender identity, or socio-economic circumstance, will have unfettered access to high quality, life-extending care, free from stigma and discrimination.

KEY STEPS IN IMPLEMENTING THE STRATEGY

The National HIV/AIDS Strategy is just a collection of words on paper, unless it provides a strategic vision for the country that leads to action. This document outlines key actions to be undertaken by the Federal Government.

Since taking office, the Obama Administration has worked to engage the public to evaluate what we are doing right and identify new approaches that will strengthen our response to the domestic epidemic. The White House Office of National AIDS Policy (ONAP), a component of the Domestic Policy Council, has been tasked with leading the effort to develop a national strategy. Throughout the process, ONAP has taken steps to engage as many Americans as possible to hear their ideas for making progress in the fight against HIV. ONAP's outreach included hosting 14 HIV/AIDS Community Discussions with thousands of Americans across the United States, reviewing suggestions from the public via the White House web site, conducting a series of expert meetings on HIV-specific topics, and working with Federal and community partners who organized their own meetings to support the development of a national strategy. A report summarizing public recommendations for the Strategy, entitled Community Ideas for Improving the Response to the Domestic HIV Epidemic, was published in April 2010.[2]

ONAP convened an interagency working group of officials from across the Federal Government to assist in reviewing the public recommendations, assessing the scientific evidence relevant to those recommendations, and making their own recommendations for the Strategy.

This National HIV/AIDS Strategy provides a roadmap for addressing the domestic HIV epidemic. It is not intended to be a comprehensive list of all activities needed to respond to HIV/AIDS, but is intended to be a concise plan that identifies a set of priorities and strategic action steps tied to measurable outcomes. The Federal Implementation Plan outlines the specific steps to be taken by various Federal agencies to support the high-level priorities outlined in the Strategy. Both the National HIV/AIDS Strategy and the Federal Implementation Plan may be accessed at www.WhiteHouse.gov/ONAP.

The quantitative targets that we have set are ambitious, and success is not assured. In the area of HIV prevention, for example, research conducted at CDC shows that while reallocation of existing resources and focusing on the most effective interventions will further improve the impact of HIV prevention efforts, there is still a strong case for making new investments in prevention, which could pay for themselves by reducing costly new infections in the future. Achieving these goals, however, requires stronger partnerships between Federal,

State, and local and tribal governments, as well as faith groups, businesses, foundations, and community-based organizations.

ONAP Oversight, Coordination and Annual Reporting

ONAP will continue to serve as the lead entity for setting the Administration's HIV/AIDS policies and will remain engaged in overseeing government-wide efforts to improve the Nation's response to the HIV epidemic. This role will include working with the Departments to support and monitor the implementation of the National HIV/AIDS Strategy. Departments will prepare and submit annual reports to ONAP.

ONAP will use this information to advise the President and produce an annual report describing the progress toward achieving goals in the Strategy. In addition, ONAP will continue to convene a Federal Interagency Working Group to foster collaboration across the Administration. ONAP will also continue to highlight important issues by convening meetings at the White House and working with Federal and non-Federal partners.

Role of Federal Departments

To support the implementation of the Strategy, the President has issued a Presidential Memorandum instructing relevant departments to provide a report to the President within the next 150 days outlining the steps they will take to ensure that they implement the recommendations in the Strategy. Federal agencies will also be tasked with establishing a responsible entity for coordinating their Department's efforts to achieve the goals of the Strategy and report on their progress. Other Departments are instructed to review their policies and identify steps that they can take to support implementation of the National HIV/AIDS Strategy. A copy of the Presidential Memorandum can be found at www.WhiteHouse.gov/Presidential-AIDS-Memo.

Role of the HHS Office of the Secretary

Implementation of the Strategy requires a new level of coordination and collaboration across agencies and among the Federal Government, States, tribes, and localities. Central to this coordination is the HHS Office of the Secretary (HHS OS)[3], which includes the Office of the Assistant Secretary for Health (ASH), who will be responsible for:

- Coordinating operational and programmatic activities for the National HIV/AIDS Strategy within the Department of Health and Human Services;
- Coordinating HIV/AIDS programs with other Departments;
- Tracking Federal programs implemented in each State or territory and working with States to ensure Federal HIV/AIDS activities are coordinated with State HIV/AIDS plans; and

- Establishing regular cross-Departmental meetings to coordinate program planning and administration of HIV/AIDS-related programs and activities.

Within ASH, the Deputy Assistant Secretary for Health will play a lead role in the supporting the implementation of the Strategy by forging collaborations across HHS and with other Federal departments and coordinating Federal efforts with States.

ROLE OF STATES AND LOCAL GOVERNMENTS

HHS will work with States to encourage the development of statewide HIV/AIDS plans. This will include encouraging the development of needs assessments and identifying specific action steps that improve coordination among State agencies, local and tribal governments, non-profits and private advocacy groups, and the activities funded by multiple Federal agencies. The purpose of State plans would be to enhance coordination between planning and resource allocation activities, which are often siloed in a way that separates prevention and care. States will also be encouraged to establish a lead entity to coordinate the development and implementation of statewide HIV/AIDS plans and be accountable for reporting regularly on progress made towards the goals of the National HIV/AIDS Strategy. To ensure effective collaboration in developing and implementing the statewide plans, the lead entity could be made up of representatives from State and local HIV/AIDS agencies, health departments, tribal governments, private advocacy groups, community-based organizations and people living with HIV. In developing their plans, States will also be encouraged to identify all Federal, State, and local resources, and to the extent feasible, private and nonprofit resources to ensure that all HIV/AIDS resources are allocated in the most efficient manner to address the full range of prevention, care, and social service needs.

ROLE OF NONGOVERNMENTAL PARTNERS

Although this document outlines initial steps the Federal Government will take after the release of the National HIV/AIDS Strategy, the job of implementing the Strategy does not fall to the Federal, State, tribal, and local governments alone. Businesses, faith communities, philanthropy, health care providers, the scientific and medical communities, educational institutions, professional organizations, and others must also do their part to support the achievement of the Strategy's goals. As we focus more attention on high-risk communities, for example, or as we consider the need to support people in meeting basic needs such as food and housing, and as we take steps to reduce stigma and discrimination, leadership is needed by people both inside and outside of government. Individuals or institutions themselves have a better understanding how they can maximally contribute to our efforts than the Federal Government. We hope that many interested parties will step forward and work together with the Federal Government to help end the HIV epidemic.

PACHA Review

The Presidential Advisory Council on HIV/AIDS (http://www.pacha.gov) will provide, on an ongoing basis, recommendations on how to effectively implement the strategy, as well as monitor the Strategy's implementation. At least once per year, a significant focus of one of the PACHA meetings will be to review the progress of Federal agencies and non-federal stakeholders in implementing the recommendations.

Annual Reporting

Progress in achieving the goals of the National HIV/AIDS Strategy will be reported by ONAP. ONAP will use information from the departments and States to publish an annual report on the Federal Government's progress.

SUMMARY NATIONAL HIV/AIDS STRATEGY TARGETS FOR 2015

Reducing New HIV Infections

- By 2015, lower the annual number of new infections by 25 percent (from 56,300 to 42,225).
- Reduce the HIV transmission rate, which is a measure of annual transmissions in relation to the number of people living with HIV, by 30 percent (from 5 persons infected per 100 people with HIV to 3.5 persons infected per 100 people with HIV).
- By 2015, increase from 79 percent to 90 percent the percentage of people living with HIV who know their serostatus (from 948,000 to 1,080,000 people).

Increasing Access to Care and Improving Health Outcomes for People Living with HIV

- By 2015, increase the proportion of newly diagnosed patients linked to clinical care within three months of their HIV diagnosis from 65% to 85% (from 26,824 to 35,078 people).
- By 2015, increase the proportion of Ryan White HIV/AIDS Program clients who are in continuous care (at least 2 visits for routine HIV medical care in 12 months at least 3 months apart) from 73 percent to 80 percent (or 237,924 people in continuous care to 260,739 people in continuous care).
- By 2015, increase the number of Ryan White clients with permanent housing from 82 percent to 86 percent (from 434,000 to 455,800 people). (This serves as a measurable proxy of our efforts to expand access to HUD and other housing supports to all needy people living with HIV.)

Reducing HIV-Related Health Disparities

While working to improve access to prevention and care services for all Americans,

- By 2015, increase the proportion of HIV diagnosed gay and bisexual men with undetectable viral load by 20 percent.
- By 2015, increase the proportion of HIV diagnosed Blacks with undetectable viral load by 20 percent.
- By 2015, increase the proportion of HIV diagnosed Latinos with undetectable viral load by 20 percent.

*All numbers based on current estimates.

REDUCING NEW HIV INFECTIONS

Reducing the number of new HIV infections is imperative. The targets below reflect our sense of urgency. From 2010 to 2015, the United States aims to:

- *Lower the annual number of new infections by 25 percent.* This would mean that the annual number of new infections would fall from 56,300 to 42,225. (*data source: CDC surveillance data*)
- *Reduce the HIV transmission rate, which is a measure of annual transmissions in relation to the number of people living with HIV, by 30 percent.* This would result in a reduction from 5 persons infected each year per 100 people with HIV to 3.5 persons each year per 100 people with HIV. (*data source: CDC surveillance data*)
- *Increase from 79 percent to 90 percent the percentage of people living with HIV who know their serostatus.* This would represent an increase from 948,000 to 1,080,000 Americans living with HIV who know their serostatus. (*data source: CDC surveillance data*)

2008 was the first year in which the United States could estimate the number of new HIV infections each year based on a direct measure of new infections. HIV incidence provides the best measure of the current state of the epidemic. Other measures, such as HIV diagnoses or AIDS cases, are also important, as they can indirectly estimate incidence. HIV diagnoses, for example, can provide some indication of the distribution of HIV in the United States, but it can also be affected by efforts to increase HIV testing. Expanded HIV testing could lead to more people learning their HIV status even if the annual number of new infections remains stable. The number of new infections (HIV incidence) provides a more current snapshot of how many people are becoming infected. We propose to lower the number of new infections by 25 percent by 2015.[4]

No measure is perfect. While stability in new infections is one sign of progress, incidence data alone cannot quantify the amount of transmission that occurs in relation to the growing population infected with HIV. The HIV transmission rate is another measure that takes both HIV incidence and the number of people living with HIV (prevalence) into account. It provides a measure of the number of new HIV infections that are transmitted in a given year for every 100 people living with HIV. It is expressed as a percentage and provides a "worst case" estimate of the number of infections occurring in relation to the number of people living with HIV. It provides a better means to assess the effects of public health efforts to promote changes in risk behavior, as well as the preventive effects of HIV diagnosis and treatment. HIV transmission rate is a useful measure because it is more sensitive to detecting progress in HIV prevention in the face of HIV flat incidence in the United States from year to year. According to CDC estimates, the HIV transmission rate in the United States was approximately 44.4 in 1984, 11.7 in 1990, 6.6 in 1991 and 5.0 in 2006.[5] We propose to lower the HIV transmission rate by 30 percent by 2015.[6]

Thirty years into the epidemic, the challenge we face is not to initiate a brand new response to HIV. As we have already acknowledged, the U.S. and the Federal Government do many things right in responding to the epidemic. To some extent, the public should hope and expect that the best ideas for prevention, care, and research are already being implemented, even if imperfectly. That does not mean, however, that the Nation cannot expect something new and better. It does mean that many of the steps we need to take may appear incremental or mundane, even if they are transformative over time.

For the first couple of years of implementing the Strategy, the focus on achieving our HIV incidence goals will be on taking the necessary steps to ensure that we have the epidemiological data we need and that we use these data to enhance efforts to ensure that resources for HIV prevention follow the epidemic. We also believe that a short-term focus needs to be on identifying and evaluating effective combinations of HIV prevention methods for specific high risk groups, as well as evaluating the success of existing programs. In future years, we expect to know more about which combinations of interventions work for which communities and then we can turn to scaling up our efforts to deploy effective prevention combinations. Specifically, our goal in the later years is to address several gaps in prevention including: 1) conducting research to improve methods for estimating the proportion of persons living with HIV who are unaware of their infections, as well as methods to reach these individuals; 2) testing and growing the portfolio of interventions that incorporate issues such as sexual networks, income insecurity, and other social factors that place some individuals and populations at greater risk for HIV infection than others; and, 3) improving methods to prevent HIV infection among women whose heightened risk for HIV is based on the risk behaviors of their male partners.

Step 1. Intensify HIV Prevention Efforts in Communities where HIV is Most Heavily Concentrated

1.1. Allocate Public Funding to Geographic Areas Consistent with the Epidemic

Governments at all levels should ensure that HIV prevention funding is allocated consistent with the latest epidemiological data and is targeted to the highest prevalence populations and communities.

Timeframe	Lead Agency/ Other Agencies	Actions to be Performed
By the end of 2010	HHS OS/CDC, SAMHSA, HRSA, and HUD	HHS OS will initiate consultations with CDC, SAMHSA, HRSA, HUD, and other departments or agencies as appropriate to develop policy recommendations for revising funding formulas and policy guidancein order to ensure that Federal HIV prevention funding allocations goto the jurisdictions with the greatest need.
	CDC	CDC will continue to evaluate all existing HIV prevention programs every five years to ensure that Federal dollars support programs that are effective and have demonstrated improved health outcomes.
By the end of 2011	HHS OS	All HHS agencies, as appropriate, will report to the HHS Office of the Secretary (OS) on baseline measures for funding allocations for their programs.
	HHS OS	HHS OS and relevant agencies will consult with States and other jurisdictions prior to allocating prevention funding to targeted populations and communities to ensure coordination of efforts.

1.2. Target High Risk Populations

Federal agencies should develop new mechanisms for ensuring that grant funding to State and local health departments and community-based organizations is based on the epidemiological profile within the jurisdiction.

Timeframe	Lead Agency/ Other Agencies	Actions to be Performed
By the end of 2011	CDC	CDC will establish new standards for reviewing State and local prevention plans to ensure that Federal funds are used in a manner addressing people living with HIV and reflecting populations with greatest need.
	CDC/HRSA, SAMHSA, HHS OS	CDC in consultation with HRSA, SAMHSA, and HHS OS will develop and implement a plan of recommended actions for reducing the proportion of HIV-positive individuals with undiagnosed HIV infectionamong target populations in high prevalence and incidence.
	CDC	CDC will update and issue guidelines on the provision of HIV counseling and testing in nonclinical settings.
	CDC	CDC will work with States to ensure that the new guidelines are incorporated into State HIV/AIDS plans

1.2.1. Prevent HIV among Gay and Bisexual Men[7] and Transgender Individuals

Congress and State legislatures should consider the implementation of laws that promote public health practice and underscore the existing best evidence in HIV prevention for sexual minorities.

Timeframe	Lead Agency/ Other Agencies	Actions to be Performed
By the end of 2010	HHS OS	HHS OS will initiate planning for a consultation with national Lesbian, Gay, Bisexual, and Transgender (LGBT) organizations to re-engage LGBT community leadership in health promotion.
By the end of 2011	CDC	CDC will develop recommendations for essential prevention activities and services provided to gay and bisexual men as part of the MSM initiative in the FY 2011 budget.
	CDC	CDC will work with States to increase capacity of STD surveillance systems to identify gender of sex partners and HIV infection status of men with reportable STDs.
	HHS OS	HHS OS will work with Congress to consider revising restrictions in thePublic Health Service Act that hinder the implementation of scientifically validated, culturally appropriate HIV prevention services
	CDC	CDC will expand its work evaluating adaptations of specific interventions for transgender populations and issue a fact sheet recommending HIV prevention approaches for transgender persons.
	CDC	CDC will work with States to ensure that State plans address deficiencies in directing the needed proportion of resources to gay male andtransgender populations—overall, and within racial/ethnic groups heavily impacted by the epidemic.

1.2.2. Prevent HIV among Black Men and Women[8]

To lower risks for all Americans, prevention efforts should acknowledge the heavy burden of HIV among Black Americans and target resources appropriately.

1.2.3. Prevent HIV among Latinos and Latinas

HIV prevention efforts that target Latino communities must be culturally appropriate and available to acculturated and nonacculturated Latino populations .

1.2.4. Prevent HIV among Substance Users

Substance use is associated with a greater likelihood of acquiring HIV infection. HIV screening and other comprehensive HIV prevention services should be coupled with substance treatment programs.

Timeframe	Lead Agency/ Other Agencies	Actions to be Performed
By the end of 2010	CDC	CDC will release an update of Act Against AIDS activities and an evaluation of successes and challenges
By the end of 2011	HHS OS	HHS OS will complete an initiative to compile and collectively assess all effective programs and initiatives for reducing HIV infections among Black Americans.
	CDC	CDC will work with States and localities with implementing the best combination of approaches to address HIV and STD prevention among Black Americans.

Timeframe	Lead Agency/ Other Agencies	Actions to be Performed
By the end of 2011	CDC	CDC will launch an evidence-based social marketing campaign targeted to the Latino community and will collaborate with nationalLatino organizations on HIV prevention efforts.
	CDC	CDC will release a report on suggestions for border states to help improve HIV surveillance and prevention interventions among migrant communities
	CDC	CDC will work States and localities with implementing the best combination of approaches to address HIV and STD prevention among Latinos.

Timeframe	Lead Agency/ Other Agencies	Actions to be Performed
By the end of 2010	SAMHSA/HHS	SAMHSA and other relevant HHS agencies will consider guidance requiring Federally funded substance abuse and mental health treatment clinics to offer voluntary routine HIV testing to their clients.
	CDC, SAMHSA	CDC and SAMHSA will complete guidance for evidence-based comprehensive prevention, including syringe exchange and drug treatment programs, for injection drug users.
By the end of 2011	SAMHSA/HHS OS	SAMHSA will consult with the HHS OS on policy recommendations for revising funding formulas for State/Territory Substance Abuse Prevention and Treatment and Mental Health Block Grants and policy guidance in order to ensure that Federal HIV prevention funding allocations follow the epidemic at the State and local levels.
	SAMHSA/HUD, DOJ, CDC, HRSA, his, HHS OS	SAMHSA will work with relevant Federal agencies, HHS OS, States, andcommunity-based service providers to implement ways to improve integration of substance abuse and mental health screening in programs that serve communities with high rates of new HIV infections. These should include risk reduction efforts to reduce sexual transmission of HIV among substance using populations.

1.3. Address HIV Prevention in Asian American and Pacific Islander (AAPI) and American Indian and Alaska Native (AI/AN) Populations

Federal and State agencies should consider efforts to support surveillance activities to better characterize HIV among smaller populations such as Asian American and Pacific Islanders (AAPI), American Indians and Alaska Natives (AI/AN).

Timeframe	Lead Agency/ Other Agencies	Actions to be Performed
By the end of 2011	CDC	CDC will provide State health departments with greater concentrations of AAPI or AI/AN populations with recommendations on effectiveHIV surveillance activities for these small populations.
	CDC/IHS, HHS OS	CDC and IHS will coordinate with HHS OS to consult with tribes to develop and implement scalable approaches for effective prevention interventions for AI/AN populations that reach those at greatest risk.
	CDC	CDC will work with States with the largest AAPI communities to implement the best combination of approaches to prevent HIV that reach AAPIs at greatest risk for infection

1.4. Enhance Program Accountability

New tools are needed to hold recipients of public funds accountable for achieving results.

Timeframe	Lead Agency/ Other Agencies	Actions to be Performed
By the end of 2011	HHS OS/CDC HRSA, SAMHSA OPHS, IHS	Relevant HHS agencies will work with States, localities, tribal governments, community-based organizations, and evaluation experts to develop standard performance measures for HIV prevention programs and provide guidance on utilizing these measures.
	CDC/SAMHSA	CDC will work with SAMHSA to make recommendations for strengthening evaluation and aligning measures and benchmarks across programs.
	HHS OS	HHS OS will devise ways to provide incentives to reward high performing Federal grantees for delivering effective prevention services.
	CDC	CDC will continue to evaluate the effectiveness of all CDC-funded HIV prevention programs to assess their impact on improving health outcomes and redirect resources to the most effective programs.

Step 2. Expand Targeted Efforts to Prevent HIV Infection Using a Combination of Effective, Evidence-Based Approaches

2.1. Design and Evaluate Innovative Prevention Strategies and Combination Approaches for Preventing HIV in High Risk Communities

Government agencies should fund and evaluate demonstration projects to test which combinations of effective interventions are costefficient, produce sustainable outcomes, and have the greatest impact in preventing HIV in specific communities.

Timeframe	Lead Agency/ Other Agencies	Actions to be Performed
By the end of 2010	NIH/CDC	NIH and CDC will continue to test mathematical models to explore thebest combinations of behavioral and biomedical prevention activities.
By the end of 2011	CDC/HRSA, SAMHSA	CDC, HRSA, SAMHSA will collaborate with States and localities on pilot initiatives for expanding the most promising models for integrating HIV testing, outreach, linkage and retention in care in high risk communities.
	NIH/CDC	NIH will work with CDC to develop and implement a plan for evaluating promising community-generated ('homegrown') HIV prevention interventions.

2.2. Support and Strengthen HIV Screening and Surveillance Activities

There is a need to support existing surveillance methods to identify populations at greatest risk that need to be targeted for HIV prevention services.

Timeframe	Lead Agency/ Other Agencies	Actions to be Performed
By the end of 2011	FDA	FDA will prioritize review of 4th generation HIV diagnostic tests andresearch in developing new tests for incident infections.

2.3. Expand Access to Effective Prevention Services

Federal funds should support and State and local governments should be encouraged to expand access to effective HIV prevention services with the greatest potential for population-level impact for high-risk populations.

2.4. Expand Prevention with HIV-Positive Individuals

Although most people diagnosed with HIV do not transmit the virus to others, there are effective approaches that support people living with HIV from transmitting HIV to others.

Timeframe	Lead Agency/ Other Agencies	Actions to be Performed
By the end of 2010	CDC/SAMHSA	CDC and SAMHSA in consultation with other agencies, will recommend necessary elements of comprehensive, evidence-based HIV prevention for injection drug using populations.
By the end of 2011	HHSOS/CDC, HRSA, SAMHSA, NIH, CMS	Relevant HHS agencies will make recommendations for scaling up access to post exposure prophylaxis (PEP), with priority given to highprevalence jurisdictions. Consideration will be given to the role of emergency departments (if any), standardized treatment guidelines, and regimen selection.
	BOP/CDC	BOP will expand access to HIV, STD, viral hepatitis screening to prisoners on entry, and CDC and BOP will promote risk reduction interventions for healthy reintegration of ex-prisoners back into community settings.
	HHS OS/CDC, HRSA, SAMHSA	Relevant HHS agencies will prioritize expanding access to combination approaches for HIV prevention, appropriate to epidemic profiles in specific localities.

Timeframe	Lead Agency/ Other Agencies	Actions to be Performed
By the end of 2010	HRSA	HRSA will work with States and localities to ensure that medical providers comply with existing HHS treatment guidelines to offer antiretroviraltherapy to HIV-positive clients in care with CD4 up to 500 cells/ml.
	CDC	CDC will work with States and localities to promote and implement scalable interventions with individuals living with HIV to lower their risk of transmitting HIV.
By the end of 2011	CDC	CDC will develop recommendations for promoting seroadaptationstrategies (strategies used by people with HIV to voluntarily adjust their behavior toward HIV-negative individuals to lower the risk of transmitting HIV).

Step 3. Educate All Americans about the Threat of HIV and How to Prevent it

3.1. Utilize Social Marketing and Education Campaigns

Outreach and engagement through traditional media (radio, television, and print) and networked media (such as online health sites, search providers, social media, and mobile applications) must be increased to educate and engage the public about how HIV is transmitted and to reduce misperceptions about HIV transmission. Efforts will be made to utilize and build upon World AIDS Day (December 1st) and National HIV Testing Day (June 27th), as well as other key dates and ongoing activities throughout the year.

Timeframe	Lead Agency/ Other Agencies	Actions to be Performed
By the end of 2010	CDC	CDC will initiate a CDC-wide review of all social marketing and education campaigns related to HIV, STI, substance abuse and risk behaviorsthat increase risk of HIV transmission and will work to expand evidence based efforts to achieve maximum impact.
By the end of 2011	CDC	CDC will work with States and localities to expand public-private partnerships to focus on reaching high risk communities and/or the general public to prevent HIV/STI infection.

3.2. Promote Age-Appropriate HIV and STI Prevention Education for All Americans

Too many Americans do not have the basic facts about HIV and other sexually transmitted infections. Sustained and reinforcing education is needed to effectively encourage people across the age span to take steps to reduce their risk for infection.

Timeframe	Lead Agency/ Other Agencies	Actions to be Performed
By the end of 2010	CDC	CDC will consider strategies for ensuring that school-based health education is providing scientifically sound information about HIV transmission and risk reduction strategies.
By the end of 2011	CDC	CDC will develop a toolkit and work with States, localities, and school boards to implement age-appropriate HIV health educationprograms.
	CDC	CDC will consider potential partnerships, such as with private businesses, to expand HIV and STI prevention education

INCREASING ACCESS TO CARE AND IMPROVING HEALTH OUTCOMES FOR PEOPLE LIVING WITH HIV

People living with HIV should receive appropriate care and treatment to manage the disease, as well as prevention services that reduce the risk they will transmit HIV. HHS treatment guidelines for treatment of HIV infection provide the rationale for our targets concerning improving access and outcomes for people living with HIV. From 2010 to 2015, the U.S. aims to:

- *Increase the proportion of newly diagnosed patients linked to clinical care within three months of their HIV diagnosis from 65 percent to 85 percent (from 26,284 to*

35,079 people). (data source: CDC surveillance data)
- *Increase the proportion of Ryan White HIV/AIDS Program clients who are in continuous care (at least 2 visits for routine HIV medical care in 12 months at least 3 months apart) from 73 percent to 80 percent (or 237,924 people in continuous care to 260,739 people in continuous care).* (data source: HRSA data)
- *Increase the percentage of Ryan White recipients with permanent housing from 82 percent to 86 percent (from 434,600 to 455,800 people).* (data source: HRSA data) (This serves as a measurable proxy of our efforts to expand access to HUD and other housing supports to all needy people living with HIV.)

Our renewed national effort to improve health outcomes for people living with HIV comes at a time when several Departments of the Federal Government are working with States and private sector partners to implement the Affordable Care Act. Supporting a successful implementation of this law is essential to improving health outcomes for people living with HIV. This work will ensure that in the future, health care access for people with HIV is more stable, affordable, and of high quality. Until that time, we must also stay focused on bolstering our current health care safety net for people with HIV. With the economic downturn that has caused many States to reduce services and with growing numbers of people with HIV in need of services, ongoing attention will be required to bridge short-term gaps in health coverage until the Affordable Care Act is fully implemented.

Over the next couple of years, our attention will need to remain on filling gaps in coverage, while also expanding coordination between Federal agencies, and across levels of government to improve linkages to care. We must also step up our efforts to address workforce shortages by taking initial steps to expand the size and diversity of the clinical and nonclinical HIV workforce. Addressing workforce challenges, however, is necessarily, a long-term effort. As we recognize the extent to which individuals with HIV have other co-occurring health conditions or other challenges in meeting their basic needs, our initial focus will be on enhancing collaboration. This will encompass coordination across agencies that provide HIV services, as well as enhancing programmatic and policy linkages between HIV programs and other health care programs, mental health and substance abuse prevention and treatment programs, STI prevention and treatment programs, as well as increasing collaboration with HUD, the VA, and other departments and agencies. In addition, the Federal Strategic Plan to End Homelessness will focus Federal efforts to reduce homelessness and increase housing security. Implementation of the National HIV/AIDS Strategy must entail integrating efforts to increase housing security for people living with HIV.

In addition to increased program collaboration, there are opportunities to use technology to improve care delivery and strengthen linkages to care. As more health information is collected electronically, it will be necessary to develop applicable standards for using electronic records systems to facilitate linkage coordination and care management for people living with HIV, in order to manage patient confidentiality while facilitating the sharing of information.

Step 1. Create a Seamless System to Immediately Link People to Continuous and Coordinated Quality Care when They Learn they are Infected with HIV

1.1. Facilitate Linkages to Care

HIV resources should be targeted to include support for linkage coordinators in a range of settings where at risk populations receive health and social services.

Timeframe	Lead Agency/ Other Agencies	Actions to be Performed
By the end of 2010	HRSA	HRSA will begin to develop information templates to enable health departments to provide customized, local information on where to access care and support services; such information could be disseminated online at community health centers and other facilities.
By the end of 2011	HRSA/CDC, VA, HUD	HRSA in collaboration with CDC, VA, HUD and other relevant agencies will develop plans that support health care providers and other staff who deliver HIV test results to conduct linkage facilitation to ensure clients access appropriate care following a positive diagnosis.
	SAMHSA	SAMHSA will issue guidance for providers to increase linkages to substance abuse treatment and mental health services for people living with HIV and offer voluntary routine HIV testing to all persons diagnosed with an STD.
	CDC, HRSA, SAMHSA	CDC, HRSA, SAMHSA and other relevant HHS agencies will work with States, tribal governments, localities, and CBOs to promote co-location of providers of HIV screening and care services as a means of facilitating linkages to care and treatment, and to enhance current referral systems within CBOs.

1.2. Promote Collaboration among Providers

All levels of government should increase collaboration among HIV medical care providers and agencies providing HIV counseling and testing services, substance abuse treatment, mental health treatment, housing and support services to link people with HIV to care.

1.3. Maintain People Living with HIV in Care

Clinical care providers should ensure that all eligible HIV-positive persons have access to and are maintained on a medication regimen as recommended by the HHS treatment guidelines.

Timeframe	Lead Agency/ Other Agencies	Actions to be Performed
By the end of 2011	HHS OS/HUD	HHS agencies, HUD, and other relevant Federal agencies will develop joint strategies to encourage co-location of and enhance availability of HIV-related services at housing and other nontraditional HIV care sites.
	HHS OS	HHS agencies will develop plans and work with States to implement training opportunities for health care providers that will highlight the importance of program collaboration and service integration to reduce missed opportunities for identifying HIV infection.
	CDC, SAMHSA, DOJ, HUD	HHS OS will work with CDC, SAMHSA, DOJ, and HUD to identify and develop potential programs where there can be joint grant awards

Timeframe	Lead Agency/ Other Agencies	Actions to be Performed
By the end of 2010	CMS/HRSA	CMS and HRSA will initiate a dialogue on ways to support Medicaid and Medicare providers to engage marginalized populations in HIV care.
	CMS	CMS will promote and support the development and expedient review of Medicaid 1115 waivers to allow States to expand their Medicaid programs to cover pre-disabled people living with HIV.
By the end of 2011	BOP	BOP will conduct a review of current policies and procedures and issue guidance to encourage all prisons to provide discharge planning to link HIV-positive persons to appropriate services upon release from incarceration in order to reduce interruptions in HIV treatment. This will include considering ways to promote broader adoption by nonfederal systems of BOP's standards of providing a 30-day supply of HIV medications upon release.
	NIH	NIH will continue efforts to investigate new antiretroviral therapies for HIV and treatment for its associated conditions that are safer, more effective, more tolerable, and more durable, making adherence to medication regimens easier for people living with HIV.
	NIH/CDC, HRSA, VA	NIH will work with CDC, HRSA, VA, and other relevant agencies to continue to update and disseminate the HHS treatment guidelines

Step 2. Take Deliberate Steps to Increase the Number and Diversity of Available Providers of Clinical Care and Related Services for People Living with HIV

2.1. Increase the Number of Available Providers of HIV Care
Federal agencies should provide incentives to encourage more health care clinicians including primary care providers, reproductive health care providers and providers of sexually transmitted disease treatment, mental health providers, and substance abuse treatment providers to offer HIV services.

2.2. Strengthen the Current Provider Workforce to Improve Quality of HIV Care and Health Outcomes for People Living with HIV
Federal agencies should engage clinical providers and professional medical societies on the importance of routine, voluntary HIV screening and quality HIV care in clinical settings consistent with HHS and CDC guidelines.

Timeframe	Lead Agency/ Other Agencies	Actions to be Performed
By the end of 2010	HRSA	HRSA will issue guidance encouraging medical, dental, pharmacy, physician assistant, nurse practitioner, social work, and nursing schools to implement curricula that include HIV-specific training.
By the end of 2011	HRSA	HRSA will consider opportunities to foster residency training in HIV management and care at community health centers.
	HRSA/NIH, OMH	HRSA, NIH and OMH will develop a proposal to fund training programs to increase interest, representation and competence of healthprofessionals, researchers, and racial and ethnic minority students in research, public health and HIV/AIDS care.

Step 3. Support People Living with HIV with Co-Occurring Health Conditions and Those Who Have Challenges Meeting their Basic Needs, Such as Housing

3.1. Enhance Client Assessment Tools and Measurement of Health Outcomes
Federal and State agencies should support case management and clinical services that contribute to improving health outcomes for people living with HIV and work toward increasing access to nonmedical supportive services (e.g., housing, food, transportation) as critical elements of an effective HIV care system.

Timeframe	Lead Agency/ Other Agencies	Actions to be Performed
By the end of 2010	HRSA	HRSA will work with its AETCs to expand training for HIV clinicians and provider organizations to address provider-associated factors (e.g., cultural competency, provider continuity) that affect treatment adherence.
	AHRQ	AHRQ will develop a plan for working with public and private insurersto develop common data collection and reporting systems across all health care provider settings to enable monitoring of clinical care utilization, quality indicators, and health outcomes for people living with HIV
	HRSA	HRSA will develop a proposal to increase the number of clinical providers who are engaged in innovative rural HIV/AIDS health care delivery systems (e.g. home healthcare, telehealth).
	HRSA	HRSA will develop and issue guidance promoting task shifting (transferring specific tasks to be performed by physician extenders, such as nurse practitioners or other health workers) and co-management (generalist physicians overseeing HIV care while under regular consultation with an HIV expert) as methods to improve HIV workforce efficiency
	DOL, HRSA	DOL and HRSA will work with health professions associations and collaborate on workforce training efforts to increase the number of health providers who are culturally competent.
	HRSA, AHRQ, DOL/HHS OS	HRSA, AHRQ, and DOL will coordinate with HHS OS to work with States, local governments, and state health professions associations toimplement their recommendations and guidance to strengthen the current HIV/AIDS provider workforce.

Timeframe	Lead Agency/ Other Agencies	Actions to be Performed
By the end of 2011	SAMHSA/VA	SAMHSA, VA, and other relevant agencies will collaborate and develop materials for training health care providers to conduct mental health and substance use disorder assessments and treatmentreferrals as appropriate.
	AHRQ/HRSA, VA, CMS, HHS OS	AHRQ, HRSA, VA and CMS, in coordination with HHS OS, will work withStates, localities, and CBOs to encourage the adoption of nationally accepted clinical performance measures to monitor quality of HIV care.

3.2. Address Policies to Promote Access to Housing and Supportive Services for People Living with HIV

Federal agencies should consider additional efforts to support housing assistance and other services that enable people living with HIV to obtain and adhere to HIV treatment.

Timeframe	Lead Agency/ Other Agencies	Actions to be Performed
By the end of 2011	HUD/HHS OS	HUD will lead a process with HHS OS and relevant Federal agencies toidentify ways to collaborate and increase access to nonmedical supportive services (e.g., housing, food/nutrition services, transportation)as critical elements of an effective HIV care system.

REDUCING HIV-RELATED HEALTH DISPARITIES

HIV differentially affects different groups. Making progress in lowering the number of new infections and improving access to care requires making progress toward minimizing disparities across groups. From 2010 to 2015, the United States aims to:

- Increase the proportion of HIV diagnosed gay and bisexual men with undetectable viral load by 20 percent. (data source: CDC data)
- Increase the proportion of HIV diagnosed Blacks with undetectable viral load by 20 percent. (data source: CDC data)
- Increase the proportion of HIV diagnosed Latinos with undetectable viral load by 20 percent. (data source: CDC data)

One of the challenges of reducing HIV-related health disparities is that it is easier to diagnose and document the problems than it is to implement concrete, evidence-based solutions. By expanding access to prevention and care services to high-risk communities, we will lay the groundwork for reducing inequities. Our short-term focus will be on putting in place the necessary tools to lead to improvements in health indicators for underserved communities. By working to ensure that all high-risk groups have access to the same and most appropriate diagnostic tests can help us to better monitor the health outcomes we are working to improve. Further, it is easy to see that community-level interventions are needed to respond to the magnitude of the HIV epidemic in many communities, but there are too few such interventions that reduce HIV incidence or increase access to care.

Addressing ongoing stigma and discrimination is perhaps the biggest challenge we face, as this is not about what government does as much as it is about changing hearts and minds among members of the public. At the same time, three decades of experience tell us that essential starting points for addressing stigma and discrimination include maintaining a commitment to civil rights enforcement, working to ensure that public policies are grounded in best public health practices, and supporting people living with HIV to disclose their status and promote the public leadership of community members living with HIV.

Step 1. Reduce HIV-Related Mortality in Communities at High Risk for HIV Infection

1.1. Ensure that High Risk Groups Have Access to Regular Viral Load and CD4 Tests

All persons living with HIV should have access to tests that track their health, but more must be done to make sure that these tests are available to African Americans, Latinos, and gay and bisexual men.

Timeframe	Lead Agency/ Other Agencies	Actions to be Performed
By the end of 2011	VA, CMS, HRSA, CDC, SAMHSA, NIH	VA, CMS, HRSA, CDC, SAMHSA and NIH will jointly consider and issue a report of strategies to encourage providers to collect and report standardized viral load and CD4 data from infected individuals withinpopulations at greatest risk for HIV infection.

Step 2. Adopt Community-Level Approaches to Reduce HIV Infection in High Risk Communities

2.1. Establish Pilot Programs that Utilize Community Models

In order to reduce disparities between various groups affected by the epidemic, testing community-level approaches is needed to identify effective interventions that reduce the risk of infection in high prevalence communities.

2.2. Measure and Utilize Community Viral Load

Ensure that all high prevalence localities are able to collect data necessary to calculate community viral load, measure the viral load in specific communities, and reduce viral load in those communities where HIV incidence is high.

Timeframe	Lead Agency/ Other Agencies	Actions to be Performed
By the end of 2011	HHS OS	HHS OS will collaborate with HHS agencies to engage in policy research and evaluation activities to identify effective prevention approaches to reduce disease burden in high prevalence communities.
	HHS OS	HHS OS will work with the relevant HHS agencies to consider ways toenhance the effectiveness of prevention and care services provided for high risk communities, including services provided through the Minority AIDS Initiative
	HHS OS/HUD	HHS OS and HUD will explore potential demonstration projects of bundled/braided funding across agencies to address HIV and other issues in high prevalence communities
By the end of 2010	CDC	CDC will identify which States and localities collect CD4 and viral load data.
By the end of 2011	HRSA, CDC	HRSA and CDC will convene a consultation with clinical providers and community-based organizations to develop recommendations for gathering and reporting necessary data to calculate community viral load.
	CDC	CDC, in consultation with States, will provide technical assistance to localities, particularly those with a heavy disease burden, to collect necessary data to calculate community viral load.

2.3. Promote a More Holistic Approach to Health

Promote a more holistic approach to health that addresses not only HIV prevention among African Americans, Latinos, gay and bisexual men, women, and substance users, but also the prevention of HIV related co-morbidities, such as STDs and hepatitis B and C.

Timeframe	Lead Agency/ Other Agencies	Actions to be Performed
By the end of 2010	HRSA/CDC, SAMHSA	HRSA, CDC, and SAMHSA will include language in grant announcements requiring the integration of prevention and care services, including referrals to clinical services
By the end of 2011	HHS OS/CDC, HRSA, NIH, AHRQ	HHS OS will coordinate among HHS agencies to mine existing databases to explore associations between HIV infection and socialdeterminants of health.

Step 3. Reduce Stigma and Discrimination against People Living with HIV

3.1. Engage Communities to Affirm Support for People Living with HIV

Faith communities, businesses, schools, health care providers, community-based organizations, social gathering sites, and all types of media outlets should take responsibility for affirming nonjudgmental support for people living with HIV and high risk communities.

Timeframe	Lead Agency/ Other Agencies	Actions to be Performed
By the end of 2010	HHS OS/DOJ, DOL	HHS OS, DOJ, and DOL Offices of Faith Based and Community Initiatives will develop a plan for engaging more faith leaders to promote nonjudgmental support for people living with HIV.
By the end of 2011	DOL	DOL will consider ways to increase supports for employers to hire andmaintain employment of people with HIV and how to integrate them in broader employment initiatives for people with disabilities.
	HHS OS/DOL	HHS OS will coordinate with DOL to develop standardized occupational guidelines for outreach workers, health educators, hotline operators, peer counselors, and testing/counseling personnel.
	DOL/SSA, DOJ, HHS OS	DOL, SSA, DOJ, and HHS OS will develop a joint initiative to consider ways to help individuals living with HIV access income supports, including job skills and employment.

3.2. Promote Public Leadership of People Living with HIV

Governments and other institutions (including HIV prevention community planning groups and Ryan White planning councils and consortia) should work with people with AIDS coalitions, HIV services organizations, and other institutions to actively promote public leadership by people living with HIV.

3.3. Promote Public Health Approaches to HIV Prevention and Care

State legislatures should consider reviewing HIV-specific criminal statutes to ensure that they are consistent with current knowledge of HIV transmission and support public health approaches to screening for, preventing and treating HIV.

3.4. Strengthen Enforcement of Civil Rights Laws

The Department of Justice and other Federal agencies must enhance cooperation to facilitate enforcement of Federal antidiscrimination laws.

Timeframe	Lead Agency/ Other Agencies	Actions to be Performed
By the end of 2011	HRSA/CDC, HHS OS	HRSA, CDC, and HHS OS will develop recommendations for strengthening the parity, inclusion, and meaningful representation of peopleliving with HIV on planning and priority-setting bodies.
By the end of 2011	HHS	The CDC/HRSA HIV/AIDS Advisory Committee will solicit public input and make recommendations for normalizing and promoting individuals' safe, voluntary disclosure of their HIV status. HRSA will publish therecommendations.
	DOJ/HHS OS	DOJ and HHS OS will identify a departmental point of contact and provide technical assistance resources to States considering changes to HIV criminal statutes in order to align laws and policies with public health principles.
	PACHA	The Presidential Advisory Council on HIV/AIDS (PACHA) will be tasked with developing recommendations for ways to promote and normalize safe and voluntary disclosure of HIV status in various contexts and circumstances.

Timeframe	Lead Agency/ Other Agencies	Actions to be Performed
By the end of 2010	DOJ/HHS OS	DOJ and HHS OS will enter into a Memorandum of Understanding deferring complaints of discrimination on the basis of HIV to the Department of Justice for investigation and prosecution.
By the end of 2011	DOJ/EEOC, DOL, HUD	DOJ, the Equal Employment Opportunity Commission, DOL's Officeof Federal Contract Compliance Programs, and HUD's Fair Housing Enforcement Office will prioritize and fast track investigations of discrimination charges involving HIV, as necessary and appropriate under relevant statutes, and consider additional policies to prevent discrimination from occurring.
	DOJ	DOJ will examine and report on HIV-specific sentencing laws and implications for people living with HIV.

ACHIEVING A MORE COORDINATED NATIONAL RESPONSE TO THE HIV EPIDEMIC IN THE UNITED STATES

This implementation plan delineates initial steps for addressing each of the President's goals for the National HIV/AIDS Strategy. Progress in reaching the Strategy's goals will be publicly reported annually by ONAP. We believe that this plan is ambitious, and success at completing all of these activities is not assured. We are committed to acting with the urgency that the epidemic requires to push Federal agencies to do more and achieve better results, and regularly assess and refine our activities.

Improving coordination of HIV programs is both the simplest and hardest task ahead of us. In recent years, various Federal agencies have already taken steps to increase collaboration and coordination. The HIV Federal Interagency Working Group, which has been central to the development of the National HIV/AIDS Strategy, has also helped to foster a new level of collaboration across disparate agencies. These efforts will continue. The challenge, however, lies in moving beyond the mechanics of having agency leaders talk to each other on a regular basis to creating a culture where agencies are naturally more interconnected and their programs are better aligned. In the short-term, our focus will be on strengthening the mechanisms for Federal agencies to work together more closely about policy issues, as well as the operational aspects of their programs. We also intend to encourage similar efforts at the State and local levels. Longer term, we hope to get to the next level of improved coordination and tackle issues that may require years of sustained planning and effort, such as initiating joint funding initiatives and streamlining data collection and reporting requirements. Beyond government, health care providers, affected communities, businesses, philanthropy, faith communities, and others are also encouraged to increase their own level of collaboration and coordination with other partners.

Step 1. Increase the Coordination of HIV Programs across the Federal Government and between Federal Agencies and State, Territorial, Local, and Tribal Governments

1.1. Ensure Coordinated Program Administration

The Federal Government will increase its focus on coordinated planning for HIV services across agencies. States and tribal and local governments will also be encouraged to collaborate and develop coordinated planning models, including coordinated prevention and care planning and resource allocation activities.

1.2. Promote Equitable Resource Allocation

The Federal Government should review the methods used to distribute Federal formula grants or project implementation funds and take steps to ensure that resources go to the States and localities with the greatest need.

Timeframe	Lead Agency/ Other Agencies	Actions to be Performed
By the end of 2010	HHS OS/HUD, VA, DOL, SSA, and DOJ	HHS OS will work with HUD, VA, DOL, SSA, DOJ, and other relevant Departments or agencies to establish an ongoing process to discusscoordination of planning and services delivery for domestic HIV programs.
	HHS OS	HHS OS will coordinate *National HIV/AIDS Strategy*efforts with HealthyPeople 2020, the U.S. Preventive Services Task Force, and the Task Force on Community Preventive Services in order to make sure that recommendations are aligned across groups to the maximum extent possible
By the end of 2011	HHS OS/HUD, VA, DOL, SSA, and DOJ	HHS OS, HUD, VA, DOL, SSA and DOJ and other relevant agencies will produce a joint progress report on HIV/AIDS program collaboration. This report will highlight key deliverables, areas for consolidating grant awards, successes and current challenges, and proposed measurable outcomes
	HHS OS/HUD	HHS OS, HUD, and other relevant agencies will consider ways to work with State and local health officials to improve coordination of Federal, state, and local programs.States will also be encouraged to submit, in consultation with localities and CBOs, to HHS OS progress reports on State HIV/AIDS plans and on efforts to improve coordination of Federal, state, and local programs.
	SAMHSA	SAMHSA will collect and report to HHS OS (and its agency partners) on how States are using Block Grant HIV set aside funding and report it annually to HHS and its agency partners.
	OGAC	OGAC will take specific actions to facilitate the exchange of best practices and lessons learned between domestic and international HIV/AIDS programs funded by the U.S. government.
	HHS	HHS agencies including CDC, HRSA, and SAMHSA will collaborate to examine the use of the same unique identifier across federal reportingto allow better coordination at the local, state, and federal levels.)

Timeframe	Lead Agency/ Other Agencies	Actions to be Performed
By the end of 2011	HUD	HUD will work with Congress to develop a plan (including seeking statutory changes if necessary) to shift to HIV/AIDS case reporting as abasis for formula grants for HOPWA funding.
	HHS OS	HHS OS will work with Congress and HHS agencies to shift from AIDS cases to HIV infections case reporting as a basis for formula grants for HIV prevention and to ensure that resources go to States and localitieswith the greatest need.

1.3. Streamline and Standardize Data Collection

The Federal Government should take short-and long-term efforts to simplify grant administration activities, including work to standardize data collection and grantee reporting requirements for Federal HIV programs.

Timeframe	Lead Agency/ Other Agencies	Actions to be Performed
By the end of 2010	HHS OS/HUD, OMB	HHS OS, HUD, and OMB will convene a working group to consider recommendations for streamlining data collection requirements.
By the end of 2011	HHS OS/HUD, OMB	HHS OS, HUD, and OMB will consult with State and local health officials and consider changes to lessen grantee reporting burden.

Step 2. Develop Improved Mechanisms to Monitor, Evaluate, and Report on Progress toward Achieving National Goals

We need to measure the results of our efforts to reduce incidence and improve health outcomes to chart our progress in fighting HIV and AIDS nationally, and refine our response to this public health problem over time. This requires a monitoring system that evaluates the implementation of the Strategy, its progress, and the impact of the Strategy efforts. A system of regular public reporting will help to sustain public attention and support.

2.1. Provide Rigorous Evaluation of Current Programs and Redirect Resources to the Most Effective Programs

Prioritize programs that are 1) scientifically proven to reduce HIV infection, increase access to care, or reduce HIV-related disparities, 2) able to demonstrate sustained and long lasting (>1 year) outcomes toward achieving any of these goals, 3) scalable to produce desired outcomes at the community-level, and 4) cost efficient.

Timeframe	Lead Agency/ Other Agencies	Actions to be Performed
By the end of 2010	HHS OS	HHS OS will task relevant agencies to assess their programs and report to ONAP and OMB, on which programs and initiatives satisfy this requirement, as well as those that both do not meet evidence-based criteria and should be phased-out and those that may requireadditional review.
By the end of 2011	ONAP/HHS OS	ONAP and HHS OS will work with Federal partners to establish a monitoring system to evaluate the implementation of the Strategy, its success at completing key actions, and demonstration of impact through achieving specified targets.

2.2. Provide Regular Public Reporting

Progress in reaching Strategy goals will be reported by the Federal Government through an annual report at the end of each year.

Timeframe	Lead Agency/ Other Agencies	Actions to be Performed
By the end of 2011	HHS OS/DOJ, DOL, HUD, VA, and SSA	HHS OS, DOJ, DOL, HUD, VA, and SSA will submit data, as requested, to ONAP on successes and challenges in achieving the goals of the *National HIV/AIDS Strategy*.
	PACHA	PACHA will establish a mechanism to monitor progress toward achieving the *National HIV/AIDS Strategy* goals
	ONAP/HHS OS	Relevant Federal departments and agencies will work with ONAP andHHS OS to review progress annually and identify remediation steps (if any) to achieve *National HIV/AIDS Strategy* goals. This will include considering key action steps for the coming year

2.3. Encourage States to Provide Regular Progress Reports

The Federal Government will encourage States to provide annual reports to ONAP and HHS OS on progress made implementing their comprehensive HIV/AIDS plans. ONAP will incorporate the State reports into the national progress report at the end of each year.

Timeframe	Lead Agency/ Other Agencies	Actions to be Performed
By the end of 2011	HRSA, CDC/ HHS OS	HRSA and CDC, and other relevant Federal departments, in coordination with HHS OS, will work with States to encourage them to produceannual reports on progress made implementing their comprehensive State HIV/AIDS plans and that outline successes and challenges in achieving the goals of the *National HIV/AIDS Strategy*.
	ONAP, HHS OS	ONAP, HHS OS, and relevant Federal departments and agencies will review progress annually and identify recommended remediation steps(if any) to assist States in achieving *National HIV/AIDS Strategy*goals

EVALUATING THE NATIONAL HIV/AIDS STRATEGY

Evaluation is the systematic acquisition and assessment of information to provide useful feedback of a situation. In 2004, CDC proposed a framework for HIV/AIDS monitoring and evaluation.[9] The framework proposes three tiers for a national monitoring and evaluation plan and provides useful questions for each of these tiers:

1. Are we doing the right things?
2. Are we doing them right?
3. Are we doing them on a large enough scale?

These questions are useful guides in evaluating the U.S. response to the domestic HIV epidemic and the degree to which our national efforts align with the President's goals for the Strategy. The first evaluation step is to determine what is currently being done. The U.S. is doing many things to address the HIV epidemic, but there has not been a concerted effort across all Federal agencies to determine which activities are grounded in evidence, produce sustainable outcomes, and target those populations or areas with the greatest disease burden. Furthermore, our efforts are not always well coordinated. In recent years, key Federal leaders have taken important steps to promote collaboration. Nonetheless, individual efforts must give way to more sustained and consistent integration across programs and agencies.

The second evaluation step is to determine how evidence-based approaches are being implemented. Identifying and utilizing the right approaches to address the HIV epidemic are only useful if these approaches are being implemented correctly. An effort must be made to evaluate the application of effective behavioral and biomedical interventions, and the capacity and technical assistance required to implement these interventions. In the area of care delivery, more work is needed to measure quality of care, and assess measures such as whether individuals are being offered therapy consistent with current clinical practice standards. It is also important to evaluate whether policies that have been put in place to address the epidemic are being followed appropriately, including enforcement of civil rights laws that are such a critical part of any effort to reduce stigma and discrimination.

Last, we must ensure that enough people receive critical services to have an impact. After identifying the right approaches and implementing them correctly, these important efforts can be undermined if they are not taking place on a large enough scale to make a difference. To effectively monitor our progress, we plan to:

- By the end of 2010, release information to more clearly delineate the implementation and monitoring roles and responsibilities of ONAP, Federal agencies, the Federal HIV Interagency Working Group, and the Presidential Advisory Council on HIV/AIDS (PACHA).
- By March 2011, ONAP, in consultation with the Federal Interagency Working Group and PACHA, will prepare an evaluation plan that will include a timetable for reporting across agencies, and a framework for evaluating progress toward reaching Strategy goals.
- By the end of 2011, ONAP will issue its first annual progress report on Federal implementation efforts and describe specific action steps for 2012.

CONCLUSION

HIV is a complex epidemic that requires all of us to address this critical national public health issue. This Federal Implementation Plan includes timelines for actions supporting the high-level priorities outlined in the strategy. This approach reflects a commitment to act with the urgency that the HIV/AIDS epidemic requires. Federal agencies will strive to take the steps described in this plan and take other steps to work with other partners to advance the goals of the National HIV/AIDS Strategy. The Federal Government, however, is only one of component of the broad effort needed to improve our response to the domestic epidemic. New partnerships and a commitment to better coordination and improved accountability will help us move forward.

With governments at all levels doing their parts, a committed private sector, and leadership from people living with HIV and affected communities, the United States can dramatically reduce HIV transmission and better support people living with HIV and their families.

The United States will become a place where new HIV infections are rare and when they do occur, every person, regardless of age, gender, race/ethnicity, sexual orientation, gender identity, or socio-economic circumstance, will have unfettered access to high quality, life-extending care, free from stigma and discrimination.

End Notes

[1] The National HIV/AIDS Strategy for the United States and the National HIV/AIDS Strategy: Federal Implementation Plan are available at www.WhiteHouse.gov/ONAP.

[2] See www.WhiteHouse.gov/ONAP.

[3] Throughout this document, we assign responsibilities to 'HHS OS', as they are being given new responsibilities for improving coordination across the Department. As appropriate, the Secretary will delegate responsibilities to specific offices or agencies

[4] Please refer to http://cdc.gov/hiv/topics/surveillance/incidence.htm for more information on HIV incidence calculations.

[5] Holtgrave DR, Hall IH, Rhodes PH, Wolitski RJ. Updated annual HIV transmission rates in the United States, 1977-2006. *J. Acquir. Immune Defic. Syndr.* 2009; 50 (2): 236–8.

[6] For more information on the transmission rate, please refer to http://www.cdc.gov /hiv/topics/surveillance/resources/factsheets/transmission.htm.

[7] Throughout this document we use the terms "gay and bisexual men" and "gay men" interchangeably, and we intend these terms to be inclusive of all men who have sex with men (MSM), even those who do not identify as gay or bisexual.

[8] Throughout this document we use the terms "Black" and "African American" interchangeably, and we intend these terms to be inclusive of all individuals from the African Diaspora who identify as Black and/or African American.

[9] Rugg D, Peersman, Carael M. Global advances in HIV/AIDS monitoring and evaluation. *New Directions for Evaluation.* 2004;103:36.

In: Responding to HIV/AIDS
Editor: Lawrence T. Jensen

ISBN: 978-1-61324-618-4
© 2011 Nova Science Publishers, Inc.

Chapter 3

COMMUNITY IDEAS FOR IMPROVING THE RESPONSE TO THE DOMESTIC HIV EPIDEMIC: A REPORT ON A NATIONAL DIALOGUE ON HIV/AIDS[*]

White House Office of National Aids Policy

EXECUTIVE SUMMARY

At the beginning of his Administration, President Obama instructed the White House Office of National AIDS Policy (ONAP), a component of the Domestic Policy Council (DPC), to develop a National HIV/AIDS Strategy and re-focus our response to the HIV epidemic in the United States. The President directed that this strategy be driven by three primary goals:

1) Prevent new HIV infections.
2) Increase access to care and optimize health outcomes.
3) Reduce HIV-related health disparities.

From the beginning, ONAP recognized that community involvement was essential in creating a more effective strategy for combating HIV/AIDS in America. To achieve this undertaking, ONAP developed a comprehensive approach for gathering public input and ensuring that ideas from individuals living with HIV, as well as other stakeholders and interested parties, were reflected in the Nation's roadmap for moving forward. ONAP conducted 14 community discussions in locations across the United States and its territories and spoke with more than 4,200 people. ONAP also solicited recommendations for the strategy through the White House Web site.

Over 1,000 written recommendations for the National HIV/ AIDS Strategy were submitted to ONAP from the community discussions or Web-related submissions.

---

[*] This is an edited, reformatted and augmented version of White House Office of National Aids Policy publication, dated April, 2010 and is available at www.whitehouse.gov/onap.

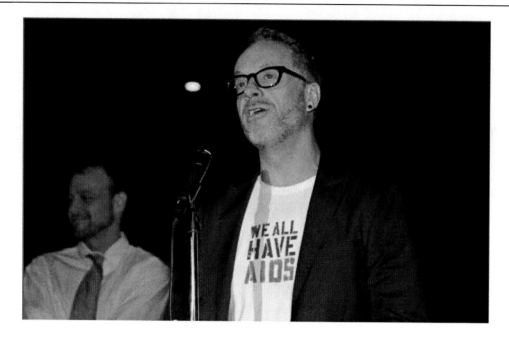

This report is a summary of these community recommendationsRecommendations related to prevention were made against a backdrop of growing HIV prevalence in the United States. People commonly suggested that we need a broad-based, public information campaign. Individuals told us that this campaign should be vast in scope and should educate a public that remains highly vulnerable to HIV infection. Participants at the community discussions noted that population-specific interventions are crucial. Moreover, they said that any public action must address the numerous social, economic, and behavioral factors that fuel HIV transmission.

Public comments and written testimonies related to improving access to care shared common themes with those related to prevention and health disparities. In particular, consumers of HIV/AIDS services, as well as services providers and advocates, warned about defining populations too broadly and not recognizing the depth or diversity that exist within subpopulations disproportionately affected by the epidemic. Participants primarily discussed access to care in terms of the broad array of health and social services that are necessary for chronic disease management and long-term wellbeing. They spoke passionately about the need for comprehensive health insurance coverage, culturally competent providers, and a greater number of HIV care providers in underserved rural and urban communities. Perhaps because, comparatively speaking, more people access primary medical care than other services, many testimonies focused on how to make these other services more accessible, including transportation, housing, and job training.

Participants suggested that expanding access to care could help reduce HIV transmission rates and alleviate health disparities. Advocates from or representing vulnerable populations discussed many of the disparities evident in today's epidemic, ranging from racial and ethnic disparities to sex and gender, sexual orientation, age, immigration status, and geographic disparities. Nearly all of the comments referenced the structural inequalities that contribute to these issues. The President's three goals are interconnected, and many participants' recommendations regarding issues, opportunities, and challenges spanned the topics of prevention, access to care, and health disparities. These recommendations most commonly focused on the need for more streamlined funding processes and greater collaboration among Federal, State, and local agencies to facilitate more efficiency. They also addressed the need to increase specificity in the Nation's surveillance data and inequities in the Nation's public and private insurance markets. People also expressed concerns about the shortage of health professionals, specifically of those qualified to address HIV/AIDS, and called for remedies to address this problem.

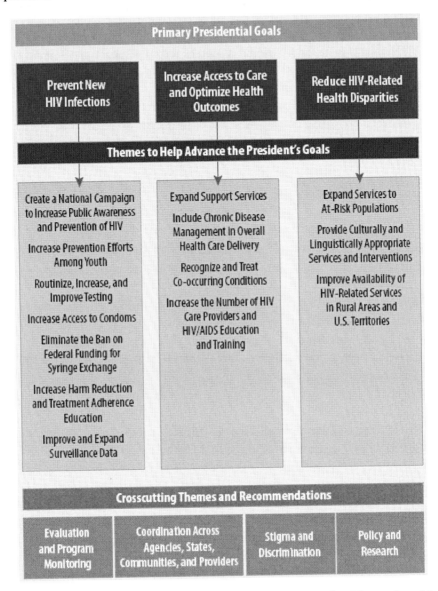

Figure 1. The National Conversation for an HIV/AIDS Strategy for America: Themes from 14 Community Discussions and Submissions to the White House.

INTRODUCTION

"When one of our fellow citizens becomes infected with HIV every nine-and-ahalf minutes, the epidemic affects all Americans."

—President Barack Obama

Participants in our national conversation about HIV/AIDS devoted significant attention to this public health crisis and invested a great deal of time crafting public testimony and writing recommendations. Community members presented thoughtful testimony that drew from real life experiences. Their recommendations and personal stories are embodied in this report. They are invaluable tools as ONAP and the Administration work toward drafting an effective strategy that addresses HIV/AIDS in America.

This report summarizes and organizes oral testimony, as well as written and Web-based submissions, in categories that reflect the President's three goals. It also highlights overarching and crosscutting issues related to funding, evaluation, and program integration.

The NHAS will likely identify a small number of targeted, high-payoff actions that can be taken to achieve the President's goals. The Strategy is not intended to be a comprehensive list of all of the actions, policies, and programmatic priorities needed to respond to the domestic HIV epidemic. Rather, it is intended to build upon ongoing public and private initiatives, determine areas where targeted attention can produce results, and identify programs that may benefit from better inter-agency coordination.

METHODOLOGY

From the outset, achieving public input and counsel has been critical to ONAP's approach to creating an NHAS. To foster participation from as many perspectives as possible, ONAP created three mechanisms through which people's voices could be heard: (1) community discussions, (2) written submissions and, (3) online/email submissions to the White House Web site. Each of these mechanisms is described below.

Community Discussions

ONAP conducted 14 community forums and invited the public to discuss its concerns, recommendations, and ideas. The locations for these forums were geographically and demographically diverse. The purpose of these discussions was to hear the unique challenges affecting both large and small communities, and to facilitate meaningful dialogue and recommendations. The community discussions were not designed to be a scientific research study with formal, structured data collection methods.

Community discussions were hosted in the following cities: Atlanta, Georgia; Washington, D.C.; Minneapolis, Minnesota; Albuquerque, New Mexico; Houston, Texas; San Francisco, Los Angeles, and Oakland, California; Columbia, South Carolina; Jackson, Mississippi; Fort Lauderdale, Florida; New York City, New York; Puerto Rico; and the U.S. Virgin Islands. (See Figure 2.) Over 4200 individuals attended the discussions.

Local planning groups comprising State health organizations and local community-based organizations assisted with locating venues and moderators and developing the format of discussions. The meetings were advertised in the communities in which they were held in a variety of ways. The White House issued press releases for each of the meetings, and President Obama referenced the discussions in various speeches, including his speech at the bill signing for the reauthorization of the Ryan White Program.

> **Diversity in Geography, Diversity in Needs**
>
> Many common themes emerged across all community discussions, yet each location highlighted some unique issues to its location:
>
> - In Jackson, Mississippi, the unmet need for transportation services in this predominantly rural State was given significant attention.
> - In San Francisco, California, the need for affordable housing in one of the Nation's most-costly housing markets was strongly emphasized.
> - In New York City, New York, discussions highlighted growing disparities among infection rates in boroughs like Brooklyn and the Bronx.
> - In Albuquerque, New Mexico, there were many Native Americans present while in Oakland, California, participants were predominantly African-American and Latino.
> - HIV infection among immigrant communities was a common theme among Africans in Minneapolis and Latinos in Los Angeles.

Moreover, to encourage participation from all members of the community, most discussions provided translation services that included American Sign Language interpretation and Spanish-language translation. Each location was also accessible by public transportation and in compliance with the Americans with Disabilities Act (ADA).

Each of the 14 community discussions was scheduled to last two hours; however, some discussions lasted longer. In an effort to hear as many participants as possible, people were invited to provide remarks for one-and-a-half to two minutes. The specific time allotment depended on the audience size and was established during the ground rules at the beginning of each discussion.

The intent of the community discussions was to collect input for the NHAS and to serve as a vehicle for community members to gather, listen, and share their ideas and experiences. The community discussions were video recorded and uploaded onto the White House Web site.

Written Submissions

Individuals who spoke at the community discussions were also encouraged to submit hard copies of their prepared remarks. This gave people an opportunity to provide more comprehensive and detailed suggestions than the oral comment period may have allowed.

In many instances, advocacy organizations created and distributed worksheets before the discussion to assist participants in organizing and presenting their input in order to maximize their limited time at the microphone. ONAP received a total of 267 hard-copy written submissions.

Web Submissions

ONAP created a Web-submission mechanism entitled "Call to Action: Americans Speak about HIV/AIDS" that was housed on the ONAP page located on the White House Web site. This allowed ONAP to receive input from individuals across the country regardless of their proximity to the 14 community discussions. The online "Call to Action" also facilitated submissions from people who may have been unwilling or unable to present their comments and recommendations during the community discussions. To maximize participation, the "Call to Action" was included in White House press releases, advertised on various Federal Web sites and listservs, and announced on membership lists of various community advocacy organizations and coalitions.

Individuals were encouraged to complete specific information before they could submit their recommendations to the White House Web site. This included their State or Territory, and affiliation (individual, community-based organization, health care/medical organization, research entity, or State/Federal agency; See Figure 3). Recommendations could be typed directly into a field that accepted 5,000 characters or uploaded as a word processing or PDF file.

Because it was not always possible to hear from all participants at the community discussions, participants at the community meetings were encouraged to use the Web-submission mechanism to provide additional recommendations. The "Call to Action" submission process lasted from October 2, 2009, through November 23, 2009, but additional submissions were accepted until early December via the ONAP email address. We received more than 700 Web submissions from 46 States, 3 U.S. territories, and the District of Columbia (See Figure 4.)

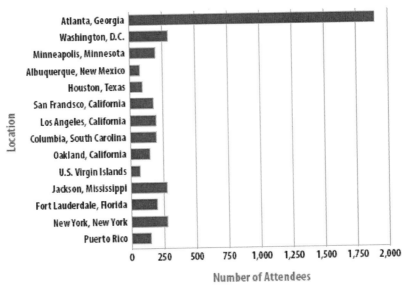

Note: The Atlanta Community Discussion took place during CDC's 2009 National HIV Prevention conference, which had several thousand attendees.

Figure 2. Community Participation, N= 4,285.

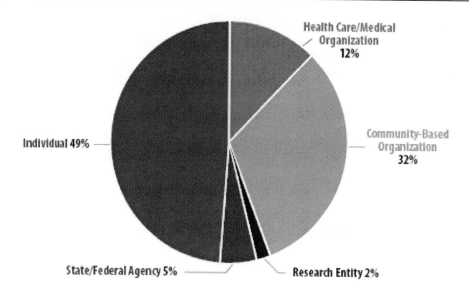

Figure 3. Web site submissions by affiliation, N=719.

Other Email Submissions

An additional 103 individuals or organizations bypassed the "Call to Action" and submitted recommendations directly to ONAP's email or provided hard-copy recommendations from community-initiated meetings. In some instances, these recommendations were from organizations that submitted more than one document or a particular document with a long list of signatories.

Organizing the Material

A total of 1089[#] written submissions were received from the community discussions, and from email, Web, and hard-copy submissions. These submissions were integrated into a single list to organize and highlight key findings across communities. ONAP reviewed and organized all of the recommendations put forward for consideration.

An outline of major topic areas was created after reading through the material and for the purposes of organizing this report.

Submissions have been organized and discussed in this report with the objective of providing a comprehensive written record and creating a planning tool for the NHAS development process.

[#] Tallies were created from counting individual comments or group submissions where possible; those numbers are reflected in the tables and charts in this chapter. Please note these numbers are approximate. In cases where identical recommendations were submitted through multiple channels, those recommendations were counted only once and through the channel from which they were first received.

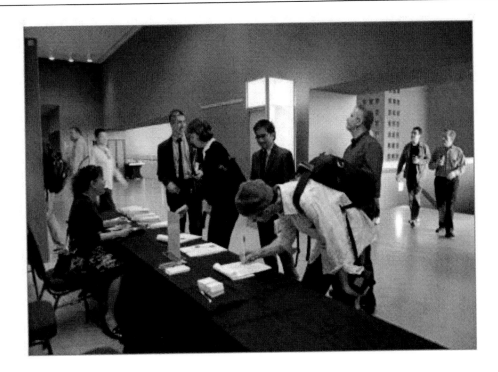

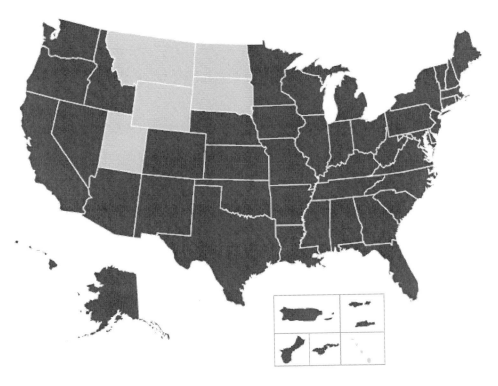

Figure 4. Web site submissions by state/U.S. territory, N=719.

Alabama	7	Hawaii	3	Mississippi	9	Rhode Island	4
Alaska	3	Idaho	1	Missouri	8	Puerto Rico	9
American Samoa	1	Illinois	22	Nevada	2	South Carolina	13
Arizona	9	Indiana	7	Nebraska	2	Tennessee	9
Arkansas	9	Iowa	6	New Hampshire	2	Texas	23
California	102	Kansas	3	New Jersey	8	Vermont	1
Colorado	6	Kentucky	7	New Mexico	12	Virginia	14
Connecticut	7	Louisiana	20	New York	109	Virgin Islands	6
Delaware	1	Maine	2	North Carolina	10	Washington	21
District of Columbia	19	Maryland	13	Ohio	26	West Virginia	4
Florida	56	Massachusetts	16	Oklahoma	7	Wisconsin	2
Georgia	22	Michigan	6	Oregon	13		
Guam	1	Minnesota	22	Pennsylvania	34		

+No Web-based submissions were received from individuals or organizations in Montana, North Dakota, South Dakota, Utah, Wyoming, or the U.S. Territory Northern Mariana Islands.

■ Blue indicates a State or territory where comments have been received.

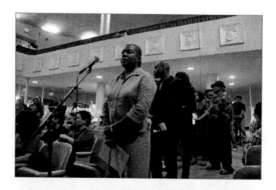

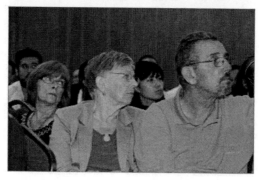

PREVENTING HIV TRANSMISSION

The first cases of what later became known as AIDS were reported in June of 1981.[9] Otherwise healthy men were diagnosed with rare infections including Pneumocystis pneumonia—a disease seen only in immunosuppressed patients.[10] By 1990, more than 100,000 individuals had died of AIDS.[11]

We have come a long way since the beginning of the epidemic and, thankfully, there have been many successes in preventing HIV since the 1980s. The Centers for Disease Control and Prevention (CDC) has reported that the number of new infections dropped from more than 130,000 per year in the mid-1980s to just over 56,000 per year by 2006.[12,13] In 1994, findings from the Pediatric AIDS Clinical Trial Group 076 showed that an AZT (Zidovudine) regimen reduced perinatal transmission of HIV by two-thirds.[14] AZT was quickly recommended for use in all HIV-positive pregnant women, and mother-to-child transmission plummeted. Today, with proper treatment throughout pregnancy, perinatal HIV transmission cases have declined.[15]

In 1995, combination therapy, also known as highly active antiretroviral therapy (HAART), was introduced.[16,17,18] HAART dramatically increased survival rates and improved quality of life for people living with HIV, while also reducing infectiousness among people living with HIV and the probability of HIV transmission to uninfected persons. Moreover, because of comprehensive prevention efforts, including needle exchange programs and provision of sterile equipment, CDC recently reported that HIV incidence has decreased by 80 percent among injection drug users.[19]

Despite these successes, the HIV epidemic continues to place various populations at high risk. Today, men who have sex with men (MSM), are the only transmission group where HIV incidence is markedly increasing. Additionally, communities of color, especially Black and Latino communities, remain disproportionately affected by HIV.

During the community discussions, participants often mentioned that the HIV/AIDS epidemic in the United States has been increasingly forgotten or ignored. Despite the diminishing mainstream media coverage, and a shrinking presence of HIV in the public consciousness, the HIV epidemic remains a reality for many individuals across the country. We heard that HIV prevention in the United States must be bold, address the complex risks and vulnerabilities of diverse communities, and streamline inefficiencies across Federal agencies.

Participants in the community discussions called for a strategy that maximizes available tools to reduce transmission rates. The recommendations submitted to ONAP were straightforward and often crosscutting. Common themes that we heard include:

A. Create a National Campaign to Increase Public Awareness and Prevention of HIV

> "...a national social marketing campaign that states the facts about condoms and their ability to prevent HIV just like the seatbelt campaign that we all saw in the 1980s."
>
> — Houston, Texas community discussion

There is a lack of knowledge related to HIV risk and transmission across broad segments of the American public. "I hear from middle and high school students that having or living with STDs is just the way it is going to be....There is a lot of misconceptions in the media that is leading them to believe it is no big deal," explained an AIDS activist in New Mexico. The absence of information related to HIV/AIDS, and only a partial understanding of HIV risk, is fueling new infections in the United States every year.

The participants called for a far-reaching, more comprehensive approach to increasing public awareness about HIV/AIDS.

Audiences

"[Our] interactions with other AIDS service organizations keeps awareness of HIV high [among our congregants]...so we can continue to be on the forefront of responding...and ministering to those whom it affects."

— Episcopal Church representative Web submission

Participants in public forums across the country emphasized that a single message and approach will not evoke the desired response among all target audiences. "Begin a coordinated education campaign with identified individuals...and definitely connect to the African-American community," recommended one participant. "People seem to have forgotten middle-class White women who have been divorced recently, and who do not have a clue that HIV exists. Education needs to be given to them too," added another.

The target audiences for a national campaign must be segmented to reflect population-specific barriers to information and behavior change. "I am an Asian Pacific Islander transgender woman. I face different issues than my gay brothers, and I have different needs," explained one respondent.

Many participants suggested that culturally-appropriate messages and message delivery strategies be crafted to address diverse populations. They recommended that unique messaging, messengers, and delivery mechanisms be developed for audiences defined by the following characteristics:

- *Risk category.* Participants requested messaging that addresses the risks of specific communities.
- *Age.* These messages should be unique and crafted for specific age brackets, beginning with youth still in school and ranging to older adults. Participants noted the need to reach people early in life, and to continue to tailor risk reduction messages for individuals as they age. Several participants highlighted the need to address HIV prevention messages for people over the age of 50, as well as HIV care services for people living with HIV as they age or those who seroconvert as seniors.
- *Race/ethnicity.* Participants said that these messages should also be crafted for the five racial categories currently tracked in CDC surveillance reports (White, Black, Latino, Asian/ Pacific Islander, American Indian/Alaska Native) and for other racial and ethnic populations as well, such as Arab Americans and Africans who have recently immigrated to America.
- *Gender.* In addition to establishing culturally-appropriate approaches to target males and females, participants also voiced how important it is to craft a national HIV education campaign targeting transgender individuals, many of whom are not reached by current messaging.

Messages, Messengers, and Message Placement

"Effective health education and HIV/AIDS prevention education has been proven to work when methods are used that are science and research based."

— Los Angeles, California community discussion

Many participants called for science-driven prevention messages. They urged that information regarding issues like safer sex and risk reduction be defined by scientifically-proven—rather than ideologically-driven—approaches to reducing HIV incidence.

However, even the best messages are only as effective as the messenger. Participants suggested that potential messengers include:

- Peers within each of the risk behavior groups,
- Peers from LGBTQ communities,
- Key influencers with whom at-risk groups identify, including parents, teachers, faith-based leaders, and community leaders, and
- Opinion leaders, such as political and other publicly recognized officials.

Many of the comments advocated for enlisting trusted community leaders and stakeholders to help engage community members and spotlight public health needs. "Bring education to Native Tribes and Native American community-based organizations and get buy-in from leaders," suggested one Albuquerque man. Take "our hip hop community and utilize it to disseminate information to the people who are most prevalent in catching [HIV] disease," recommended a Houston resident.

"There is no education in our tribes," said an Albuquerque man. Stressing the need for culturally-specific efforts, he explained, "There are over 300 tribes or nations…We are different people. I myself am an Apache, [and] cannot speak up [for] a Pueblo or a Navajo here in New Mexico. [We] have different ways."

The difficulty of reaching out to young people was emphasized repeatedly, with many participants urging parents and schools to become actively involved in delivering risk-reduction messages to youth. There was widespread support for providing information about male and female condoms to audiences of all ages.

The need to embed HIV prevention within a cultural context was repeatedly noted at locations across the country. As one San Francisco resident explained,

"A/PI's [Asian and Pacific Islanders] are not one ethnic or racial group. They are 40 different ethnicities speaking over 100 different languages. As long as they do not see pictures of people living with HIV who are also A/PIs, they will never realize that HIV is something that will affect their community adversely."

Participants also highlighted the importance of distributing risk-reduction information in specific locations, such as schools, faith-based institutions, and social-services organizations. HIV prevention efforts should be visible wherever people at high risk for infection can be found. "Women that are incarcerated both in jails and prisons need this information," stated a Jackson, Mississippi resident.

Respondents urged broader use of print, radio, mail, and, especially, television in a more widespread and far-reaching campaign. "Do what Surgeon General Koop did in 1988 and mail each U.S. household an updated brochure on HIV/AIDS and include current trends, statistics, myth busters, HIV prevention and treatment information, and information to online resources," suggested a Sacramento, California woman. A more public and more visible platform for HIV prevention efforts was also discussed.

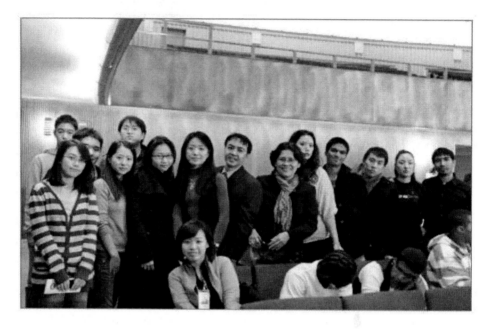

Participants recommended that a national campaign be visible on television and employ new media platforms that harness the power of virtual communities.

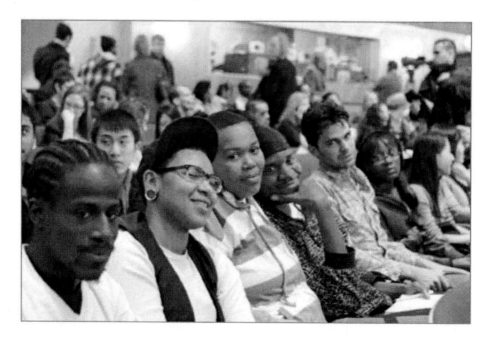

B. Increase Prevention Efforts among Youth

"I am tired of telling teenagers that their HIV test is positive.... Every 17-year-old I diagnose with HIV represents 60 to 80 years of transmission potential [and] each represents nearly a million dollars in health care costs over their lifetime."

—Minneapolis, Minnesota community discussion

Written submissions and public testimonies across the country highlighted the need for population-specific approaches to HIV prevention and care efforts to reduce health disparities. Participants discussed the unique challenges faced by racial and ethnic minorities, sexual minorities, and women. They gave significant attention to the needs of young people and emphasized the importance of preventing HIV infections as early as possible.

Participants repeatedly highlighted how critical prevention efforts are among young people. Young people[20] accounted for an estimated 29 percent of new HIV infections in 2006.[21] Youth also represent one of the most medically underserved populations in the United States, and they are often unaware of their HIV status.

A student in St. Croix wrote, "We need the U.S. Government to keep youth informed on the facts about HIV and AIDS...and to get more serious about our behaviors." The majority of HIV-positive youth become infected through behaviors like drug use or sexual intercourse. Although there are relatively few annual perinatal infections in the United States, we heard from several community members that prevention of perinatal infection should remain a priority. As one participant stressed,

"I was born HIV positive....[at] a time when we did not have medications to prevent mother-to-child transmission....That is not the case anymore. We can prevent it...there is absolutely no reason why more children should be infected and a generation should continue going forward being HIV positive."

Participants discussed the need to reach youth early and often, and called for comprehensive sexuality education to take place both in school settings and in other venues where youth are found. Many advocated that this education be science-based and include information pertinent to all sexual orientations, condom use, and HIV and other STDs. Virtually whenever community members spoke about HIV prevention for young people, they advocated for comprehensive, evidence-based sexuality education.

Many people demanded that the Federal Government stop funding abstinence-only education initiatives. As one respondent summarized,

"Teach...the benefits of abstinence without demonizing those who are sexually active."

"HIV/AIDS prevention education does not need to be reinvented, but such efforts do need teeth in mandating laws to ensure that programs are really provided by qualified teachers as designed and evaluated to maintain effectiveness," asserted one respondent.

An Albuquerque, New Mexico resident stated, "It is important that our youth get correct and factual messages for them using all types of media and technical methods of communication."

C. Routinize, Increase, and Improve Testing

"The first step toward HIV treatment is getting tested, knowing your status."

— Columbia, South Carolina community discussion

An estimated 21 percent of HIV-positive persons in the United States do not know their status.[22] Besides compromising their long-term health outcomes due to delayed care, undiagnosed individuals may unknowingly place their sexual partners at risk for HIV transmission. According to a CDC study, between 54 to 70 percent of new HIV transmissions in the United States are due to people with unrecognized HIV infection.[23]

Studies indicate that people who are diagnosed with HIV reduce their risk behaviors with HIV-negative partners to minimize the possibility of transmission.[24] "I have not infected anyone and I am undetectable now," said a California man on the prevention value that HIV-testing has for reinforcing responsible behaviors.

Access to HIV testing should also be expanded to help individuals learn their HIV status earlier in the course of their illness. According to a CDC analysis of 34 States with confidential name-based reporting, 38.3 percent of persons with a new HIV diagnosis developed AIDS within one year.[25] Without treatment, most people live for close to a decade from the time of infection until they are diagnosed with AIDS. This high percentage of people who are diagnosed with AIDS so soon after learning their HIV status suggests that we are not reaching many people until they have been living with HIV for many years. Many factors cause late testing, including underestimating HIV risk. This leads to delayed care, poorer health outcomes, increased morbidity and mortality, and more opportunities for HIV transmission.

Participant recommendations related to HIV testing largely fall into four categories:

- Routinize HIV testing.
- Encourage HIV testing.
- Locate HIV testing in nontraditional settings.
- Improve the content of the testing encounter.

Routinize HIV Testing

To increase overall testing, diagnose HIV infection early, and engage HIV-positive persons in appropriate medical treatment, CDC recently revised its testing recommendations to include routine screenings of 13- to 64-year-olds in health care settings.

(To learn more, visit http://www.cdc.gov/hiv/topics/testing/healthcare/index.htm.) In short, CDC recommends that all adults and adolescents get tested for HIV as part of their regular medical care.

Community discussion participants emphasized putting existing CDC guidelines into practice. "I'd recommend providing adequate funding for implementing the CDC guidelines and making this approach a program of national priority just like the prevention of perinatal transmission in the late 1990s," suggested one Web respondent who was referencing the AIDS Clinical Trial Group 076 that proved perinatal transmission could be cut dramatically.

Participants also stated that testing should continue to be accompanied with referrals and counseling, and that the government should assist organizations in expanding HIV testing.

Several participants advocated for co-locating HIV testing in primary care settings to encourage seamless linkage to care. Although some pushed for universal HIV testing, others advocated HIV testing for targeted groups. There was consensus that HIV testing should be voluntary.

Encourage HIV Testing

"Psychological science has shown if we don't talk about it... people feel it must not matter."

— Newburgh, New York Web submission.

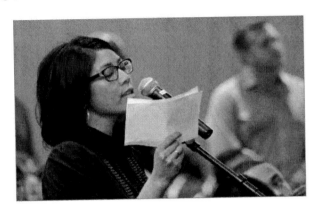

Participants advised that a population-specific approach be designed to ensure that messages, messengers, and distribution mechanisms reflect the needs and realities of diverse demographic groups. They noted that risk factors are not the only elements that should drive the creation of testing promotion strategies, and they stated other demographic characteristics such as race and gender are also critical.

Participants reminded ONAP that to provide a framework for promoting HIV testing among the general population, stigma must be considered and addressed. They also noted that routinization of HIV testing, coupled with visible involvement and encouragement from well-known individuals, community leaders, and peers, is critical. Public comments also stressed separating HIV testing from other issues, such as immigration and fear of deportation, as well the importance of partner notification.

Partner notification involves trained public health specialists locating and contacting any person whose name has been supplied by an HIV-positive partner or his/her health provider. Utilizing partner notification is sometimes the best—and quickest—way to ensure partners are contacted.[26] As one social worker in Minneapolis, Minnesota described, "There needs to be an overhaul of partner notification services nationally to address antiquated and underperforming systems, health campaigns to sell the importance of partner notification services to the public, update training, and incorporate new technologies to more effectively and efficiently notify individuals of their possible exposures...When conducted effectively, partner notification services are a proven method to reduce HIV incidence and increase access to care for those at risk."

Locate HIV Testing in Nontraditional Settings

"People in our community [were] deciding to die rather than get tested—so great was the stigma in some parts of our community."

— Washington, D.C. community discussion

The theme of making testing more widely available was also prevalent in many discussions and submissions. This included a call for continued outreach with mobile vans or peers on foot to find hard-to-reach individuals who are often the last to enter care. Other recommendations included increasing access and reducing the cost barrier to at-home testing devices; making testing more widely available and encouraged in corrections institutions; incorporating testing into dental visits; and allowing testing in nonclinical settings where at-risk populations frequent.

Improve the Content of the HIV Testing Encounter

"Geriatric specialists must include HIV testing as a routine test…Taboos in this generation, such as not speaking about sex, have to be addressed diligently."

— San Juan, Puerto Rico Web submission.

Comments suggested the importance of using every encounter to provide as much information and support as possible. There is a divide within the community over whether we need to re-emphasize pre- and post-test counseling as we expand HIV testing or whether this serves as a barrier to expanded testing, or even whether this stigmatizes HIV testing. Many participants noted that some individuals who test for HIV never return for test results. Participants also discussed the need to provide negotiating skills for individuals at risk for contracting HIV/AIDS.

D. Increase Access to Condoms

"[T]he effect of Black American heterosexual men who do not use condoms and engage in concurrent relationships or have multiple sex partners, plays a most significant role in the exposure of Black American women."

— Oakland, California community discussion.

Over 80 percent of new HIV/AIDS diagnoses among adults and adolescents in the United States in 2007 were related to sexual activity.[27] Virtually all of these cases could have been prevented. "The Federal Government needs to sponsor and fund the broad based availability of male and female condoms in HIV and STD impacted communities across America," urged a San Francisco woman representing one of a number of participants calling for increased access to condoms in prevention efforts.

Several individuals recommended expanding access to safer sex materials and needle exchange programs. Many people advocated for the distribution of condoms in schools, as well as in prisons and jails. Several people also stated that we must lower financial barriers to condoms and make them easier to access in pharmacies.

> **Sexual Transmission of HIV**
>
> Eighty-five percent of new infections result from sexual transmission.
>
> Men who have sex with men (MSM), account for an estimated 4 percent of the male population in the United States, but 53 percent of all new HIV infections, making them both the single largest risk group and the group most disproportionately at risk for HIV infection.
>
> MSM are more than 44–86 times more likely to become infected than other men in the United States, and 40–77 times more likely to become infected compared to women. Within this at-risk population, Black and Latino MSM are more likely than Whites to become infected with HIV.
>
> Among the 26 percent of cases among women, Black women account for an estimated 60 percent of all new infections. The majority of HIV cases among women are due to sexual behavior with men.
>
> Sources: CDC. (2009, August). *HIV/AIDS in the United States: CDC HIV/AIDS facts*. Retrieved from the CDC Web site: *http://www.cdc.gov/hiv/resources/factsheets/PDF/us.pdf*. CDC. (2009). *HIV/AIDS Surveillance Report*. 2007,19, Table 3.
> CDC. (2010), *CDC Analysis Provides New Look at Disproportionate Impact of HIV and Syphilis Among U.S. Gay and Bisexual Men*. Retrieved from the CDC Web site: *http://www.cdc.gov/nchhstp/Newsroom/msmpressrelease.html*.

As one participant summarized, "Teaching people how to use condoms is no longer [enough]....They need to have their positive self identity improved so that they feel like they are important and they need to take care of themselves." Building self esteem and increasing access to information about condoms was echoed throughout submissions and community discussions.

E. Eliminate the Ban on Federal Funding for Syringe Exchange

> "Understand that syringe exchange is the gateway to treatment and we need to take the obstacles and hurdles out of people getting into [care]."
>
> — Washington, D.C. community discussion

Injection drug use (IDU) accounted for 17 percent of new HIV diagnoses among adults and adolescents diagnosed in 2007.[28] An additional 3 percent of newly diagnosed cases were attributed to MSM/IDU.[29] IDU also accounts for the most hepatitis C (HCV) infections in the United States, and co-infection of HIV/HCV can complicate both treatment and health outcomes.[30]

Research indicates that syringe exchange programs are cost effective and have positive impacts in reducing the spread of HIV. According to a cohort study published in the *Journal of Acquired Immune Deficiency Syndromes*, IDUs involved in syringe-exchange programs are up to six times less likely to put themselves at risk of HIV infection.[31] Access and funding for such programs, however, have been limited by both State laws and a Federal ban on funding for such programs. Many participants recommended eliminating the ban on Federal funding for syringe exchange programs. Another recommendation was to expand access to syringe exchange programs in pharmacies.

In November 2009, Congress lifted the ban on using Federal funding for needle and syringe exchange programs. The lifting of this ban was welcomed by the Administration and seen as another step toward policy informed by science and not ideology.

F. Increase Harm Reduction and Treatment Adherence Education

> "We must have more comprehensive harm reduction programs available across the Nation that includes needle exchange."
>
> — Asheville, North Carolina Web submission

Harm Reduction

In the context of HIV prevention, harm reduction commonly refers to minimizing risk associated with one's behavior. This may include condom use, although it often refers to the reduction of drug-related harm, such as syringe exchange programs (described in section E) and medication-assisted drug therapy. A guiding principle of harm reduction interventions is to meet people where they are and to work with them to decrease risk to the fullest extent possible. The phrase "where they are" can refer to individuals and their struggles with addiction or unprotected sexual activity. It also refers to where people are in a literal sense, such as corrections institutions, substance abuse treatment facilities, health clinics, or other key points of entry in the medical system.

"Jails are a perfect opportunity to offer evidence-based prevention interventions …it is less expensive to be proactive in our prevention efforts [and] to foster behavior change among those at high risk for HIV transmission," expressed a respondent from Wilkinsburg, Pennsylvania, emphasizing the need to intervene among those at highest risk for HIV infection and among those already living with the disease.

Treatment and Adherence

Medical treatment and adherence are two of the many services for people living with HIV that can help reduce HIV transmission. People living with HIV who take antiretroviral therapy have lower viral loads and are less infectious than those not on therapy, and they also have better health-related outcomes.

Many participants discussed the importance of working with people living with HIV to help stop HIV transmission. "Treatment education is a crucial tool for the success of antiretroviral therapy and long-term adherence," stated one Web respondent. These are important components of any strategy to secure the health of people living with HIV. As nonadherence increases risk for drug resistance and viral replication, it is imperative that once people living with HIV begin a particular medication regimen, that regimen remains stable.[32]

Participants also made specific recommendations related to working with those at high risk for HIV infection and those already living with HIV/AIDS. These included expanding activities that target people living with HIV for primary and secondary prevention, building the skills of HIV positive individuals to disclose their HIV status, and improving negotiation skills for safer sex practices with drug-using partners.

G. Improve and Expand Surveillance Data

> "Health data on race and ethnicity must be collected uniformly throughout the United States. To date, one-third of all States throughout our country have yet to break out Asian and Pacific Islanders as a separate category. Until this happens, we will never know the true extent of the epidemic in our communities."
>
> — San Francisco, California community discussion

HIV/AIDS surveillance is critical to HIV prevention efforts: The more we know about populations affected by HIV, the more effective our approach for targeted HIV prevention and improved health outcomes. Recommendations regarding HIV surveillance focused primarily on increasing the specificity in which data are gathered. This includes:

- Increasing demographic categories for race and gender, and
- Collecting a detailed history during testing encounters.

More detailed surveillance categories across local, State, and national data was repeatedly echoed in Web and hard-copy submissions, as well as community discussions. These data are recognized as important tools for creating better strategies for preventing HIV and improving outreach to bring infected persons into care. Many individuals recommended that surveillance data better target specific demographic groups.

Several participants remarked upon improving the accuracy of HIV surveillance information. Statements like, "Include transpeople in collected data on HIV" and "Do not mis-categorize transgender women as MSM," were common across community discussions. We heard from Native Americans and Asian and Pacific Islanders requesting they not be categorized as "other" in surveillance data. Arab Americans asked that they be recognized separately and not classified as "White." African immigrants discussed their unique challenges that set them apart from African-Americans.

H. Summary

We received a variety of specific proposals for reducing HIV incidence. By far, we heard most about the need for a wide-scale and multifaceted HIV prevention campaign to engage the American public.

Targeted efforts for specific populations were also championed during the community discussions, including comprehensive sex education for youth, clean injection equipment for injection drug users, and greater availability of condoms for all groups. It was also a common recommendation that targeted prevention efforts should be accompanied with more accurate surveillance that reflects the diversity of communities.

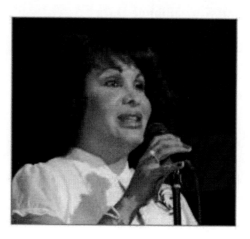

INCREASING ACCESS TO CARE AND OPTIMIZING HEALTH OUTCOMES

Increasing access to care and improving health outcomes requires coordination in a number of arenas. When people enter care late and have problems staying in care, they suffer poorer health outcomes. There are social, economic, and other factors that affect access to appropriate care. For example, a lack of permanent or stable housing may result in missed appointments and inadequate adherence.[33] Cultural differences and language skills may equate to difficulty navigating the health care system.[34,35] Workforce shortages, particularly in HIV/AIDS and primary care, may mean fewer available providers, longer waiting times for medical appointments, and more obstacles to accessing care.[36,37,38,39]

For many people living with HIV, access to the services needed for improving health is hampered by entrenched barriers to services. ONAP received recommendations drawn from individuals' personal experiences and knowledge concerning removing common barriers to care. Recommendations commonly fell in the following categories:

A. Expand Support Services

"I find that my clients are underserved and lack the needed support services and medical care that affects their health and wellbeing."

— Long Beach, California Web submission.

It is not surprising that, given the high rates of poverty among people living with HIV, the public urged the Administration to examine the role of support services in optimizing health outcomes for people living with HIV. Considering the combination of poverty and high rates of co-occurring conditions, many people commented that HIV/AIDS treatment extends beyond treating HIV infection, to addressing care for the whole person and the entire range of his or her health and support needs.

Across venues, people living with HIV explained how access to housing, food, and legal services ensured they could focus on managing the disease; how child care and transportation allowed them to keep appointments; how case managers, social workers, and interpreters helped them navigate the health and social services systems; and how support groups and job training meant they could focus not on where they are but on where they wanted to go.

Health Insurance and Access to Treatment

Participants reported that insurance costs remain an extraordinary barrier to prevention and care services for many people living with HIV. A number of individuals stressed the role of cost containment in reducing pressures on public and private insurance programs. Participants also focused on the need to make the Nation's patchwork of public and private programs easier to navigate. They also cited obstacles inherent to enrolling in some programs. "Populations, including homeless U.S. citizens, formerly incarcerated individuals, and legal immigrants have trouble accessing appropriate HIV medical care because they do not possess personal identification documents," noted the Ryan White Medical Providers Coalition in its written recommendations. "Such documents should be made easier to acquire," the group suggested, adding that "jurisdictions that release individuals from incarceration should provide personal identification documents upon release."

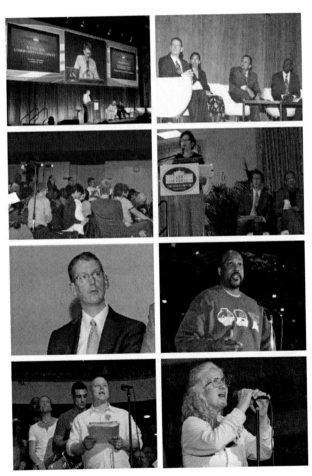

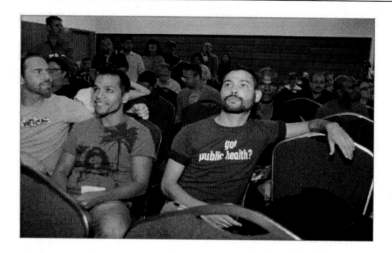

Participants advocated for the removal of coverage limits for particular services such as substance abuse treatment, dental care, and mental health services. In several communities, participants also asked for coverage for hormone therapy treatments that have not been covered historically. Pre-existing conditions and their potential to negatively impact health coverage and health outcomes was also echoed across community discussions. As the Staten Island Ryan White Part B HIV CARE Network wrote, "[We] support language in health insurance reform legislation prohibiting companies from refusing coverage for an individual based on their medical history or health risk."

One of the most frequently repeated policy recommendations was to address the Medicare Part D coverage gap, often referred to as the Medicare "donut hole." Once Part D enrollees surpass the prescription drug coverage limit, they are responsible for 100 percent of the total drug costs until they reach the "catastrophic coverage threshold."[40] As a Florida HIV pharmacist described, "Many Medicare D clients self ration their drugs because of the donut hole. They split tablets. They skip days. They skip drugs. This can lead to viral resistance. It can lead to secondary infections. It can lead to infecting others with the resistant virus all of which could cause or increase health costs later on."

Some community discussion attendees called for a more rapid FDA approval process for HIV treatments. Other health care advocates asked for additional policies to improve access to the Ryan White AIDS Drug Assistance Program (ADAP) and Medicare Part D.

Participants also asked for less stringent eligibility requirements and for shorter waiting periods for some programs. "Patients…must wait 24 months after qualifying for SSDI [Social Security Income Disability Insurance] for their Medicare coverage to come into force. The waiting period creates gaps in care for these patients and Ryan White funds are not always readily available to fill these gaps. Such waiting periods should be abolished so that individuals have seamless access to care."

Housing

"[W]hen we talk about housing first, it really is housing first. If you do not have a place to live it is really difficult to even think about medication, to think about medical appointments, to think about behavior changes."

— San Francisco, California community discussion

According to the National AIDS Housing Coalition, an estimated 50 percent of persons infected with HIV will need some sort of housing assistance over the course of their illness.[41] Lack of stable housing can pose enormous barriers to staying in care and treatment adherence. Thus, housing is often viewed as a health care issue. "Acquiring and maintaining stable housing has long been recognized as an important component in the response to HIV/AIDS," noted one New York State resident. "The lack of a home undermines sound nutrition and HIV treatment adherence, makes contact with health care providers difficult, and makes employment problematic."

Many persons who are homeless, in transitional housing, in shelters, and assisted living came out to the community discussions. In urban areas, they voiced their concerns about the high cost of living. In San Francisco, for example, people discussed the challenges of living in the country's second-highest-priced housing market and making ends meet with current levels of Federal income support.

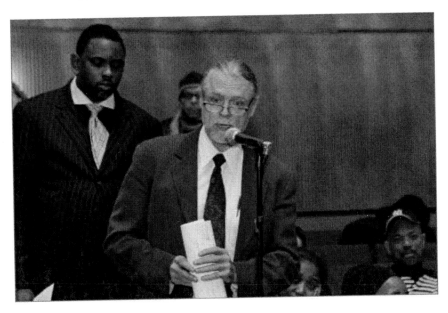

Others discussed the need for longer grace periods before eviction for persons who are sick or recently disabled. "One thing that we can do is have a national standard of 120 days notice to evict a senior, disabled, or catastrophically ill tenant," said one speaker.

Around the Nation, many members of the public have called for greater funding for housing assistance. In addition, many called for a more streamlined application process for the Housing Opportunities for Persons with AIDS (HOPWA) program. The public also requested that housing policy reflects the unique needs of populations such as at-risk youth or youth living with HIV, persons recently released from correctional settings, and transgender individuals.

Job Training/Employment Services

"Resources should be committed to enhance economic stability through education, jobs, and leadership training."

— Washington, D.C. Web submission

HIV affects the most vulnerable in our society. Nearly 60 percent of individuals receiving care from the Ryan White HIV/AIDS Program had household incomes at or below the Federal poverty level.[42] Moreover, studies have shown that among individuals living with HIV, educational attainment has a direct correlation with health outcomes.[43]

Participants at various community discussions advised the Administration that these results underscored the need for increased access to job training and employment services. Participants made specific suggestions to capitalize on the unique experiences many have acquired through their work as peer counselors. They also noted that while many would like to work, HIV compromises their ability to do so on a regular basis.

Others explained the employment dilemma faced by persons currently receiving disability benefits who fear entering the workforce and losing needed disability benefits. "I want to continue to contribute as much as possible by working," explained a Seattle, Washington man. "But work is largely an either/or situation. I am considering returning to disability."

Participants also voiced worries about being unable to afford private health insurance or being denied health insurance due to a pre-existing condition. They called for:

- An end to insurance coverage limitations related to pre-existing conditions,
- More affordable health care coverage,
- Programs and incentives to help people living with HIV who are working, but unable to afford co-payments and medications, and
- Employer incentives to hire people living with HIV and to offer flexible, part-time opportunities.

Comments highlighted that employment and job training services are especially important for people transitioning from corrections institutions. Research indicates that each year, about one in four people living with HIV spend time in a correctional facility,[44] and participants at the community discussions frequently referenced the unique employment challenges of ex-offenders. Participants discussed the importance of re-entry programs that help ex-offenders succeed and that keep them from returning to the environment and circumstances that resulted in their initial incarceration.

One New York State man explained his recommendation through his life experience in a study group:

"[The doctor] studied two approaches to re-entry of formerly incarcerated [people living with HIV]. One group received minimal transition planning. They relied on welfare and safe houses once released. The other was provided with comprehensive transitional support, including access to education, job training, and transitional housing. Ten years later all the members of the first group are dead. The second group, we are still here. I was part of that second group. I am now a successful community advocate and a retired health educator for the State. I am proof of the success of a holistic approach to HIV."

Some respondents called for job training to begin while individuals are still incarcerated. Others recommended training as part of a re-entry program. Many participants pleaded for government incentives for businesses to hire ex-offenders and for apprenticeships to train this population for long-term employment.

Transportation

"People in rural areas may face tremendous barriers to health care. Two of those barriers are stigma and transportation. Transportation would not be as big an issue if we had more doctors trained to treat HIV."

— Finger Lakes Region, New York recommendation

Transportation issues in many rural and suburban areas involve lack of infrastructure, and people living with HIV in urban areas face unique challenges related to transportation as well. Since people living with HIV are disproportionately poor, even accessible public transportation systems may be too expensive for indigent individuals and families.

The need for transportation support has long been a factor affecting access to care. Transportation services for accessing medical care are funded through Medicaid and can be funded through the Ryan White Program. Since Ryan White prioritizes funding core medical services, however, rising prevalence in many communities has forced cuts in funding for transportation and other nonmedical support services.

Many individuals have called for increasing funding for transportation services for people living with HIV. Still others have recommended improving the country's transportation infrastructure and public transit systems, especially in more rural and suburban communities. These areas have fewer providers, often requiring patients to travel long distances for care. As a Columbia, South Carolina resident explained, "There is just not enough means of getting from point A to point B."

Legal Services

"Many experts now recognize that law and legal counseling can play a pivotal role in stemming the spread of HIV by ensuring access to public and private resources essential to preventing and managing HIV effectively."

— Washington, D.C. Web submission

From rural residents to those living in the country's most populated cities, advocates explained the critical role legal services play in helping clients gain access to and stay in care, remain in their homes, and counter discriminatory employment practices and other issues people living with HIV face.

One New York City-based organization stated, "Since the creation of the Ryan White CARE Act,[45] thousands of [people living with HIV] have accessed legal services that have enabled them to obtain medically appropriate housing, access to medical benefits and services, fight discrimination, and make appropriate end-of-life care decisions." Several individuals spoke critically of current Ryan White policies that limit the scope of legal services that can be funded through the Ryan White HIV/AIDS Program. Some individuals called for States to expand the legal services they cover through Ryan White, whereas others advocated for clearer guidance from HRSA that explicitly defines a broad range of legal services that can be covered.

"The unnecessarily narrow definition of the scope of legal services is depriving PLWHAs [people living with HIV/AIDS] of crucial support services, including such fundamental assistance as eviction prevention," asserted South Brooklyn Legal Services. One individual added, "We have the capacity to represent people in asylum cases who have been forced to leave their own country for being tortured because of HIV and because of their...sexual relationships ... [but under the current Ryan White definition] we are not allowed to do so."

Translation Services

"There must be a plan [that] ensures translation is always accessible and available to all people with HIV/AIDS."

— Philadelphia, Pennsylvania Web submission

Access to language services and translated documents can help facilitate effective communication between people living with HIV and their providers. The capacity to communicate with clients in the language in which they are most comfortable is an important component of cultural competency. Individuals identified language and translation services as critical needs associated with optimizing health outcomes.

Language Line

While many urban areas have access to an array of interpreters and some larger medical facilities have them or bilingual staff on hand, smaller or more traditional settings cannot afford this luxury. Many are, therefore, turning to Language Line, an organization offering live, confidential medical interpretation services by telephone in over 170 languages.

(To learn more, visit *http://www.languageline.com/page/industry_healthcare/* or call 1-800-752-6096.)

A Rochester, New York man stated, "I am an Asian gay man who is deaf. I am speaking to you through an interpreter. When I was diagnosed, I went to the doctor's office. The sign language interpreter didn't know the medical words used for HIV. Besides being emotionally distraught over being HIV positive, a non-English speaking person faces confusion and frustration from not being able to communicate with the people who are trying to help."

As a project manager at the Asian and Pacific Islander Coalition explained, "New York [City] is a city of immigrants. Asian and Pacific Islanders make up 12 percent of the population. Seventy-two percent of this population group is foreign born and...49 percent speak English less than very well...[and need] access to culturally and linguistically competent services."

According to a New England Journal of Medicine study, 22.3 million Americans have limited English proficiency—a number that has grown in recent years.[46] According to one study, nearly one-half (46 percent) of emergency room cases of patients with limited English proficiency had no interpreter assistance.[47] This lack of available interpreters is directly related to workforce shortages, lack of clinician training with interpreters, and lack of reimbursement for interpreter services. Yet access to these services has shown to have a positive improvement in patient satisfaction and overall health outcomes.[48,49]

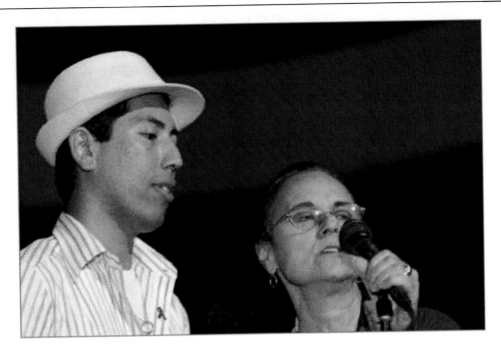

Case Management

"AIDS case management services allow people to access primary health care and to maintain their dignity and respect."

— Los Angeles, California community discussion

Case managers are an important resource for linking people to services, coordinating care, and ensuring retention in care. Case managers are often the persons with whom people living with HIV have the most direct contact. They are involved in making referrals, tracking follow-up, and monitoring patient utilization and outcomes, and they can play a significant role in determining if patients stay in care. Case managers often work closely with HIV/AIDS and primary care providers as part of a comprehensive team approach.[50]

As a Long Island, New York man explained,

"HIV/AIDS medical care often involves a complex continuum of care. Even those of us who have been living with the disease for decades require the assistance of a case manager to help navigate the system. In addition, as we live longer, new issues emerge that we need guidance on. We cannot stress enough the importance of our case managers, of having someone who knows us, knows our needs, and knows the continuum of care. We urge the Federal government to continue the support of community-based case management programs for all people living with HIV, not just the newly diagnosed. We also recognize that there is very high turnover rates among case managers and encourage the Federal government to support programs to increase retention and continuing education for our case managers."

Case managers can also link patients to population-specific services, such as assisting HIV-positive mothers in identifying and gaining access to child-care services, or helping to enroll clients in programs like WIC (the Special Supplemental Nutrition Program for Women, Infants, and Children). Many participants at the community discussions called for increased access to supportive services like these as a step toward both decreasing no-show rates for medical appointments and increasing patient adherence to treatment. Availability of child care services for mothers may help improve patient retention,[51] while access to nutritional services can play an important role in improving medication absorption and malnutrition.[52]

Case managers may be able to help assess patient needs and work to ensure patient access of necessary services. These services may range from oral health care to housing assistance and anything in between.[53] Whether they are medical or nonmedical case managers, these individuals play an important role in assisting people living with HIV. As a Fort Lauderdale community discussion participant summarized, "Without the support that I have gotten from my case manager...I probably would not be here today."

B. Include Chronic Disease Management in Overall Health Care Delivery

> "Our nationally recognized medication management program has resulted in...the prevention of chronic disease progression."
>
> — Smyrna, Georgia Web submission

Many participants at the community discussions urged the Government to seize the opportunity presented by health care reform legislation to cover all Americans and create a framework for chronic disease management. "All too often, people suffering from multiple chronic conditions receive little to no coordination of their health care from the various specialists that they regularly interact with. Adapt chronic health care models that emphasize outpatient primary care, patient education, and multiple-condition health care coordination," urged a Harlem, New York organization.

Chronic disease management is a comprehensive, coordinated approach for addressing the health care needs of the patient. Such an approach is intended to improve health, lower incidence of comorbidities and medical complications, slow disease progression, and potentially reduce health disparities among people living with HIV. "Part C [of the Ryan White HIV/AIDS Program] clearly needs more funding to provide direct medical care in the chronic disease model," mentioned an Albuquerque, New Mexico medical director.

In addition to expressing support for chronic disease management coverage in general, many recommendations focused on specific services that such an approach could encompass. In particular, the importance of preventive health care was repeatedly highlighted. Participants at the community discussions promoted the use of peer counselors, noting the proven value of this approach in educating patients about living with HIV disease and its comorbidities, as well as supporting treatment adherence. "We need more prevention-with-positives interventions," said one participant. "Utilize peer-based models to retain women living with HIV in care," added another.

At the Puerto Rico community discussion as well as many others, individuals discussed how improved treatment has helped HIV evolve into a chronic disease. As the Services & Advocacy for Gay, Lesbian, bisexual & Transgender Elders organization explained, "If current trends in infection rates remain stable, in less than 10 years, one-half of all people living with HIV in the United States will be over age 50." The AIDS Community Research Initiative of America (ACRIA) added that, "As people with HIV grow older, they become prey to the same ailments faced by their HIV-negative brothers and sisters, such as arthritis, cardiovascular disease, diabetes, and dementia." As the HIV population ages—whether as long-term survivors or from contracting the disease later in life—participants called for increased care coordination with conditions that commonly occur with aging.

> **High Rates of Co-Occurring Conditions among People Living with HIV Requires Improved Access to Care**
>
> The rates of some health conditions among people living with HIV are related to the long-term effects of HIV and its treatment such as lipoatrophy and lipodystrophy. But high rates of poverty and stigma and poor access to regular medical care also contribute to HIV-related disparities as well.
>
> The prevalence of hepatitis C among people living with HIV may be as high as 30 percent and as high as 90 percent among people infected with HIV through injection drug use.
>
> Studies on post-traumatic stress disorder in people living with HIV have found prevalence rates from between 30 and 50 percent; approximately 60 percent of individuals meeting diagnostic criteria were untreated for their condition.
>
> People living with HIV have high rates of oral health problems, a contributor to poor nutrition and the capacity to adhere to treatment regimens, and they are at disproportionate risk for medical concerns associated with the aging process.
>
> Sources: Gennaro, S., Naidoo, S., & Berthold, P. (2008). Oral health and HIV/AIDS. *American Journal of Maternal/Child Nursing, 33(1),* 50-7.
> Israelski, D.M., Prentiss, D.E., Lubega, S., Balmas, G., Garcia, P., Muhammad, M.,... Koopman, C. (2007). Psychiatric co-morbidity in vulnerable populations receiving primary care for HIV/AIDS. *AIDS Care,* 19(2), 220-5.
> School of Dentistry, Louisiana State University Health Sciences Center. (2007). *HIV+ outpatient overview.*
> Sherman, K.E., Rouster, S.D., Chung, R.T., & Rajicic, N. (2002). Hepatitis C virus prevalence among patients infected with human immunodeficiency virus: a cross-sectional analysis of the US adult AIDS Clinical Trials Group. *Clinical Infectious Diseases 34(6),* 831-837.
> Sulkowski, M.S., & Thomas, (2003). D.L.. Hepatitis C in the HIV-infected person. *Annals of Internal Medicine 138(3),* 197-207.
> Thomas, D.L.(2002). Hepatitis C and human immunodeficiency virus infection. *Hepatology 36 (5 suppl 1),* S201-9.

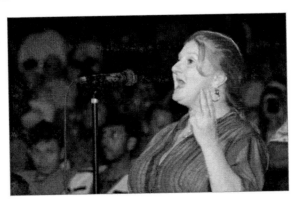

Comments frequently included the need for increasing access to a multidisciplinary team of specialists to ensure providers can address the unique needs of not only the older population but of all persons managing HIV.

C. Recognize and Treat Co-Occurring Conditions

"Many Americans who are at risk of contracting HIV are also at risk of contracting viral hepatitis...Viral hepatitis is the most common cause of liver cancer, which is one of the most lethal, expensive, and fastest rising cancers in the United States."

— Hepatitis C Appropriations Partnership Web submission

HIV/AIDS services providers are working in a world with growing medical need. While treatment of HIV/AIDS with antiretroviral therapy has been a success, the incidence of comorbidities associated with aging and long-term survival has increased. Moreover, people living with HIV may be at heightened risk for other conditions, including addiction, mental illness, tuberculosis, and hepatitis C, as well as certain metabolic and other disorders such as heart disease. These conditions fuel a high level of demand for services.

In the HIV Costs and Services Utilization Study (HCSUS), one-half of adults with HIV had symptoms of a psychiatric disorder; 19 percent had signs of substance abuse, and 13 percent had co-occurring substance abuse and mental illness.[54] Yet approximately one-half of people living with HIV who have depression have undiagnosed and untreated conditions.[55] The implications of untreated mental illness are severe. Psychiatric disorders can pose barriers to medical care and negatively affect medication adherence. Several studies have found that depression, trauma, stress, and anxiety can lead to increased disease progression and mortality.[56,57,58,59]

Recent research on people living with HIV being treated for depression found that use of selective serotonin reuptake inhibitors (SSRIs) not only improved mental health but had a direct correlation on improved antiretroviral adherence and decreased viral load.[60] These findings echo the calls of many respondents for increased screening for—and access to—mental health services for people living with HIV, which they stated is highly disproportionate among this population. "Treatment of mental illnesses has to be one of the top priorities in the fight against HIV/AIDS," said a Web respondent from San Juan, Puerto Rico. "[There is] a dire need for psychiatric, substance abuse, and other mental health services in the community," wrote a doctor from Chicago, Illinois. "There are no resources for mental health or counseling with respect to HIV/AIDS. I asked my doctor after I was diagnosed over a year-and-a-half ago for a referral to some sort of counseling. He had none to offer," explained a Mississippi man. We need more mental health and substance abuse treatment and funding for those treatments," added a Fort Lauderdale, Florida physician.

Some drugs, such as methamphetamine, can a cause cognitive impairment,[61] lead to depression (due to damage of dopamine receptors),[62] increase HIV viral replication,[63] and remove protective mucosa making people susceptible to a variety of pathogens including HIV.[64,65] Other drug-taking activities, like injection drug use, have long been recognized for its role in HIV transmission.[66] Injection drug use has also been shown to fuel health conditions like hepatitis C.

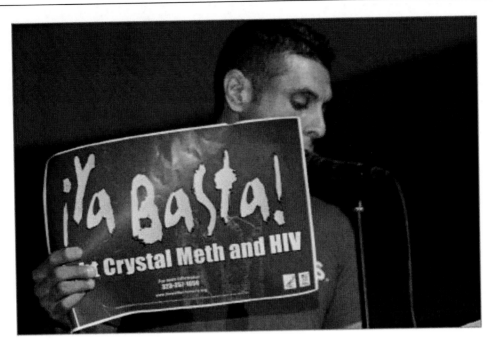

Hepatitis C may interfere with HIV treatment and may lead to increased progression of liver disease.[67] End stage liver disease is now a major cause of death among persons infected with HIV.[68,69,70] Infection with HIV is also the strongest known risk factor for progression from latent tuberculosis to active (or contagious) tuberculosis.[71,72]

As a Providence, Rhode Island respondent wrote, "Prisoners face an enormous burden of co-occurring disorders such as mental illness, addiction, viral hepatitis, and sexually transmitted diseases. Another person said, "Correctional settings represent a major opportunity…[for] prison and jail-based screening, treatment, and linkage to care." This comment came from one of the many participants who stressed the need to better utilize key points of entry[73] to identify, address, and treat co-infections. In many recommendations, respondents emphasized the risk of infection with multiple sexually transmitted diseases. Sexually transmitted diseases such as syphilis infection are shown to increase HIV viral load and heighted transmissibility of HIV.[74] People living with HIV may also experience more severe reactions to particular sexually transmitted infections, such as gonorrhea and herpes, due to their weakened immune systems.[75]

D. Increase the Number of HIV Care Providers and HIV/AIDS Education and Training

"As an internist who just completed residency, I feel very comfortable treating the complications of HIV in a hospital setting but have limited knowledge in treating outpatient HIV. In my residency program, patients who were diagnosed with HIV were transferred to the Infectious Disease clinics. As a new physician I am excited and honored to work with this population, but I do feel overwhelmed at times by all of the information I need to learn."

— Virgin Islands Web submission

This doctor's experience reinforces findings from a 2004 HIV Medicine Association survey. The survey included 729 first-year internal medicine residents in the 10 States with the highest HIV prevalence. One-half (51 percent) of respondents said their residency had not prepared them for HIV medicine.[76] The need to increase the breadth of HIV training was an issue raised across community discussions. Participants stressed the importance of improving capacity, increasing the number of providers, and creating a workforce where HIV education extends to all health professions.

Increase Capacity in Minority Communities

"Community-based organizations are in the position to directly address issues prevalent [in] their own communities," said one respondent from Stockton, California. Access to technical assistance and training can ensure that community-based organizations (CBOs) have increased capacity to address local challenges and barriers to care.

Organizations based within the communities they seek to serve may be uniquely positioned to garner community buy-in and local leadership support. This factor is of particular importance to communities that have been disenfranchised and suffered discrimination, such as racial and ethnic minorities. "Let people of color develop their own messages that work, not outside people telling them how and what they need to do. Help develop and educate grassroots CBOs and ASOs about how to serve the community they are in," emphasized a Stratford, Connecticut resident.

"Accessing and building the capacity of faith-based organizations is also necessary," advised a Cleveland, Ohio minister. The emphasis on training faith-based leaders and engaging faith-based organizations in the fight against HIV/AIDS was stressed as a critical step in reaching minorities, particularly Black and Latino communities.

Many minority communities in both urban and rural areas have few health care providers due to challenges in recruiting and retaining health care professionals. According to a 2008 survey of Ryan White HIV/AIDS-funded clinics, lack of reimbursement and lack of providers were cited as leading causes preventing recruitment.[77] Although it is unknown what proportion of these surveyed clinics are based in communities of color, Ryan White HIV/AIDS Program clients are overwhelmingly from these communities: 72 percent of clients are racial or ethnic minorities and 89 percent are either uninsured or on a public insurance plan.[78]

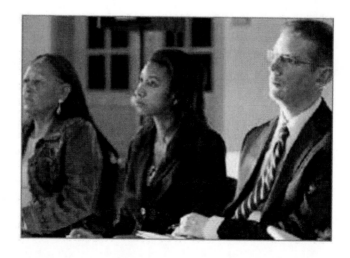

In minority neighborhoods, community organizations often serve as the pathway into the health care system. It is no surprise, then, that many participants at the community discussions called for increased HIV/AIDS training for organizations providing social services.

"Build capacity for community-based organizations that work primarily with women and support providers that have demonstrated core competence in working with [this population]," requested one San Francisco Web respondent. "As part of the consultation and community engagement, ONAP should ensure that tribes and Native American CBOs receive technical and capacity building assistance," suggested another participant.

Build a Bigger, Better Workforce

"…Patients need HIV medication. They also need access to the health care providers that can prescribe the medication."

— Birmingham, Alabama Web submission

"More than a third of U.S. physicians in practice are age 55 or older and likely to retire in the next 10 to 15 years. The aging of the physician workforce will be a key factor limiting future growth of the health care system."[79] Several comments discussed how the shortage of providers working in HIV/AIDS and primary care stands to pose significant barriers to people living with HIV and the health infrastructure in place to care for these persons. A hospital worker in St. Thomas explained that after 30 years of hospital work, there had been no training opportunities in which she could enroll to learn about HIV specialty care. Other participants noted that increasing demands for expanding the scope of HIV/AIDS services, as well as low provider reimbursement rates, is further exacerbating this problem. While these trends exist in many States, participants reminded us that rural communities in the South, in particular, are experiencing acute provider shortages as HIV/AIDS incidence and prevalence increase in this region. A submission from Arkansas summed up many of these comments: "There is a shortage of doctors and medical professionals experienced with treating HIV and it is nearly impossible for many individuals to travel the often long distances to reach those that do exist for adequate treatment and lab work."

Participants across the 14 community discussions were very vocal about the steps the Administration could take to try to curtail the workforce shortage of providers working in HIV/AIDS or primary care. By far, the most recommendations related to government incentives for health professionals (e.g., doctors, nurses, dentists, pharmacists) to enter HIV/AIDS or primary care or to work with HIV-positive persons. Specifically, participants suggested loan repayment or loan forgiveness programs for persons entering into these fields and for those willing to work in high-need communities, including rural towns. "Nobody is going into primary care anymore or HIV, partly because of the costs [and] partly because when they graduate from medical school they owe thousands [or] hundreds of thousands of dollars," said an Albuquerque, New Mexico doctor in favor of loan forgiveness.

As an HIV/AIDS doctor explained,

"Not a lot of docs and health care providers are coming into the business. It does not actually pay terribly well for one thing…so [we need] some kind of program to support the training of physicians and other health care workers in the area of HIV medicine."

The American Academy of HIV Medicine suggested, "The Administration should provide for expanded opportunities for medical, PA [physician assistant], and NP [nurse practitioner] students to seek practice opportunities in HIV medicine as part of their training and to pursue clinical fellowships after their residency...to draw some students into HIV care that would not otherwise focus on the field." The American Association of Colleges of Nursing echoed this recommendation and highlighted the dwindling number of nurses in HIV/AIDS care because of the unavailability of training.

Curricula and Improved Education of Providers

Quality of life and life expectancy for people living with HIV have improved dramatically since the advent of highly active antiretroviral therapy. Yet treating the disease remains complex. Today, providers across a number of health disciplines are now caring for and treating people living with HIV. This factor has resulted in a call to teach all health professionals, regardless of medical specialty, about HIV/AIDS. Some participants focused on the need to provide HIV/AIDS education to individuals working in fields ranging from education, law, social work, psychology, and others.

Notwithstanding a number of training programs across the country, some participants discussed their interactions with providers who seemed not to have stayed abreast of HIV care and treatment issues.

To address this, the American Academy of HIV Medicine suggested, "Rotations in HIV care and/or exposure to populations impacted by HIV should be expanded...along with outpatient opportunities for internal medicine and family medicine residence." They added that "clinical training opportunities, satellite learning, and consultation through teleconferences and Web-based programs should be expanded and encouraged for primary care providers already in the field."

Respondents also emphasized the need for health professionals to undergo cultural competency training so they understand not only what but whom they are treating. Since the onset of the epidemic, this has been an enormous concern for gay and bisexual men, who were initially simply ignored by many health professionals.

Keeping Providers Abreast of Latest Research Findings

The debate on the optimal time to begin treatment has been ongoing for some times. A number of Web submissions highlighted recent research on earlier initiation of antiretroviral therapy and its correlation with survival rates.* This development underscores the importance of providers keeping pace with the latest research and clinical findings.

*Source: Kitahata, M.M., Gange, S.J., Abraham, A.G., Merriman, B., Saag, M.S., Justice, A.C., Moore, R.D. (2009, April 30). Effect of early versus deferred antiretroviral therapy for HIV on survival. New England Journal of Medicine, 360(18), 1815-26.

The transgender community continues to note significant levels of discrimination from a medical community that may not understand them or their needs. Cultural competency extends beyond the issue of sexual orientation or gender identification, however, to include, age, substance use, and race/ethnicity. For example, "Native peoples have distinct and unique approaches to health and wellness, based upon their respective cultural values and traditions," said one New York City resident. "Socio-cultural and individual factors contribute to the growing HIV problem among Asian and Pacific Islanders," added a Brooklyn, New York native.

E. Summary

Improving access to care and enhancing health outcomes for underserved people living with HIV can be a complex undertaking. Access to HIV/AIDS health care can often be facilitated for those lacking private health insurance through an array of public programs. However, the need for HIV/AIDS care is often just one of many needs, especially for those living in poverty and with social problems that often accompany HIV/AIDS. Left unaddressed, these nonmedical needs can affect how people access care, and, ultimately, health outcomes.

At community forums and in written submissions, individuals explored the multitude of factors that must be addressed if access to care and improved health is to become a reality for all people. Certainly, access to HIV/AIDS care is important, particularly access to care for related conditions and essential social services, like housing, transportation, and job training.

Ultimately, the particular services that are needed differ for each person, and comments conveyed that providers serving people living with HIV must recognize each individual's unique needs and circumstances. One San Francisco doctor succinctly described the issue: "Treating HIV/AIDS is not a one-size-fits-all situation."

REDUCING HIV-RELATED HEALTH DISPARITIES

HIV has had a disproportionate impact on specific populations, since the beginning of the HIV epidemic. Three quarters of HIV/AIDS diagnoses are among men in the United **States**, and men who have sex with men are particularly impacted by the epidemic. Approximately one-half of all persons living with HIV in the United States are MSM, and MSM account for 53 percent of new HIV infections each year.[80] CDC scientists have determined that MSM are 44 to 86 times more likely to become infected with HIV than other men and 40 to 77 times more likely to become infected than women.[81] Moreover, MSM is the only risk group in the United States whose estimated annual number of new infections is increasing. A disproportionate number of HIV diagnoses among MSM are MSM of color. Communities of color, especially the African-American and Latino communities, are also disproportionately impacted by HIV. For example:

- Approximately 71 percent of all HIV/AIDS cases diagnosed in 2007 were among racial and ethnic minorities.[82]
- While comprising just 13 percent of the U.S. population, African-Americans accounted for 47 percent of the estimated AIDS cases diagnosed in 2007; Latinos make up 15.4 percent of the population, yet comprise 17 percent of AIDS cases.[83,84]

- Although women account for a quarter of HIV/AIDS cases in the United States, 84 percent of HIV/AIDS cases among women are among women of color, with African-American women accounting for more than three of every five cases.[85]

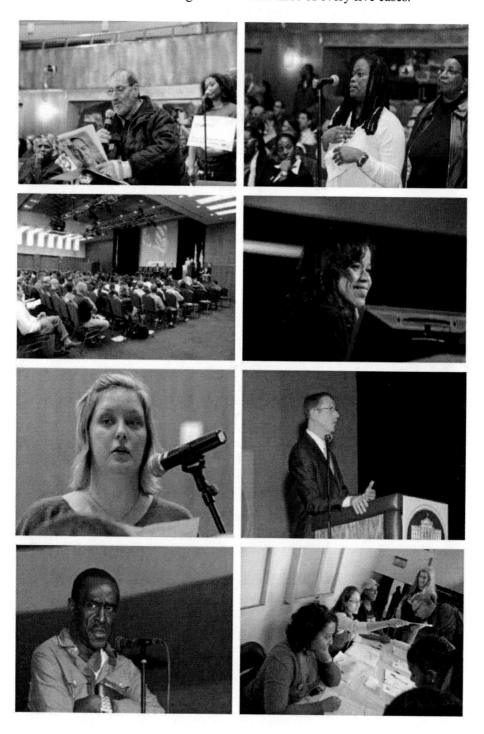

Disparities are also evident in the geographic distribution of HIV/AIDS cases in the United States with a disproportionate number of HIV cases occurring in the South as well as the Northeast. Although over 80 percent of reported AIDS cases in the United States between 1994 and 2007 occurred in large (more than 500,000 persons) metropolitan areas, the South has the largest number and percentage of AIDS cases diagnosed in nonmetropolitan areas (less than 50,000 persons) in the United States.

People participating in our national conversation about HIV/AIDS underlined that resources must be targeted to those communities most heavily affected by the epidemic. They offered specific recommendations for action:

A. Expand Services to at-Risk Populations

> "[We need] to ensure that communities with small populations have access to resources, and to develop strategies for emerging communities."
>
> — New York City, New York community discussion

Racial and Ethnic Minorities

The call for swift action to address health disparities among racial and ethnic minorities was an overarching theme throughout the community discussions and in the many submissions made to ONAP.

As the National Medical Association wrote in its submission to ONAP, "Persons of color living with HIV/AIDS are more likely to experience a myriad of social and economic challenges that inevitably exacerbate the conditions known to be associated with this disease." They added, "The negative impact of HIV infection will become increasingly salient over time."

Given the disproportionate burden of HIV among African-Americans, many people advocated for a declaration of a national state of emergency regarding HIV/AIDS in the African-American community. In San Francisco, we heard this plea:

> "African-Americans have been disproportionately affected by HIV/AIDS since the epidemic's beginning and that disparity has deepened over time...we must do something about it. I would like to ask you to please consider recommending, implementing, and declaring a national state of emergency within the African-American community and allocating resources accordingly."

Significant public attention was given to other racial and ethnic minority groups as well. A number of individuals, particularly at the New York City and Minneapolis meetings, discussed the unique challenges faced by African immigrants. Discussions also emphasized the particular needs of Asian/Pacific Islanders, Native Americans, and Latinos.

Latinos are the fastest growing minority group in the Nation. As of 2008, Latinos continue to represent a growing proportion of HIV cases.

Nearly one out of five HIV/AIDS cases diagnosed in the United States in 2007 were among this population.[86] Puerto Rico was among the top 10 States and Territories in terms of AIDS cases in 2007.[87]

Policy Recommendation to Address HIV Disease among Black Americans

Across several community discussions and Web submissions, individuals expressed a need for policy makers to speak with stakeholders from communities of color. In particular, many people asked for a more focused response targeting the African-American community. They asked that the National HIV/AIDS Strategy include provisions for funding grants and initiatives in the African-American community and create periodic reports on the work being done and the outcomes achieved.

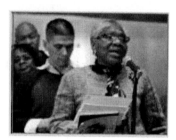

Health Disparities among Racial/ Ethnic Minorities Living with HIV/AIDS

- Immigrants are more likely than native-born U.S. residents to present for care with an AIDS-defining illness.
- African-Americans accounted for approximately 49 percent of new HIV infections diagnosed in 2007. African-Americans suffer disproportionate rates of diabetes, heart disease, and stroke and are more likely than their White counterparts to die from cancer.
- Racial/ethnic minorities in care are less likely than their White counterparts to be taking antiretroviral therapy.

Sources: Weiwel E, Nasrallah H, Hannah D, et al. HIV diagnosis and care initiation among foreign-born persons in New York City, 2001-2007. Presentation at the 16th Conference on Retroviruses and Opportunistic Infections; February 8-11, 2009; Montreal, Quebec.
CDC HIV/AIDS Surveillance Report. 2007; 19. Table 1.
U.S. Department of Health and Human Services, Office of Minority Health. African American profile. n.d. Available at: http://minorityhealth.hhs.gov/templates/browse.aspx?lvl=2&lvlID=51. Accessed December 15, 2009.
Stone VE. Physician contributions to disparities in HIV/AIDS care: the role of provider perception regarding adherence. Curr HIV/AIDS Rep. 2005 Nov; 2(4): 189-93.

"Negative cultural influences and stigma are big challenges for [Latinos], and we need interventions that will address core family values among the Hispanic community as well as traditionalism and machismo," said a Laredo, Texas Health Department employee. Many participants added stigma to the list of barriers impeding HIV testing and care within the Latino population.

One common suggestion for improving health disparities, particularly among Blacks and Latinos, was to involve religious leaders and faith-based organizations. "Religiosity plays an important role in the life of most Hispanics or Latinos. It is estimated that 75 percent of Latinos arriving in the United States consider themselves Catholic," explained a Miami, Florida community participant. She added, "In our experience, for the majority of Latinos—no matter their country of origin or whether recently arrived or living in the United States for many years—the church represents a safe, nonthreatening place to go for services beyond spiritual counseling."

Recognizing spirituality as well as traditional health practices were highlighted as important aspects of culturally competent care for a range of racial and ethnic minorities. As a New York community discussion respondent suggested, "Support the integration of traditional health care practices, which includes the use of traditional medicine practitioners within the HIV/AIDS service delivery system...for Native Americans."

American Indian/Alaska Native advocates and consumers expressed concern that misperceptions about their community were a cause of health disparities. They noted that many Native Americans live in urban areas, not just on reservations, and they highlighted the diversity of tribes and cultures.[88,89] Participants asserted that such diversity should be considered when devising prevention and care strategies.

One person suggested consulting with the 13 U.S. Indigenous Epidemiology Centers to create a broader, more tailored approach. Similar sentiments were echoed by a Ohio man: "Prevention messages must be available in multiple Asian languages (including over 100 languages), and be culturally sensitive."

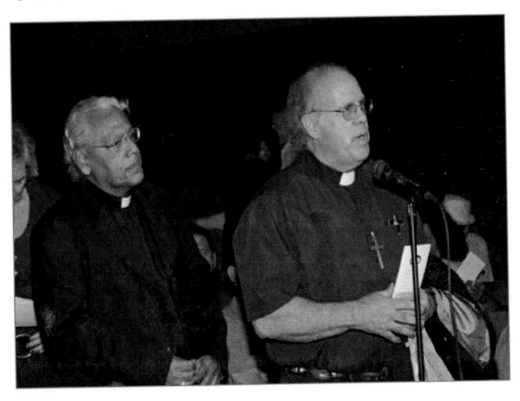

Women

"The face of HIV is changing and [we] need to be target[ing] women," explained a Jackson, Mississippi resident. Women represent 26 percent of HIV/AIDS cases diagnosed in 2007, of which 83 percent were attributed to heterosexual contact.[90] "A heterosexual woman's biggest infector is a man, whether that man is heterosexual, gay, down low or in prison," wrote a woman from Pennsylvania. "I am not HIV-positive," wrote a woman from Florida, "but I have been myself a woman at risk. I have lost friends and co-workers because of HIV/AIDS, and for the past eleven (11) years I have shared my life with my husband, who now has AIDS." ONAP heard from numerous women living with HIV who were infected by their male partners. As a woman from Kansas explains,

> "I was very much like so many people ... I thought that AIDS did not affect me. I am a college educated African American Female who had been married for 15 years with 3 small children when I began this unexpected journey and received an HIV+ diagnosis. Of course I had no risk factors, I knew my risk but I did not know my husband's risk."

Among women, there are diverse sets of challenges. For some women living with HIV, the responsibilities of care giving, or working two jobs, is the primary impediment to ongoing health care. Among others, trauma, violence, and stigma inhibit health care seeking behaviors and give rise to comorbidities associated with HIV/AIDS. As one participant explained, "We learned that a lot of these females have dual diagnoses. They are substance users.

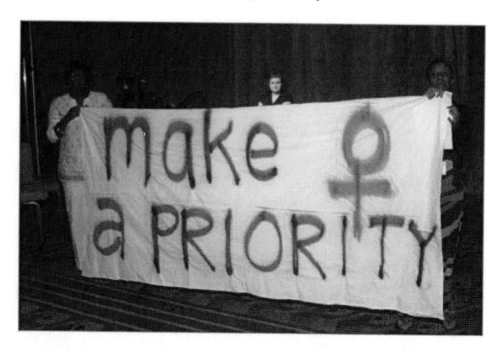

They have mental health issues and a lot of them are in treatment facilities…and they are not knowledgeable of the disease."

Participants cited gender-based inequities, underestimated HIV risk, and lower socioeconomic levels as some of the issues undercutting women's ability to access appropriate health care.

Participants advocated for peer-based approaches in outreach, messaging, and service delivery targeting women. "Actively recruit and fund more communal, cultural, homegrown interventions by women of color for women of color," said a Houston, Texas woman. "When we train women to be peer educators, they exhibit a lot more ownership of the prevention messages that we teach them and they often adopt them in their own lives and then go on to adopt safer behavior [and] communicate [that] to their communities," added an Albuquerque, New Mexico woman.

Men Who Have Sex with Men

Several recommendations reflected concern over Federal policies that discouraged health promotion activities that target gay and bisexual men and the de-emphasis of men who have sex with men overall as a priority population for HIV-prevention activities. One Washington, D.C. resident commented:

> "I am particularly speaking from the standpoint of a gay man here this evening, one who has lived with HIV for 27 years, that first and foremost in the legislative agenda we need to end the restrictive provisions of Section 2500 Public Health Service Act. It is ridiculous that we cannot have frank, adequate, explicit education aimed at our communities. [And] rolled up within that is the inadequacy of CDC interventions aimed at gay and bisexual men… at this time only 4 of 17 of the approved interventions target us, but yet we represent over half of the new HIV infections."

Other comments pointed to the diversity among MSM populations and the need for prevention responses that recognize this diversity. For example:

- Some MSM may culturally identify as bisexual or heterosexual and not respond to messaging or care approaches targeting "out" gay men.
- The influence of culture on HIV risk should be recognized. Culture can be a protective factor. Among Latino MSM, greater acculturation into U.S. culture has been associated with increased risk behaviors for HIV infection.[91,92]
- A greater proportion of Black and Latino MSM become infected with HIV between ages 13 and 29 than do White MSM.[93]
- Noninjection drug use is associated with HIV risk behavior and HIV infection among MSM, but substance use patterns differ markedly across MSM by race and ethnicity, and geography.[94]

Many participants called for increased prevention education and more targeted efforts, including tapping into online social and dating venues for risk reduction messages, and utilizing positive role models to reach various segments of MSM. A great deal of public attention was given to young MSM. In a written submission, the Gay Men's Health Crisis called for:

> "School interventions that promote tolerance and acceptance of LGBT [lesbian, gay, bisexual, transgender] youth. Gay/straight alliances and anti-bullying curricula correlate with lower HIV risk behavior…and better health and school performance outcomes. HHS and CDC should [also] promote parental acceptance as a public health imperative."

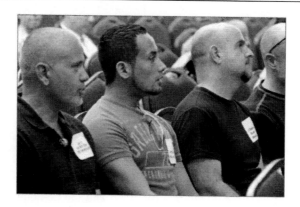

Transgender Persons

Many participants stated that transgender populations have been overlooked by HIV prevention programs. The Los Angeles County HIV Prevention Planning Committee Transgender Task Force stated that, "The transgender population, while estimated to be relatively small compared to other populations, is disproportionately affected by HIV, and has among the highest seroprevalence rates of any group."

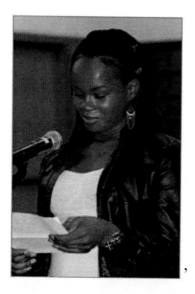

According to a recently published CDC study, estimates of HIV/AIDS prevalence among transgender populations are as high as 27 percent.[95] Other reports have documented that transgender individuals experience higher rates of abuse and institutional discrimination;[96] face unique legal challenges (e.g. qualifying for services where identification and current name do not match);[97] and may be more susceptible to HIV from survival sex or injection practices associated with hormonal therapies or silicone.[98]

Participants called for increased inclusion of transgender individuals in clinical trials and research. They asked that HIV and other health information be crafted and distributed to reach transgender individuals. Respondents also highlighted the need to better educate the public and health professions to ensure transgender individuals can receive culturally-competent care . These sentiments are summed up by a Web submission from Virginia:

"[Government agencies] have continually neglected to include transgender populations in the ways that they capture data about HIV prevalence and incidence, in the prevention interventions that they promote for health departments and community based organizations that they fund, and in making the care services accessible for HIV positive transgender persons. This is not to say that no progress has occurred, but especially considering the extremely high levels of infection among some urban transgender communities, it is clear that more needs to be done urgently."

Incarcerated Populations

Each year about one in four people living with HIV spend time in a correctional facility.[99] Some of the same socioeconomic and psychosocial factors associated with increased risk for HIV infection are also associated with incarceration. These include homelessness, poverty, substance use, and lack private insurance coverage.[100,101,102,103,104]

In the United States, Blacks and Latinos are more likely to be incarcerated than other racial or ethnic groups. Since Blacks and Latinos accounted for 63 percent of incarcerated individuals in 2002, interventions and investment specifically targeting these populations are needed.[105]

Across community discussions, individuals discussed the need to prevent both HIV and incarceration, better treat those already incarcerated, and improve re-entry programs to ensure HIV-positive individuals are connected to the services they need.

"We need...continuity of care for individuals leaving corrections facilities," said an Arkansas man. "Increas[e] health care linkages from prison," said a Pennsylvania resident. Or as a Web respondent expressed, "When patients are released, they should be given two weeks to 30-day supply of medications and community resource/provider information to schedule an appointment. Often patients are released without or with only a few days' supply of medication, and no linkage to health care." A respondent from Virginia elaborated on this point and the consequences of interrupted treatment:

"Because of medication/drug resistance, you cannot stop and start HIV medication as people do with diabetes, cholesterol and blood pressure treatment. Lack of treatment, delayed treatment, and treatment interruption, negatively impact an HIV-infected person's health status and can limit their treatment options in the future. The result is greater costs incurred in the medical care of an infected person who is less well than someone who had consistent access to treatment and health care."

B. Provide Culturally and Linguistically Appropriate Services and Interventions

"We should start looking [at] individuals, their cultures, and what the underlying needs are."

— Brooklyn, New York Web submission

Many participants at the community discussions spoke emphatically about the importance of culturally and linguistically appropriate services for people living with HIV.

A New York City man recommended messages be developed that are "specific to individual ethnic populations in their language and/or culture." A California resident explained,

> "L.A. County sprawl[s] over 4,800 square miles. We come from diverse cultures and ethnicities. We speak many languages. We are Asian/Pacific Islander, Middle Eastern, African-American; we are White, and yes we are Latino. Los Angeles is home to the largest population of Mexicanos outside of Mexico City. It has the highest concentration of people from El Salvador than any other place in this Nation. We have many unique differences and many unique needs when it comes to HIV and AIDS."

Many people told us that greater funding and more interventions targeting sexual and racial and ethnic minorities are needed. Participants noted the importance of utilizing minority-run, community-based organizations to help remove barriers associated with distrust of the health system, misinformation, stigma, and immigration status. Participants also discussed cash-strapped organizations that struggle to survive. Participants at the community forums emphasized using minority-run organizations to reduce cultural insensitivity or compromised health care. According to one organization, "[W]e found that in primary care, 30 percent of transgender people do not go to see health care [providers] because of discrimination and disrespect that they have had in the past." "Target research interventions and funding to underserved populations, including aboriginal groups, linguistic minorities, adolescents, women, active drug users, and persons who come late into HIV care," a Florida man recommended. "We need free, confidential, small, open forums culturally sensitive regardless of immigration status or sexual orientation to address our differences as women and as Latinas," added one Web respondent.

C. Improve Availability of HIV-Related Services in Rural Areas and U.S. Territories

> "[HIV/AIDS] is exacerbated by poverty, lower levels of education which are correlated with lack of information about HIV and AIDS, and fewer jobs in rural areas especially for the kinds of jobs that would provide health benefits."
>
> — Columbia, South Carolina community discussion

The need for increased health and social services in rural areas and U.S. Territories is clear:

- Nearly one-half of rural residents suffer from at least one chronic illness;[106]
- Rural residents are more likely to live below the Federal poverty level than their urban counterparts;[107] and
- HIV-positive rural residents are less likely to receive highly active antiretroviral therapy than those in urban areas.[108]

HIV/AIDS care delivery in rural geographic areas is a challenge often because of stigma and a shortage of trained providers willing to treat people living with HIV.

"Most consumers must travel to larger cities for dental services, and even then many dentists don't accept ADAP, or Medicaid. The same is true of mental health services," explained a person living with HIV from upstate New York. "Due to these limitations placed on us, we as rural consumers have not been able to lead normal, productive, healthy lives around and within our communities. We need more providers willing to treat those infected with HIV/AIDS and willing to accept the medical coverage afforded to us."

"In addition, the government must recognize that rural residents average fewer medical appointments than their urban areas and the need for increased technology infrastructure in rural areas including high speed Internet," suggested a Minneapolis, Minnesota participant.

Respondents concerned with reducing health disparities in rural areas recommended telemedicine programs and CME conferences that give rural providers an opportunity to discuss best practices. They voiced strong support for loan forgiveness programs as incentives for clinicians in areas with a shortage of health care providers. Participants also supported a national education campaign that would decrease HIV stigma and empower HIV-positive individuals in rural communities.

D. Summary

The HIV/AIDS epidemic has had a disproportionate impact on racial, ethnic, and sexual minorities in the United States. Comments from the community discussions and the Web submissions reiterated the need to expand education and prevention services to these communities to address the causes of the disparities.

Particularly high-risk groups including MSM, transgender individuals, women, Black and Latino populations, and incarcerated populations should have access to interventions tailored to each community. Moreover, participants also called for more culturally sensitive and linguistically appropriate services and interventions to eliminate barriers to care. Participants also discussed the needs of people in rural communities who have limited access to health providers, particularly those that offer HIV services. In addition to suggesting incentive programs to increase the number of providers in rural areas, they also suggested education campaigns to reduce HIV stigma.

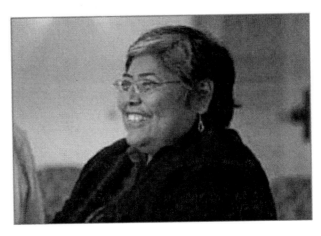

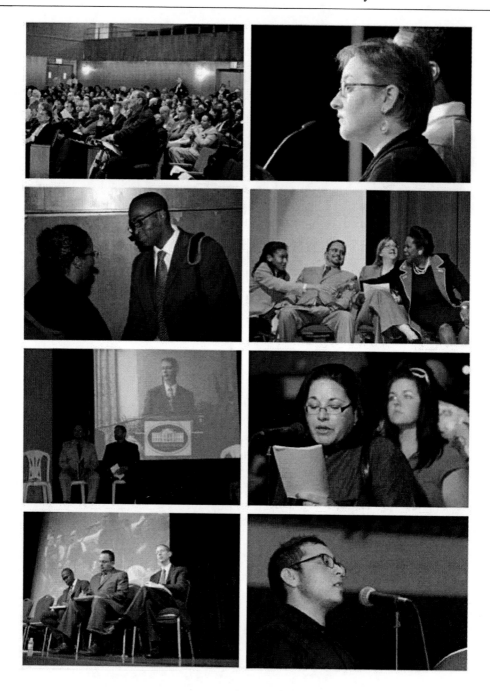

CROSSCUTTING THEMES

Many of the recommendations received do not fit neatly into one of the three key goals for the strategy, but apply to more than one or relate to crosscutting issues. Key crosscutting recommendations include:

A. Evaluation and Program Monitoring

"[Evaluation] is critical so that all of our interventions and the impact that we have on our communities are measured and sufficiently resourced."

— San Francisco community discussion

Many community discussion attendees underscored the need for tracking program performance and outcomes. "Evaluation is needed to maintain effectiveness," explained one respondent. "There needs to be a monitoring and evaluation framework so that we can be able to look back…and say [if] what we implemented has made any sense," added another.

A number of participants called for government at all levels to be held accountable for using public funds appropriately and assuring high quality public services. "Funded agencies need to be held accountable for ever[y] penny spent," said a Tennessee resident. "A funded agency that has found two new positive cases in five years is not right…If an organization or agency is not [finding] new infections, give the money to someone who is willing to do the job."

While people raised the theme of accountability at a number of community discussions, perhaps nowhere was it stressed more so than in Puerto Rico. Some of the issues related to Puerto Rico may be unique to the island. A common recommendation that we heard in Puerto Rico was for the Federal Government to consider directing funds to a third party administrator instead of sending the funds to the commonwealth government.

"I want to denounce the high level of bureaucracy that corrupts the Health Department," said one community discussion respondent. "This country…has mismanaged the delivery of care and prevention of AIDS and it is time [that] the funds are given [directly] to the agencies that provide the care," said another. Residents in Puerto Rico repeatedly stated there was a need to expedite HIV funding dissemination and remove barriers that impede care delivery. "We have a lot of frustration in getting certifications and licensing [for] detox and treatment…SAMHSA [Substance Abuse and Mental Health Services Administration] has taken so long," said one attendee. "The government receives [Ryan White HIV/AIDS Program] Part A, B, and C but many of those funds [are] not forwarded; it almost [always] stays in the northern part of the Island," stated another Puerto Rico respondent. Discrepancies in standards of care and service capacity not only varied from region to region in Puerto Rico, but between the island and the mainland U.S. A Web respondent from Puerto Rico commented, "HIV patients in Puerto Rico…lack medications because the government imposes requirements to access them that are too high… [In] the mainland, states' requirements are much lower than here. Can somebody explain that?"

The request for more equitable funding and increased standards of care, however, arose throughout the United States. In many cases, rural residents were especially likely to focus on issues related to accountability for public resources. "There needs to be [more] specificity…regarding funding priorities in order [to] address the needs of rural areas because they are different from metropolitan areas. Currently criteria mandates are not sensitive to rural needs," suggested a Jackson, Mississippi resident. But we also heard from people in large metropolitan areas who stressed the importance of evaluating available resources and how those resources are applied. "There is a lot of overlap and as the budget is being constrained [we need] to effectively see what works and what does not work," said a California woman.

B. Coordination across Agencies, States, Communities, and Providers

"We recommend that the Federal Government review the coordination of funding for HIV/AIDS, substance abuse, and mental health services on the Federal and State level, with the goal of increasing access to these services for patients with HIV."

— Ryan White Medical Providers Coalition submission

On multiple occasions, participants asked for greater coordination among the Federal, State, and local agencies addressing HIV/AIDS. "There are so many different funding [channels] and all of these disparate parts do not work together effectively," explained one public health employee. "There has really got to be a more coordinated effort...because there is just no way for all of us to meet all of the requirements from all of these different departments."

"Federal departments utilize differing income standards, definitions, age groupings, demographic categories, etc.," added another participant. "This causes confusion in matters such as reporting, setting priorities, developing objectives, understanding regulations, [and] evaluating outcomes. It can also make comparisons difficult, if not impossible, between programs."

Public Urges More Collaboration among Federal Agencies

Greater collaboration can help the Nation better address crosscutting issues ranging from rural health to workforce shortages. Examples of recent collaborations relevant to HIV/AIDS and affected populations include the following:

- CDC and the Department of Health and Human Services Office of Minority Health and the Department of Education have formed the Federal Collaboration on Health Disparities Research.
- The Substance Abuse and Mental Health Services Administration convened a national summit on methamphetamine and included HRSA, CDC, the Office of Women's Health, Indian Health Services, the Office of Minority Health, National Institute on Drug Abuse, and the Department of Justice.

In addition, respondents emphasized coordinating funding applications and reporting mechanisms so providers can streamline administrative tasks and focus attention and resources on more direct services. Some stressed the importance of better collaboration among agencies that may fund similar services to reduce duplication of services and better target financial resources.

Participants also highlighted the importance of coordination among various providers to create a more seamless transition from testing to treatment. As a Los Angeles man explained,

"I found out that I was HIV positive four blocks from here at the L.A. Gay & Lesbian Center....they took me to a case manager, a social worker, and made appointments for me for crisis counseling, for confirmatory tests, for my doctor, for treatment education, and for the medications thereafter."

Community discussion attendees explained that referrals and partnerships are vital for engagement and retention in care. They added that given the competitive funding environment, however, incentives should be created to better facilitate and improve coordination.

C. Stigma and Discrimination

"There can be no true progress without stigma reduction. Stigma is still the REAL reason so many don't want to know their status, don't get help, or are afraid to be advocates for their own health."

— Hammond, Indiana Web submission

HIV discrimination and stigma were common topics across community discussions. Many expressed frustration over the pervasiveness of HIV stigma nearly 30 years into the HIV epidemic. Studies have shown that HIV stigma is related to delayed HIV testing and care, as well as disclosure to family and friends. People living with HIV can experience violence, rejection, and even eviction from their homes because of their serostatus, and HIV-positive persons continue to report discrimination in employment and health care settings.[109]

A New York City woman discussed her inability to find a dentist who would treat her because she is HIV positive. A Jackson, Mississippi woman talked about being advised by her provider to have an abortion, merely because she was pregnant and HIV positive. A Florida man complained, "I have been refused treatment.... by medical doctors for my HIV on several counts while covered by private insurance... Imagine a world in which medical doctors do not refuse ...life saving services to people with HIV/AIDS. Is that too much to ask?"

A few community discussion participants simply asked for existing anti-discriminatory policies to be enforced. For instance, the Federal AIDS Policy Partnership suggested, "Issue an Executive Order that requires all Federal agencies [and their contractors] comply with the Rehabilitation Act by barring them specifically from using HIV infection as a basis for categorical exclusion." Participants also discussed the importance of adhering to the Health Insurance Portability and Accountability Act (HIPAA) Privacy Rule to protect personal health information. "Congress should establish stricter penalties for violating HIPAA protections that result in loss of employment, health care coverage, or breech of privacy," stated a New York organization. Enforcement of the Americans with Disabilities Act was similarly highlighted. A San Francisco man who is deaf defended his civil rights under the Americans with Disabilities Act to have access to auxiliary aids and services for effective communication. "I go to school," he noted, "[but the] school does not provide interpreters. When I go to work, they do not provide interpreting service. It is hard to get an interpreter, but we really need it for medical care to be able to speak, to go to a hospital, to get medical needs met."

Discrimination against sexual minorities was mentioned in several community discussions. We heard from those who expressed frustration over the lack of recognition of same sex relationships in visitation policies or insurance coverage.

The commonality across each of these comments is that stigma and discrimination continue to pose significant barriers to those infected or affected by HIV, and the NHAS must address these issues to be successful.

D. Policy

"There is no public policy for screening and testing youth for HIV on the island."

— Puerto Rico community discussion

ONAP received numerous recommendations related to policies that covered a range of issues. Each of these issues is briefly summarized below.

Increasing Infrastructure

Many underscored the need for policies that would address infrastructure gaps in health care and social-service systems, as well as transportation, technology, and housing. Participants called for a policy promoting greater public investment to implement widespread adoption of health information technology.

As one submission advocated, portable personal electronic health records have "the ability to transport the detailed record of medical history, drug regimens, and other treatment. They are invaluable for patients with HIV facing relocation, travel, medical emergency, and incarceration....and for [mobile patients] who move from clinic to clinic or State to State."

The challenges associated with rural areas were highlighted by many respondents, especially participants at the South Carolina, Mississippi, and New Mexico meetings.

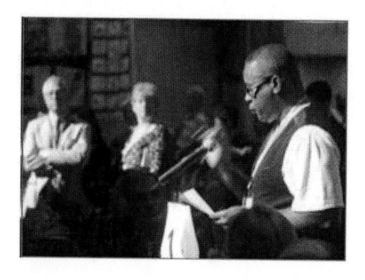

Rural residents advocated for greater investment in social services infrastructure, greater capacity to address HIV at the local level, and more transportation assistance to medical visits.

"[If you live in] the rural areas in the north part of Mississippi, you all have to drive all the way to Tennessee just to get medical care. We need help. We need transportation. We need doctors," one woman exclaimed. "How do you put sufficient infrastructure in funding so that you can maintain a minimum level of services in rural areas?" another participant asked. "It requires a model of funding other than just per capita funding because then your rural areas are always disproportionately on the losing end."

Working with Policy Makers

Many participants in community discussions stressed the importance of dialogue with policy makers because public policy must be informed by the lives and circumstances of people living with HIV. "Our senators and congressmen are responsible for making decisions regarding funding that affects the lives of those of us living with the virus, yet have no idea what living with HIV/AIDS is like," wrote a New Orleans man. "I am concerned that without this knowledge, the decisions are being made based solely on financial numbers and not on the needs of the people receiving the services."

Incentives

Participants also urged that incentives be provided to pharmaceutical companies to further invest in a vaccine, better treatments, or a cure. As one Washington, D.C. man said, "Push the foundations, especially those foundations giving money internationally, to do that here locally and nationally since we are having an economic struggle."

One of the most commonly expressed incentives were policies and programs to encourage recruitment to HIV-related health professions. "Within the past several years, we have seen an exodus of HIV-treating clinicians from the field of HIV medicine," noted a Washington, D.C. physician. "There is also a growing number of clinicians who must spend the majority of their time in non-HIV care in order to support their HIV/AIDS practices, or who take on work and stop seeing these patients altogether."

E. Research

"I have been living with HIV for at least 24 years and I am alive because of research."

— San Francisco, California community discussion

The presence of long-term HIV survivors at community discussions across the country is testament to the power and possibility of research. "I was born HIV positive. I am now 25 years old," said an Elizabeth Glaser Pediatric AIDS Foundation ambassador. "I work full time. I have a great boyfriend and am looking to go on to graduate school." Stories like this illustrate the promise of HIV medications and the role research has played in improving the lives of HIV-positive people. Individuals reminded ONAP that there is still much to do, research questions to explore, and still so much we don't know.

"What are the long-term effects of ARV [antiretroviral] treatment?" asked one respondent. "Why [are] some PLWHA long-term survivors and others suffer increased morbidity and mortality?" asked another. To be able to answer these questions, and to be equipped to address them, participants called for increased investment in research. "Invest more money and meaningful resources in medical and clinical research," said a San Antonio, Texas man.

Community members also noted that more intensive efforts are needed to ensure that women and minorities have access to clinical trials, as well as calls for intervention additional research for specific communities. On several occasions, participants underscored the need to develop and fund structural interventions that address the context of risk and move beyond individual risk behaviors. Participants noted that structural interventions such as education, employment, housing, and drug treatment programs in prisons have been shown to be successful in addressing other public health challenges[110] and that funding these types of structural factors in future research should be a priority.

F. Summary

Participants' recommendations addressed several common themes. Primarily, they called for education and anti-discrimination policy enforcement to eradicate stigma that can be a barrier to HIV prevention, diagnosis, and treatment. Comments suggested that to do this, public policy makers should work with community members and advocates to ensure that policies are based on people's medical needs as well as other service needs such as housing assistance. Participants also recommended that these policy makers streamline funding processes and ensure better coordination among Federal agencies, States, communities, and service providers. This will help make navigating the health care system more manageable for people living with HIV and for organizations applying for grants. Participants suggested that increased coordination could also help to ensure the accountability of federally-funded organizations and public resources for HIV services. Better evaluation and monitoring of these resources would help guarantee that money allocated for HIV/AIDS is being spent effectively and appropriately.

MOVING FORWARD

"Working together, I am confident that we can stop the spread of HIV and ensure that those affected get the care and support they need."

— President Barack Obama

This report will be used to inform the development of a National HIV/AIDS Strategy. The strategy will rely on proven and effective programs and practices.

ONAP has convened a Federal HIV Interagency Working Group—leaders with policy and program expertise in Federal agencies that provide HIV and other related services—to assist with the process of developing the National HIV/AIDS Strategy. The Working Group is tasked with reviewing and prioritizing the many recommendations that ONAP received for the National HIV/AIDS Strategy and analyzing them to identify those actions that hold the most potential for the greatest impact, and for which there is solid scientific evidence of their effectiveness. This report is among several key references that the Working Group will use for developing the strategy.

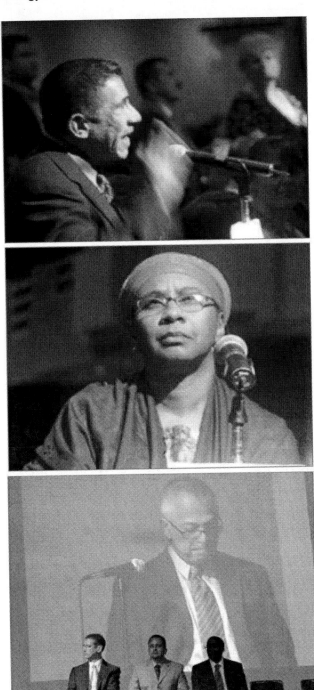

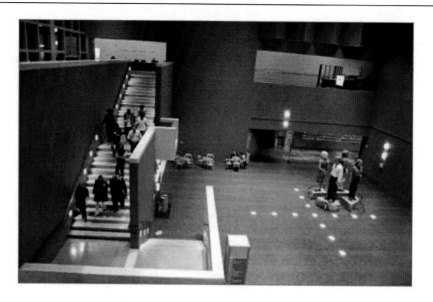

This report aggregates the most common recommendations that ONAP received from the public to provide a mechanism to understand the most commonly held views for the National HIV/AIDS Strategy. In undertaking this effort, the Presidential Advisory Council on HIV/AIDS (PACHA) will have an important role to play in supporting the effective implementation of the strategy and monitoring our progress. This report will be made available to the public via the Web site, http://www.whitehouse.gov/administration/eop/onap/, and will be circulated to the PACHA, as well as Federal agency staff.

Although this report will be among several source materials that will help inform the National HIV/AIDS Strategy, not all topics expressed in this report will be in the final strategy document. As mentioned earlier, the Strategy is not intended to be a comprehensive list of all of the actions, policies, and programmatic priorities needed to respond to the domestic HIV epidemic. Instead, the Strategy will identify a limited number of high payoff steps to address the HIV epidemic in the United States.

In addition to informing the National HIV/AIDS Strategy process, this report may also be a valuable resource for Federal, State, and local agencies, as well as other stakeholders who are working to prevent HIV infection, provide services to people living with HIV, and identify strategies to reduce HIV-related disparities. While not reflecting a scientifically-valid sample of public opinion, this report provides a fairly comprehensive summary of ideas and recommendations from a broad range of interested parties from across the country.

The Office of National AIDS Policy acknowledges and gives sincere thanks to the many individuals who devoted their time and energy to the process by contributing their ideas and sharing their personal stories included in this report.

Acknowledgments

The Office of National AIDS Policy (ONAP) thanks the moderators that facilitated the community discussions, and is grateful for the participation of many community-based organizations, business representatives, and advocates who contributed in immeasurable ways to make these discussions a success. ONAP also gives special thanks to the many people living with or affected by HIV for their courageous and frank testimony that makes this report a compelling and useful document. ONAP also thanks Capital Meeting Planning, Inc., and Impact Marketing for their contributions to the community discussions and to this report; and the State and local elected officials who participated in the community discussions, as well as the following members of Congress:

Senator Al Franken, Minnesota
Delegate Donna M. Christensen, U.S. Virgin Islands
Representative Keith Ellison, Minnesota (5th District)
Representative Eliot Engel, New York (17th District)
Delegate Eleanor Holmes Norton, District of Columbia
Representative Sheila Jackson Lee, Texas (18th District)
Representative Barbara Lee, California (9th District)
Representative John Lewis, Georgia (5th District).

We thank the following individuals for contributing photographs for this report:
Larry Bryant, Anthony Clark, Anselmo Fonseca, Samuel Johnson, Robert Kohmescher, Sofia Lee, Katrina Lewis, Roy Nelson, Daniel Sampson, Char Smullyan, Steven Underhill

This document was released April 2010 and is available at www.whitehouse.gov/onap.

End Notes

[1] CDC. (2009, August). *HIV prevention in the United States at a critical cross roads.* Retrieved from the CDC Web site: http://www.cdc.gov/hiv/resources/ reports/ hiv_ prev_ us.htm.

[2] CDC. (2008, October 3). HIV Prevalence estimates—United States, 2006. *MMWR, 57(39)*, 1073–1076.

[3] CDC. (2008, August). Estimates of new HIV infections in the United States. Retrieved from the CDC Web site: http://www.cdc.gov/hiv/topics/surveillance/ resources /factsheets/ pdf/incidence.pdf., p. 1.

[4] CDC. (2009). *HIV/AIDS surveillance report,* 2007, 19, 1–7.

[5] CDC. (2009, June 26). Late HIV testing—34 states, 1996-2005. MMWR, 58(24), 661–665.

[6] CDC. (2008, August). HIV/AIDS among Women. Retrieved from the CDC Web site: http://www.cdc.gov/hiv/topics/women/resources/factsheets/pdf/women.pdf.

[7] CDC. (2009, August). *HIV/AIDS in the United States.* Retrieved from the CDC Web site: http://www.cdc.gov/hiv/resources/factsheets/PDF/us.pdf., p. 2.

[8] CDC. (2008, February). HIV/AIDS among persons aged 50 and older. Retrieved from the CDC Web site: http://www.cdc.gov/hiv/topics/over50/resources/factsheets /pdf /over50. pdf., p. 1.

[9] CDC. (2006, June 2). Epidemiology of HIV/AIDS—United States, 1981-2005. MMWR, 55(21), 589–592.

[10] CDC. (1981, June 5). Pneumocystis pneumonia—Los Angeles. MMWR, 30(21), 1–3.

[11] CDC. Current Trends in Mortality Attributable to HIV Infection/AIDS United States, 1981–1990. January 1991: 41–44.

[12] CDC. (2008, August). Estimates of new HIV infections in the United States. Retrieved from the CDC Web site:http://www.cdc.gov/nchhstp/Newsroom/docs/Fact-Sheet-on-HIV-Estimates.pdf., p. 2.

[13] CDC. (2009, August). HIV prevention in the United States at a critical cross roads. Retrieved from the CDC Web site: http://www.cdc.gov/hiv/resources/reports/hiv_prev_us.htm.

[14] Connor, E.M., Sperling, R.S., Gelber, R., Kiselev, P., Scott, G., O'Sullivan, M.J.,and Balsley, J. (1994, November 3). Reduction of maternal-infant transmission of human immunodeficiency virus type 1 with zidovudine treatment. *New England Journal of Medicine,* 18(331), 1173–1180.

[15] CDC. (2007, October). Mother-to-child (perinatal) HIV transmission and prevention. Retrieved from the CDC Web site: http://www.cdc.gov/hiv/topics/perinatal/resources/factsheets/perinatal.htm., p. 3.

[16] HAART refers to a pharmaceutical regimen that involves taking a combination of antiretroviral medications. Initial HAART therapies included at least one protease inhibitor, but new treatment combinations exist that do not contain protease inhibitors.

[17] Baker R. (1995, December). FDA approves 3TC and saquinavir. San Francisco AIDS Foundation.Bulletin of Experimental Treatments for AIDS. 5–9.

[18] KFF. (2007, December). Global HIV/AIDS timelines. Retrieved from the KFF Web site:http://www.kff.org/hivaids/timeline/hivtimeline.cfm.

[19] CDC. (2008, August). Estimates of new HIV infections in the United States. Retrieved from the CDC Web site:http://www.cdc.gov/nchhstp/Newsroom/docs/Fact-Sheet-on-HIV-Estimates.pdf., p. 2.

[20] In this instance, young people refer to people under the age of 30.

[21] CDC. (2009, August). HIV/AIDS in the United States. Retrieved from the CDC Web site: www.cdc.gov/hiv/resources/factsheets/PDF/us.pdf., p. 2.

[22] CDC. (2008, October). New estimates of U.S. HIV prevalence, 2006. Retrieved from the CDC Web site:http://www.cdc.gov/nchhstp/newsroom/docs/prevalence.pdf., p. 1.

[23] Marks, G., Crepaz, N., & Janssen, R. (2006). Estimating sexual transmission of HIV from persons aware and unaware that they are infected with the virus in the USA. *AIDS*, 20(10), 1447–1450.

[24] CDC. (2008, August 3). HIV Testing. Retrieved from the CDC Web site: http://www.cdc.gov/hiv/topics/testing/.

[25] CDC. (2009, June 26). Late HIV testing—34 states, 1996-2005. MMWR, 58(24), 661–665.

[26] CDC. (2007, August 16). Program operations guidelines for STD prevention: partner services. Retrieved from the CDC Web site: http://www.cdc.gov/STD/Program/partner/6-PGpartner.htm.

[27] CDC. (August 2009). HIV/AIDS in the United States. Retrieved from the CDC Web site: http://www.cdc.gov/hiv/resources/factsheets/PDF/us.pdf., p. 1.

[28] Ibid., 1.

[29] CDC. (August 2009). HIV/AIDS in the United States. Retrieved from the CDC Web site: http://www.cdc.gov/hiv/resources/factsheets/PDF/us.pdf., p. 1.

[30] CDC. Hepatitis C information for the public. n.d. Available at: http://www.cdc.gov/hepatitisC/index.htm. Accessed December 3, 2009.

[31] Gibson, D.R., Brand, R., Anderson, K., Kahn, J.G., Perales, D., & Guydish, J. (2002, October 1). Two- to six-fold decreased odds of HIV risk behavior associated with use of syringe exchange. *Journal of Acquired Immune Deficiency Syndromes*, 31(2), 237.

[32] Geletko, S.M., and Poulakos, M.N. (2002). Pharmaceutical services in an HIV clinic. *American Journal of Health-System Pharmacy* 50(8),709–13

[33] National AIDS Housing Coalition. (2008). Examining the evidence: the impact of housing on HIV prevention and care. Retrieved from the NAHC Web site:http://nationalaidshousing.org/PDF/Summary-Key%20Summit%20Findings.pdf., p. 3.

[34] Flores, G. (2006, July 20). Language barriers to health care in the United States. *New England Journal of Medicine*, 355(3), 229–231.

[35] Center for Outreach Research and Evaluation, Health and Disability Working Group(2006). Making the connection: promoting engagement and retention in HIV medical care among hard-to-reach populations.Boston University School of Public Health. Retrieved from the Boston University Web site:http://www.bu.edu/hdwg/pdf/projects/LessonLearnedFinal.pdf.

[36] Carmichael JK, Deckard DT, Feinberg J et al. American Academy of HIV Medicine, HIV Medicine Association. Averting a crisis in HIV care: a joint statement of the American Academy of HIV Medicine (AAHIVM) and the HIV Medicine Association (HIVMA) on the HIV medical workforce. June 2009.

[37] Dill, M.J., and Salsberg, E.S. (2008, November). The complexities of physician supply and demand: projections through 2025. Association of American Medical Colleges, Center for Workforce Studies. Retrieved from the AAMC Web site: http://services.aamc.org/publications/showfile.cfm?file=version122. pdf&prd_id=244&prv_id=299&pdf_id=122., p. 10.

[38] Gilman B, Hargreaves M, Au M, Kim J; Mathematica Policy Research, Inc. (2009, March 6). Factors Impacting the Retention of Clinical Providers and Other Key Personnel in Ryan White HIV/AIDS Program Care Settings.

[39] HRSA Bureau of Health Professions. (2006, October). Physician supply and demand: projections to 2020. Retrieved from the HRSA Web site: ftp://ftp.hrsa.gov/bhpr/workforce/PhysicianForecastingPaperfinal.pdf.

[40] Hoadley, J., and Hargrave, E. (2009, November). Medicare Part D 2010 data spotlight: the coverage gap. KFF. Retrieved from the KFF Web site: http://www.kff.org/medicare/upload/8008.pdf., p. 1.

[41] National AIDS Housing Coalition. (2008). HOPWA 2009 need. Retrieved from the NAHC Web site:http://nationalaidshousing.org/PDF/FY09HOPWANeedPaper.pdf., p. 1.

[42] HRSA. (2008). The power of connections. Retrieved from the HRSA Web site: http://hab.hrsa.gov /publications/ progressreport08/2008ProgressReport.pdf., p. 39.

[43] Marc, L.G., Testa, M.A., Walker, A.M., Robbins, G.K., Shafer, R.W., Anderson, N.B., & Berkman, L.F. (2007, August). Educational attainment and response to HAART during initial therapy for HIV-1 infection. *Journal of Psychosomatic Research*, 63(2), 207–216.

[44] Okie, S. (2007, January 11). Sex, drugs, prisons, and HIV. New England Journal of Medicine, 356(2),106.

[45] The Ryan White Comprehensive AIDS Resources Emergency (CARE) Act is now referred to as the Ryan White HIV/AIDS Program.

[46] Flores, G. (2006, July 20). Language barriers to health care in the United States. *New England Journal of Medicine*, 355(3), 229.

[47] Baker DW, Parker RM, Williams MV, Coates WC, Pitkin K. (1996). Use and effectiveness of interpreters in an emergency department. *Journal of the American Medical Association*.275(10), 783–8.

[48] Flores, G. (2006, July 20). Language barriers to health care in the United States. *New England Journal of Medicine*, 355(3), 231.

[49] Flores, G., Laws, M.B., Mayo, S.J., Zuckerman, B., Abreu, M., Medina, L., and Hardt, E.J. (2003, January). Errors in medical interpretation and their potential clinical consequences in pediatric encounters. Pediatrics, 111(1), 13.

[50] CDC. (2006). Demonstration projects for health departments and community-based organizations (CBOs): antiretroviral treatment access study (ARTAS) II: linkage to HIV care. Retrieved from the CDC Web site:http://www.cdc.gov/hiv/topics/prev_prog/ahp/resources/factsheets/pdf/ARTASII.pdf., p. 1.

[51] CORE/HDWG. (2006). Making the connection: promoting engagement and retention in HIV medical care among hard-to-reach populations. , Boston University School of Public Health. Retrieved from the Boston University Web site: http://www.bu.edu/hdwg/pdf/projects/LessonLearnedFinal.pdf.

[52] American Dietetic Association. (2004). Position of the American Dietetic Association and the Dietitians of Canada: Nutrition intervention in the care of persons with human immunodeficiency virus infection. *Journal of the American Dietetic Association*, 104, 1427.

[53] HRSA. (2008, November). Care Action. Retrieved from the HRSA Web site:http://hab.hrsa.gov /publications /november2008/November08.pdf., p. 3.

[54] Bing, E.G., Burnman, M.A., Longshore, D., Fleishman, J.A., Sherbourne, C.D., London, A.S,and Shapiro, M. (2001, August). Psychiatric disorders and drug use among human immunodeficiency virus-infected adults in the United States. *Archives of General Psychiatry*, 58(8), 721–728.

[55] Lesser, J. (2008). Role of depression, stress, and trauma in HIV disease progression. *Psychosomatic Medicine*, 70, 539-545.

[56] Treisman, G.J., Angelina, A.F., & Hutton, H.E. (2001). Psychiatric issues in the management of patients with HIV infection. *Journal of the American Medical Society*, 286, 2857–2864.

[57] Lesser, J. (2008). Role of depression, stress, and trauma in HIV disease progression. Psychosomatic Medicine, 70, 539.

[58] Starace, F., Ammassari, A., Trotta, M.P., Murri, R., DeLongis, P., Izzo, C,& Antinori, A. (2002). Depression is a risk factor for suboptimal adherence to highly active antiretroviral therapy. *Journal of Acquired Immune Deficiency Syndromes*, 31(S136-S139), S136.

[59] Whetten, K., Reif, S., Whetten, R., Murphy-McMillian, L.K. (2008). Trama, mental health, distrust, and stigma among HIV-positive persons: implications for effective care. Psychosomatic Medicine, 70, 531.

[60] Horberg, M.A., Silverberg, M.J, Hurley, L.B.,Towner, W.J., Kelin, D.B., Bersoff-Matcha, S.,and Kovach, D.A. (2008, March 1). Effects of depression and selective serotonin reuptake inhibitor use on adherence to highly active antiretroviral therapy and on clinical outcomes in HIV-infected patients. *Journal of Acquired Immune Deficiency Syndromes*, 47(3), 384–90.

[61] Rippeth, J.D., Heaton, R.K., Carey, C.L, Marcotte, T.D., Moore, D.J., Gonzalez, R., and Grant, I. (2004). Methamphetamine dependence increases risk of neuropsychological impairment in HIV infected persons. *Journal of the International Neuropsychological Society*, 10(1), 1–14.

[62] National Institute of Drug Abuse. (2006, September). Methamphetamine abuse and addiction. Retrieved from the NIDA Web site: www.nida.nih.gov/PDF/RRMetham.pdf., p. 5.

[63] Gavrilin, M.A., Mathes, L.E., Podell, M. (2002). Methamphetamine enhances cell-associated feline immunodeficiency virus replication in astrocytes. *Journal for Neurovirology*, 8(3), 240–249.

[64] CDC (2007, January). Methamphetamine use and risk for HIV/AIDS. Retrieved from the CDC Web site: http://www.cdc.gov/hiv/resources/factsheets/meth.htm.

[65] Yeon, P.and Albrecht, H. (2008, February). Crystal methamphetamine and HIV/AIDS. AIDS Clinical Care, 20(2), 2–4.

[66] National Institute of Drug Abuse. (2006, March). Research report series: HIV/AIDS. Retrieved from the NIDA Web site: http://www.drugabuse.gov/PDF/RRhiv.pdf., p. 3.

[67] CDC. (2005, November). Coinfection with HIV and hepatitis C virus. Retrieved from the CDC Web site:http://www.cdc.gov/hiv/resources/Factsheets/coinfection.htm.

[68] Sherman, K.E., Rouster, S.D., Chung, R.T., and Rajicic, N. (2002). Hepatitis C virus prevalence among patients infection with human immunodeficiency virus: a cross-sectional analysis of the US adult AIDS Clinical Trial Group. *Clinical Infectious Diseases*, 34, 831.

[69] Sulkowski, M.S.,and Thomas, D.L. (2003). Hepatitis C in the HIV-infected person. *Annals of Internal Medicine*, 138(3), 197.

[70] Thomas Thomas, D.L. (2002). Hepatitis C and human immunodeficiency virus infection. Hepatology, 36(supplement 5), S201–9.

[71] CDC. (2009, June 1). Tuberculosis (TB): general information. Retrieved from the CDC Web site:http://www.cdc.gov/tb/publications/factsheets/general/tb.pdf., p. 2.

[72] CDC. (2009, June 1). Tuberculosis (TB): TB and HIV coinfection. Retrieved from the CDC Web site:http://www.cdc.gov/tb/topic/TBHIVcoinfection/default.htm.

[73] Key points of entry include emergency rooms, substance abuse treatment programs, detoxification centers, adult and juvenile detention facilities, sexually transmitted disease clinics, HIV counseling and testing sites, mental health programs and homeless shelters.

[74] Buchacz, K., Patel, P., and Taylor, M. (2004). Syphilis increases HIV viral load and decreases CD4 cell counts in HIV-infected patients with new syphilis infections. *AIDS*, 18(15), 2075–2079.

[75] Sowadsky R. (2009, March). The HIV-STD connection. The Body. Retrieved from the Body Web site:http://www.thebody.com/content/prev/art2283.html

[76] Lubinski C. What We Know About the Workforce in HIV/AIDS. Presentation at the HIV/AIDS Workforce Meeting of HRSA, HIV/AIDS Bureau, Rockville, MD, September 15–16, 2008.

[77] Infectious Diseases Society of America. (2009). Report: Federal HIV policies need to keep pace with scientific advancements. ISDA News.19(4). Available at: http://news.idsociety.org/idsa/issues/2009-04-01/12.html.

[78] HRSA. (2008). The power of connections. Retrieved from the HRSA Web site:http://hab.hrsa.gov /publications /progressreport08/2008ProgressReport.pdf., p. 38.

[79] HRSA. HRSA moves to head off health care workforce shortages. (2009, January). Inside HRSA. Retrieved from the HRSA Web site: http://newsroom.hrsa.gov/insidehrsa/jan2009/. Accessed November 2009.

[80] CDC. (2009, August). HIV and AIDS among gay and bisexual men. Retrieved from the CDC Web site:http://www.cdc.gov/NCHHSTP/newsroom/docs/FastFacts-MSM-FINAL508COMP.pdf., p. 1.

[81] .CDC. (2010), CDC Analysis Provides New Look at Disproportionate Impact of HIV and Syphilis Among U.S. Gay and Bisexual Men. Retrieved from the CDC Web site: http://www.cdc.gov /nchhstp /Newsroom /msmpressrelease.html

[82] CDC. (2009, August). HIV/AIDS among African Americans. Retrieved from the CDC Web site:http://www.cdc.gov/hiv/topics/aa/resources/factsheets/pdf/aa.pdf., p. 1.

[83] U.S. Census Bureau. (2008). State and county quick facts: USA. Retrieved from the Census Bureau Web site: http://quickfacts.census.gov/qfd/states/00000.html.

[84] CDC. (2009). HIV/AIDS surveillance report, 2007, 19, 1.

[85] CDC. (2009). HIV/AIDS surveillance report, 2007, 19, 1, 17.

[86] CDC. (2009, August). HIV/AIDS among Hispanics/Latinos. Retrieved from the CDC Web site:http:// www.cdc.gov/hiv/hispanics/resources/factsheets/hispanic.htm.

[87] CDC. (2007). Basic statistics. Retrieved from the CDC Web site:http://www.cdc.gov /hiv /topics/ surveillance /basic.htm.

[88] Office of Minority Health. (2009, October 21). American Indian/Alaska Native profile. Retrieved from the Minority Health Web site: http://minorityhealth.hhs.gov/templates/browse.aspx?lvl=2&lvlID=52.

[89] HRSA. (2008, August). American Indians, Alaska Natives, and HIV/AIDS. Retrieved from the HRSA Web site:ftp://ftp.hrsa.gov/hab/Native.Amer.pdf., p. 1.

[90] CDC. (2009, August). HIV/AIDS in the United States. Retrieved from the CDC Web site:http://www.cdc.gov /hiv/resources/factsheets/PDF/us.pdf., p. 1.

[91] Marks, G, (1998). Is acculturation associated with sexual risk behaviours? An investigation of HIV-positive Latino men and women. AIDS Care, 10, 283 295.

[92] Rojas-Guyler, L., Ellis, N, and Sanders, S. (2005). Acculturation, health protective sexual communication, and HIV/AIDS risk behavior among Hispanic/Latino women in a large midwestern city. *Health Education and Behavior*, 32,767, 779.

[93] CDC. (2009, August). HIV and AIDS among gay and bisexual men. Retrieved from the CDC Web site:http://www.cdc.gov/NCHHSTP/newsroom/docs/FastFacts-MSM-FINAL508COMP.pdf., p. 2.

[94] CDC. CDC fact sheet: HIV and AIDS among gay and bisexual men. August 2009. Available at:http://www.cdc.gov/NCHHSTP/newsroom/docs/FastFacts-MSM-FINAL508COMP.pdf. Accessed January 29, 2010.

[95] Herbst, J.H., Jabocs, E.D., Finlayson, T.J., McKleroy, V.S., Neumann, M.S., and Crepaz, N. (2008). Estimating HIV prevalence and risk behaviors of transgender persons in the United States: a systematic review. AIDS and Behavior, 12(1), 1–17.

[96] HRSA. (2009, September). HRSACareAction: Intimate Partner Violence. Retrieved from the HRSA Web site:http://hab.hrsa.gov/publications/september2009/September2009.pdf., p. 4.

[97] Ibid., p. 4.

[98] Xavier, J., Honnold J.A., and Bradford, J. (2007). The health, health-related needs, and lifecourse experiences of transgender Virginians. Community Health Research Initiative Center for Public Policy, Virginia Commonwealth University and Virginia HIV Community Planning Committee and Virginia Department of Health.

[99] Okie, S. (2007, January 11). Sex, drugs, prisons, and HIV. New England Journal of Medicine, 356(2), 106.

[100] Cho, Richard, Corporation for Supportive Housing. (2008, March). Overlap and Interaction of Homelessness and Incarceration: A Review of Research and Practice. NAHC Research Summit.

[101] National Health Care for the Homeless Council. (2008). Incarceration, homelessness, and health. Retrieved from the NHCHC Web site: http://www.nhchc.org/Advocacy/PolicyPapers/Incarceration2008.pdf.

[102] National Mental Health Association. (2007). Position statement 52: In support of maximum diversion of persons with serious mental illness from the criminal justice system. Retrieved from:http://www.mentalhealthamerica.net/go/position-statements/52.

[103] CDC. (2009). HIV/AIDS surveillance report, 2007, 19, Table 3.

[104] HRSA. (2008). The power of connections. Retrieved from the HRSA Web site:http://hab.hrsa.gov/publications/progressreport08/2008ProgressReport.pdf., p. 25.

[105] Human Rights Watch. (2002, February). Race and incarceration in the United States. Retrieved from the Human Rights Watch Web site: http://www.hrw.org/legacy/backgrounder/use/race.

[106] HHS. (2006). HHS programs to protect and enhance rural health. Retrieved from the HHS Web site:http://www.hhs.gov/news/factsheet/rural.html.

[107] National Rural Health Association. (n.d.) What is different about rural health care? Retrieved from the NRHA Web site: http://www.ruralhealthWeb.org/go/left/about-rural-health/what-s-different-about-rural-health-care/what-s-different-about-rural-health-care.

[108] RAND Corporation. (2006) Research brief: Disparities in care for HIV patients: results of the HCSUS study. Retrieved from the RAND Web site: http://www.rand.org/pubs/research_briefs/2006/RAND_RB9171.pdf.

[109] Herek, G.M., Capitanio, J.P., Widaman, K.F. (2002). HIV-related stigma and knowledge in the United States: prevalence and trends, 1991-1999. *American Journal of Public Health*, 92(3), 371.

[110] Blankenship, K.M., Bray, S.J, Merson, M.H. (2000). Structural interventions in public health. AIDS, 14(Supplement 1), S11–21.

In: Responding to HIV/AIDS
Editor: Lawrence T. Jensen

ISBN: 978-1-61324-618-4
© 2011 Nova Science Publishers, Inc.

Chapter 4

THE RYAN WHITE HIV/AIDS PROGRAM[*]

Judith A. Johnson

SUMMARY

The Ryan White HIV/AIDS Program makes federal funds available to metropolitan areas and states to assist in health care costs and support services for individuals and families affected by the human immunodeficiency virus (HIV) or acquired immune deficiency syndrome (AIDS). The Ryan White program currently serves more than half a million low-income people with HIV/AIDS in the United States; 33% of those served are uninsured, and an additional 56% are underinsured. The program is administered by the Health Resources and Services Administration (HRSA) of the Department of Health and Human Services (HHS). Its statutory authority is Title XXVI of the Public Health Service (PHS) Act, originally enacted in 1990.

The Ryan White program is composed of four major parts and several other components. Part A provides grants to urban areas and mid-sized cities. Part B provides grants to states and territories; it also provides funds for the AIDS Drug Assistance Program (ADAP). Part C provides early intervention grants to public and private nonprofit entities. Part D provides grants to public and private nonprofit entities for family-centered care for women, infants, children, and youth with HIV/AIDS. The other components, sometimes referred to as Part F, include the AIDS Dental Reimbursement (ADR) Program, the Community-Based Dental Partnership Program, the AIDS Education and Training Centers (AETCs), the Special Projects of National Significance (SPNS) Program, and the Minority AIDS Initiative (MAI). In October 2009, the 111th Congress passed and President Obama signed the Ryan White HIV/AIDS Treatment Extension Act of 2009 (P.L. 111-87), which reauthorizes the Ryan White program through September 30, 2013. P.L. 111-87 maintains the hold-harmless provision for Part A and Part B and provides a continuation of the transition period for states that do not have a fully mature name-based HIV reporting system. The new law requires that the Secretary establish a national HIV/AIDS testing goal of 5 million tests annually through programs administered by HRSA and the Centers for Disease Control and Prevention (CDC). It requires the Part A Planning Councils to develop a strategy for identifying

---

[*] This is an edited, reformatted and augmented version of a Congressional Research Service publication, 7-5700, www.crs.gov, RL33279, dated January 5, 2011.

individuals with HIV/AIDS who do not know their HIV status, making them aware of their status and connecting them with health care and support services. It also requires the Part B grant application to provide a comprehensive plan for the identification of such individuals and enable their access to medical treatment.

The Patient Protection and Affordable Care Act (PPACA, P.L. 111-148) contains general provisions to increase access to health insurance and which, therefore, will increase coverage for people living with HIV/AIDS. PPACA includes prohibitions on the cancellation of coverage by an insurer due to a preexisting condition, elimination of lifetime caps on insurance benefits and annual limits on coverage, and eligibility for tax subsidies to assist low- and middle-income individuals in the purchase of coverage from state health insurance exchanges. In addition, Medicaid eligibility will be broadened to include single adults, and PPACA phases out the Medicare Part D doughnut hole for HIV/AIDS individuals who are Medicare eligible.

Ryan White programs received $2.266 billion for FY2010 in the Consolidated Appropriations Act, 2010 (P.L. 111-117). In July 2010 HHS announced the reallocation of $25 million in funds for ADAP from dozens of programs throughout HHS. The additional funds were targeted for states with ADAP waiting lists or other cost containment strategies. The Obama Administration's request for Ryan White programs in FY2011 is $2.305 billion, an increase of $39.513 million over the FY2010 appropriation. The House Labor-HHS-Education Appropriations Subcommittee held a markup session in July 2010, but the full committee did not report a bill. The Senate Committee on Appropriations reported S. 3686 (S.Rept. 111-243) in August 2010, but the bill did not receive any further action. The Continuing Appropriations Act, 2011 (P.L. 111-242), as amended, provides temporary FY2011 funding through March 4, 2011, at the FY2010 rate of operations.

The Ryan White HIV/AIDS Program makes federal funds available to metropolitan areas and states to provide a number of health care services for HIV/AIDS patients including medical care, drug treatments, dental care, home health care, and outpatient mental health and substance abuse treatment. The program currently serves more than half a million low-income people with HIV/AIDS in the United States; 33% of those served are uninsured, and an additional 56% are underinsured.[1]

The Ryan White program was established in law in 1990 (P.L. 101-381) and reauthorized and amended in 1996 (P.L. 104-146), 2000 (P.L. 106-345), 2006 (P.L. 109-415), and 2009 (P.L. 111- 87). It was enacted as Title XXVI of the Public Health Service (PHS) Act and codified as Parts A, B, C, D, E, and F under 42 U.S.C. § 300ff-11 et seq. The program is administered by the HRSA HIV/AIDS Bureau. Most Ryan White funding is distributed to eligible entities based on formulas that take into account living cases of HIV/AIDS. Funding for the individual grant programs (Parts A, B, C, D, and F), appears in Table 1 at the end of this report.

P.L. 109-415 had reauthorized the Ryan White program through September 30, 2009.[2] On September 9, 2009, the House Energy and Commerce Subcommittee on Health held a hearing to consider draft legislation that would reauthorize the Ryan White program. H.R. 3792 (Pallone), the Ryan White HIV/AIDS Treatment Extension Act of 2009, was introduced on October 13, 2009.

The House Energy and Commerce approved H.R. 3792 on October 15, and a report was filed on October 20, 2009 (H.Rept. 111-305). S. 1793 (Harkin), the Ryan White HIV/AIDS Treatment Extension Act of 2009, was introduced on October 15 and passed the Senate by voice vote on October 19, 2009. The House passed S. 1793 on October 21, 2009, by a vote of 408-9. President Obama signed the legislation on October 30, 2009 (P.L. 111-87).

Table 1. Federal Funding for the Ryan White Program, FY1991-FY2011
($ in millions)

	Part A	Part B	(ADAP) (non-add)	Part C	Part D	Part E	Part F AETC	Part F ADR	Total
FY1991	87.8	87.8	—	44.9	19.5	0	17.0	—	257.0
FY1992	121.6	107.6	—	48.7	19.3	0	16.9	—	314.1
FY1993	184.8	115.3	—	48.0	20.9	0	16.4	—	385.4
FY1994	325.5	183.9	—	48.0	22.0	0	16.4	7.0	602.8
FY1995	356.5	198.1	—	52.0	26.0	0	16.3	6.9	655.8
FY1996	391.7	260.8	(52)	57.0	29.0	0	12.0	6.9	757.4
FY1997	449.8	417.0	(167)	69.6	36.0	0	16.3	7.5	996.3
FY1998	464.7	542.8	(285.5)	76.2	40.8	0	17.2	7.8	1,150.2
FY1999	505.0	737.8	(461.0)	94.3	46.0	0	20.0	7.8	1,410.9
FY2000	546.3	823.8	(528.0)	138.4	51.0	0	26.6	8.0	1,594.2
FY2001	604.2	910.9	(589.0)	185.9	65.0	0	31.6	10.0	1,807.6
FY2002	619.4	977.2	(639.0)	193.8	71.0	0	35.3	13.5	1,902.2
FY2003	618.7	1,053.4	(714.3)	198.4	73.6	0	35.6	13.4	1,993.0
FY2004	615.0	1,085.9	(748.9)	197.2	73.1	0	35.3	13.3	2,019.9
FY2005	610.1	1,121.8	(787.5)	195.6	72.5	0	35.1	13.2	2,048.3
FY2006	603.6	1,119.7	(789.0)	193.5	71.7	0	34.6	13.1	2,036.3
FY2007	604.0	1,195.5	(789.5)	193.7	71.8	0	34.7	13.1	2,112.8
FY2008	627.1	1,195.2	(794.4)	198.8	73.7	0	34.1	12.9	2,141.8
FY2009	663.1	1,223.8	(815.0)	201.9	76.8	0	34.4	13.4	2,213.4
FY2010[a]	679.1	1,275.8	(860.0)	206.4	77.6	0	34.7	13.6	2,287.2
FY2011[b]	679.1	1,283.8	(855.0)	211.9	77.8	0	37.4	15.4	2,305.4

Sources: Appropriations Committee conference reports on Labor-HHS appropriations legislation. Amounts for FY2011 are from the HRSA, FY2011 Justification of Estimates for Appropriations Committees, p. 210-241. May not add due to rounding.

Note: Totals for FY2003 through FY2011 do not include $25 million for SPNS provided via the PHS program evaluation tap (section 241 of the PHS Act).

[a]. Amounts for FY2010 reflect $25 million reallocation for ADAP as identified in S.Rept. 111-243. However, final funding levels for FY2010 are not currently available.

[b]. Amounts for FY2011 were proposed by the Obama Administration (request levels).

P.L. 111-87 provides specific authorization levels for Parts A, B, C, D, and F for each fiscal year through FY2013, resulting in a four-year reauthorization for the Ryan White program. P.L. 111-87 requires that the Secretary establish a national HIV/AIDS testing goal of 5 million tests annually through programs administered by HRSA and CDC. The Secretary must submit an annual report to Congress on the progress made in achieving the testing goal, including any barriers to meeting the goal, the amount of funding necessary to meet the goal, and the most cost-effective strategies for identifying individuals who are unaware of their HIV status. The Secretary is also required to review each of the programs and activities conducted by CDC as part of the Domestic HIV/AIDS Prevention Activities. The other provisions of P.L. 111-87 are discussed below in the sections of this report on the various parts of the Ryan White program.

The Patient Protection and Affordable Care Act (PPACA, P.L. 111-148) contains general provisions to increase access to health insurance and which, therefore, will increase coverage for people living with HIV/AIDS.[3] They include prohibitions on the cancellation of coverage by an insurer due to a preexisting condition, elimination of lifetime caps on insurance benefits and annual limits on coverage, and eligibility for tax subsidies to assist low- and middle-income individuals in the purchase of coverage from state health insurance exchanges. In addition, Medicaid eligibility will be broadened to include single adults, and PPACA phases out the Medicare Part D doughnut hole for HIV/AIDS individuals who are Medicare eligible. The long-range impact of the new health care law on HRSA's Ryan White program (meaning the replacement of health and treatment services provided under Ryan White with access to such services through health insurance via PPACA) remains to be determined.

PART A. GRANTS TO URBAN AREAS

Part A provides funds to urban areas with high numbers of people living with HIV, as well as mid-sized cities that have emerging needs for assistance with their HIV-infected populations. The boundaries of the areas are based on the Metropolitan Statistical Areas of the U.S. Census Bureau and may range in size from a single city or county to multiple counties that cross state boundaries. According to HRSA, "more than 70% of all people living with HIV/AIDS in the U.S. reside in metropolitan areas served by Part A."[4] In April 2010, grant awards for Part A were announced for FY2010.[5]

EMAs and TGAs

Part A provides funds to eligible metropolitan areas (EMAs) with a population of at least 50,000 that have had more than 2,000 reported AIDS cases in the prior five years. An EMA would stop being eligible if it failed for three consecutive years, to have (a) a cumulative total of more than 2,000 reported cases of AIDS during the most recent five calendar years, and (b) a cumulative total of 3,000 or more living cases of AIDS as of December 31 of the most recent year.[6]

The 2006 reauthorization (P.L. 109-415) established a grant program for transitional grant areas (TGAs), defined as metropolitan areas with at least 1,000 but fewer than 2,000 cumulative AIDS cases during the most recent five calendar years.[7] Unless a TGA became an EMA, it would continue to be eligible as a TGA until it failed for three years to have (a) at least 1,000 but fewer than 2,000 cases of AIDS during the most recent five calendar years, and (b) 1,500 or more living cases of AIDS as of December 31 of the most recent calendar year. P.L. 111-87 permits a metropolitan area with a cumulative total of at least 1,400 but less than 1,500 living cases of AIDS to continue to be eligible as a TGA provided that not more than 5% of the TGA grant award is unobligated as of the end of the most recent fiscal year.[8]

Under P.L. 109-415, total amounts reserved for Part A EMAs and TGAs would be adjusted based, in part, on the changing eligibility status of metropolitan areas.[9] P.L. 111-87 contains provisions that modify the transfer of Part A grant funds to Part B for metropolitan areas that lose TGA eligibility. Specifically, if a metropolitan area were to lose TGA eligibility, the state containing the TGA would receive 75% of the TGA formula grant in the first year after the loss of TGA eligibility, 50% in the second year, and 25% in the third year. The remainder in each year is made available for Part B grants, as is the entire amount of the former TGA's formula grant in the fourth year after the loss of eligibility.

Core Medical Services

Seventy-five percent of Part A funds must be spent on core medical services, defined as outpatient and ambulatory health services, AIDS Drug Assistance Program (ADAP) treatments and pharmaceutical assistance, oral health care, early intervention services, health insurance premium and cost-sharing assistance, home health, medical nutrition therapy, hospice, home and community-based health services, mental health and substance abuse outpatient services, and medical case management. The requirement may be waived if (1) there was no waiting list for receiving treatment (under the Part B ADAP program), and (2) core medical services were available to all individuals with HIV/AIDS who were eligible to receive such services under Part A. The remaining 25% of funds may be used for support services, such as outreach services, medical transportation, language services, respite care for persons caring for individuals with HIV/AIDS, and referrals for health care and support services.

Formula Grants, Supplemental Grants, and Number of Living HIV/AIDS Cases

Two-thirds of the Part A appropriation is distributed through formula grants, and the remaining one-third is distributed via competitive supplemental grants awarded on the basis of need.[10] The awarding of supplemental Part A grants is based on weighting factors. Under P.L. 111-87, success in testing for HIV/AIDS and making individuals aware of their HIV status is counted as one-third in making such determinations.

CDC collects the statistics used in the Ryan White formula. In the past, some states reported their cases by name, while others used a code-based system to protect privacy.[11] CDC initially indicated its preference for name-based reporting in 1999 in order to avoid double counting. In 2005, the agency recommended that all jurisdictions transition to name-based reporting.

In contrast to EMA and TGA eligibility definitions that are based on cumulative AIDS cases, grant award amounts are based on living HIV/AIDS cases. Prior to the 2006 reauthorization, formula grants had been distributed to EMAs in proportion to an estimate of the number of living AIDS cases in each EMA.[12] Under P.L. 109-415, funding distribution is based on the number of living HIV and AIDS cases in each EMA or TGA for states that use a name-based HIV reporting system. The requirement for name-based HIV reporting influenced states to change from code-based reporting to name-based reporting.

P.L. 109-415 provided a transition period for states that did not have a fully mature name-based reporting system.[13] P.L. 111-87 provides a continuation of the transition period for states that do not have a fully mature name-based HIV reporting system.[14] Under the new law, these jurisdictions incur a 5% reduction in the number of non-AIDS HIV cases reported for the eligible area (to account for duplicate cases caused by code-based reporting) in making Part A grant determinations for fiscal years prior to FY2012 and a 6% reduction for FY2012. Beginning with FY2013, only living name-based cases of HIV/AIDS would be used in making Part A grant determinations. In addition, as was the case under P.L. 109-415, the amount of the formula grant in these areas may not exceed that of the preceding fiscal year by more than 5%.

For the purpose of determining Part A grant amounts, P.L. 111-87 would allow an increase of 3% in the number of living HIV/AIDS cases in an area for FY2010 through FY2012 if the area switched to name-based reporting in 2007 and had experienced a decrease in funding of more than 30% in FY2007 compared with FY2006.

Hold-Harmless Provision

P.L. 111-87 maintains a hold-harmless provision for Part A.[15] Formula grants for FY2010 will be an amount equal to 95% of funding in FY2009, funding in FY2011 and FY2012 will be an amount equal to 100% of FY2010, and funding in FY2013 will be an amount equal to 92.5% of FY2012. The hold-harmless provision is funded with money that would have been distributed through Part A supplemental grants. If in a given year the supplemental funds are insufficient to fund the hold-harmless in a year, the Secretary would reduce on a pro rata basis the grant amount for each EMA other than those eligible for the hold-harmless provision, though the reduction would not be allowed to result in any additional EMA becoming eligible for the hold-harmless provision.

In September 2009, GAO released a report on the impact of several funding provisions on Ryan White grant awards.[16] One of the provisions the 2009 GAO report focused on was the distribution of hold-harmless funding among Part A EMAs. GAO found that 17 of 24 (71%) EMAs received hold-harmless funding in FY2009, compared with 21 of 51 (41%) EMAs in FY2004.[17] The total amount of hold-harmless funding distributed among the EMAs was larger in FY2009 ($24,836,500) than in FY2004 ($8,033,563).[18] GAO looked at the amount of funding (including hold-harmless) per HIV/AIDS case, which for FY2009 ranged from $645 in San Diego to $854 in San Francisco; for FY2004, the amount of funding per case ranged from $1,221 in most EMAs to $2,241 in San Francisco. GAO determined that the smaller funding range in FY2009 "resulted from San Francisco receiving less hold-harmless funding in FY2009 than in FY2004. In both years, San Francisco received the most hold-harmless funding per case. However, in FY2009, San Francisco received $208 in hold-harmless per case while in FY2004 it received $1,020 in hold-harmless funding per case."[19]

GAO also noted that "hold-harmless funding accounted for a larger percentage of San Francisco's total base funding than it did for any other EMA in FY2009 and FY2004, but the percentage was smaller in FY2009 (24%) than in FY2004 (46%)."[20] However, GAO found that for FY2009, "because of its hold-harmless funding, San Francisco, which had 17,173

HIV/AIDS cases, received a base grant equivalent to what an EMA with approximately 22,713 cases (32% more) would have received without hold-harmless funding."[21] GAO stated that "a significant portion of the difference in funding per case between San Francisco and the other EMAs results from how metropolitan area whose formula funding is based on both living and deceased AIDS cases."[22] GAO explains that this is due to the hold-harmless calculations that in part, for San Francisco alone, refer back to case counts in FY1995 that included both living and deceased AIDS cases.

The hold-harmless provision is funded with money that would have been distributed through Part A supplemental grants. Without the hold-harmless provision, in FY2009 most Part A grantees would have received more funding. GAO notes that "although 17 EMAs received hold-harmless funding in FY2009, only 7 (New York, San Francisco, San Juan, West Palm Beach, Newark, New Haven, and Nassau-Suffolk) received more funding because of the hold-harmless provision than they would have received through supplemental grants in the absence of the hold-harmless provision."[23]

Stop-Loss Provisions

Like the hold-harmless provision, stop-loss provisions in appropriations bills have had an impact on the funding of Ryan White grants. A stop-loss provision in the FY2008 Consolidated Appropriations Act (H.R. 2764, P.L. 110-161) affected the FY2008 funding of Ryan White Part A grants to metropolitan areas by setting aside some FY2008 funds to make up for losses in FY2007 grants to certain areas.[24] A similar stop-loss provision in the FY2009 Omnibus Appropriations Act (H.R. 1105, P.L. 111-8) affected the FY2009 funding of Ryan White Part A grants to metropolitan areas.[25] The FY2009 provision set aside $10.853 million, which was divided among five EMAs and seven TGAs; 58% of the set-aside went to the San Francisco EMA.[26]

The stop-loss provision in the Consolidated Appropriations Act, 2010 (P.L. 111-117), set aside $6.021 million for increasing supplemental grants for FY2010 to EMAs and TGAs "to ensure that an area's total funding under [part A] for FY2009, together with the amount of this additional funding, is not less than 92.4% of the amount of such area's total funding under part A for FY2006." This is the same as language contained in the House Labor-HHS Appropriations bill for FY2010, H.R. 3293.[27] An August 3, 2009, Government Accountability Office (GAO) analysis of the stop-loss provision in the House version of H.R. 3293 indicated that two EMAs and four TGAs would receive funds; 85% of the stop-loss funds would go to San Francisco, CA.[28]

Planning Councils

Part A grants are made to the chief elected official of the city or county in the EMA or TGA that administers the health agency providing services to the greatest number of persons with HIV. The official must establish an HIV Health Services Planning Council, which sets priorities for care delivery according to federal guidelines. Planning Councils are not mandatory for TGAs, unless the TGA was an EMA in FY2006. The Council may not be directly involved in the administration of any Part A grant. Membership of the Council must reflect the ethnic and racial make-up of the local HIV epidemic.

P.L. 111-87 requires the Part A Planning Councils to develop a strategy for identifying individuals with HIV/AIDS who do not know their HIV status, making them aware of their status and connecting them with health care and support services. Particular attention is given to "reducing barriers to routine testing and disparities in access and services among affected subpopulations and historically underserved communities."

Unexpended Funds

The 2006 reauthorization introduced restrictions on the use of unexpended funds. Starting in FY2007, if an eligible area did not obligate all supplemental grant funds within one year of receiving the award, the eligible area is required to return any unobligated funds. Similarly, starting in FY2007, if an eligible area did not obligate all formula grant funds within one year of receiving the award, the eligible area is required to return any unobligated funds. However, the eligible area may request a waiver of the cancellation of formula grant funds, explaining how the eligible area intends to spend the funds. If the waiver is approved, the eligible area will have one additional year in which to spend the funds. This is called the carryover year. If the funds are not spent by the end of the carryover year, the eligible area will be required to return the unexpended funds.

Under P.L. 109-415, regardless of whether the waiver for carryover was granted, the eligible area's formula grant funds would be reduced for the following year by an amount equal to the unobligated balance, the reduction would not be taken into account in applying the hold-harmless provision for the subsequent fiscal year and the grantee is ineligible for supplemental grants. Under P.L. 111-87, the amount of the reduction would not include any unobligated balance that was approved by HRSA for carryover. Under P.L. 109-415, the reduction in formula grant funds did not apply if the unobligated balance was 2% or less; this is changed by P.L. 111-87 to 5%. Any returned grant funds will be additional amounts available for supplemental grants, subject to both (1) the mandatory transfer of funds from Part A to Part B when a Part A area loses eligibility, and (2) the hold-harmless provision for Part A formula grants.

PART B. GRANTS TO STATES

Part B provides grants to all 50 states, the District of Columbia, Puerto Rico, the U.S. Virgin Islands, Guam, and five jurisdictions in the Pacific. Grant funds can be used for drug treatments, home and community-based health care and support services or health insurance coverage for low-income persons through Health Insurance Continuation Programs. Currently about two-thirds of Part B funding is set aside by Congress for the AIDS Drug Assistance Programs (ADAPs). ADAPs provide drug treatments for individuals with HIV who cannot afford to pay for drugs and have limited or no coverage from private insurance, Medicaid, or Medicare Part D. In April 2010, grant awards for Ryan White Part B grants were announced.[29]

P.L. 111-87 requires that the Part B grant application provide a comprehensive plan for the identification of individuals with HIV/AIDS who are unaware of their HIV/AIDS status and enable such individuals access to medical treatment for HIV/AIDS. The comprehensive plan must include efforts to remove any legal barriers, including states laws and regulations, to routine testing.

Formula Grants and Number of Living HIV/AIDS Cases

The Part B formula is based on three factors: (1) 75% of the award is based on the state's proportion of the nation's HIV/AIDS cases; (2) 20% is based on the state's proportion of HIV/AIDS cases outside Part A-funded areas (EMAs and TGAs); and (3) 5% is based on the state's proportion of HIV/AIDS cases in states with no Part A funding.[30] Prior to the 2006 reauthorization, formula grants had been distributed to states in proportion to an estimate of the number of living AIDS cases in each state.[31] Under P.L. 109-415, funding distribution is based on the number of living HIV and AIDS cases for states that use a name-based HIV reporting system. The requirement for name-based HIV reporting influenced states to change from code-based reporting to name-based reporting. P.L. 109-415 provided a transition period for states that did not have a fully mature name-based reporting system.

According to the September 2009 GAO report, 47 of the 59 Part B grantees had HRSA use their name-based HIV case counts to determine FY2009 formula funding, and the remaining 12 grantees had HRSA use code-based HIV case counts.[32] Of the 12 grantees, 7 were collectin name-based HIV case counts as of December 31, 2001, and 5 were not.[33] GAO indicated that "each of the 12 grantees could require 4 years from the date they began collecting name-based HIV case counts for such reporting systems to be considered reliable and accurate. However, grantees can determine that their reporting systems are accurate and reliable in less than 4 years."[34] If the transition period for states that do not have a fully mature name-based HIV reporting system was not extended, some grantees might not receive funding in proportion to their number of HIV/AIDS cases, "which is the intended basis of the formula grant."[35]

P.L. 111-87 provides a continuation of the transition period for states that do not have a fully mature name-based HIV reporting system. Under the new law, these jurisdictions incur a 5% reduction in the number of non-AIDS HIV cases reported for the eligible area (to account for duplicate cases caused by code-based reporting) in making Part B grant determinations for fiscal years prior to FY2012 and a 6% reduction for FY2012. Beginning with FY2013, only living name-based cases of HIV/AIDS would be used in making Part B grant determinations.

For the purpose of determining Part B grant amounts, P.L. 111-87 would allow an increase of 3% in the number of living HIV/AIDS cases in an area for FY2010 through FY2012 if the area switched to name-based reporting in 2007 and had experienced a decrease in funding of more than 30% in FY2007 compared with FY2006.

As is the case for Part A grants, 75% of Part B funds must be spent on core medical services and 25% may be spent on support services (defined above). Two-thirds of the Part B appropriation (non-ADAP) is used for the Part B base awards.

Supplemental Grants and Hold-Harmless Provision

One-third of the Part B appropriation (non-ADAP) is reserved for a supplemental grant program created by P.L. 109-415.[36] Eligible states must have a demonstrated need for supplemental financial assistance and no cancelled grant funds or waivers permitting carryover of funds (see "Unexpended Funds"). Priority in making supplemental grants is given to states with a decline in funding under Part B due to the changes in the distribution formula. Supplemental grant funds must be used for core medical services. Not later than 45 days after awarding supplemental funds under Part B, HRSA must submit a report to Congress concerning such funds P.L. 111-87 would maintain a hold-harmless provision for Part B.[37] Formula grants for FY2010 would be an amount equal to 95% of funding in FY2009, funding in FY2011 and FY2012 would be an amount equal to 100% of FY2010, and funding in FY2013 would be an amount equal to 92.5% of FY2012. The hold-harmless provision is funded by reducing the amount reserved for the Part B supplemental grant program and by any unobligated funds repaid by the states (see "Unexpended Funds"). If there are insufficient funds for the hold-harmless provision, then current law allows for a pro rata reduction of all Part B state grants, excepting those states receiving hold-harmless funds. However, such reductions will not be made in an amount that results in other states becoming eligible for the hold-harmless.

Unexpended Funds

Starting in FY2007, states are required to obligate grant funds by the end of the grant year for Part B formula grants, supplemental grants, emerging communities grants, ADAP grants, and supplemental ADAP grants. For supplemental ADAP grants, supplemental grants, and emerging communities grants, if there is an unobligated balance at the end of the grant year, the state must return the amount and the funds will be used for additional supplemental grants (subject to the hold-harmless provision).

For Part B formula grants and ADAP grants, if there is an unobligated balance the state must either return the unexpended funds or apply for a waiver to use the funds in the next year. If the waiver is approved, the funds would be available for one more year, called the carryover year. If the state fails to use the funds in the carryover year, the state must return the funds, which will be used for supplemental grants (subject to the hold-harmless provision).

However, for states with an unobligated balance for their Part B formula grant or an ADAP grant, under P.L. 109-415 the amount of the grant for the next year would be reduced by the amount of the unobligated balance, regardless of whether a waiver was approved, and the state would not be eligible for supplemental grants in the following year. Under P.L. 111-87, the amount of the reduction would not include any unobligated balance that was approved by HRSA for carryover. Under P.L. 109-415, if the amount of the unobligated balance was 2% or less, the grant reduction would not apply; this is changed to 5% by P.L. 111-87. The funds from grant reduction are used for supplemental grants (subject to the hold-harmless provision).

Drug rebates are received by Part B grantees from pharmaceutical manufacturers following the purchase of drugs for the ADAP program. There is a federal requirement that drug rebate funds be spent before federal funds are obligated. Because rebates may be received by the state late in the year, this requirement may result in some states incurring an unobligated balance penalty. Under P.L. 111-87, if an expenditure of ADAP rebate funds would trigger a penalty, the Secretary may deem the state's unobligated balance to be reduced by the amount of the rebate. Any unobligated amount returned to the Secretary would be used for ADAP supplemental grants or Part B supplemental grants.

A September 2009 GAO report found that nine states and seven territories received reduced Part B grant amounts in the 2009 grant year because they had unobligated balances over 2% in the 2007 grant year.[38] "Part B base funding penalties ranged from $6,433 in Palau to $1,493,935 in Ohio. ADAP base funding penalties ranged from $26,233 in Maine to $12,670,248 in Pennsylvania."[39] According to GAO, grantees "had varying reasons for their unobligated balances, some of which they said were beyond their control."[40] Almost half of the grantees interviewed by GAO said the 2% threshold was too low, and some suggested that 5% would be more reasonable. However, GAO noted that "only 2 of the 16 Part B grantees that received penalties for unobligated balances had unobligated balances of less than 5%."[41] The GAO reported that both grantees and HRSA stated that a requirement to spend drug rebate funds before obligating federal funds makes it more difficult to avoid unobligated balances. According to GAO, HRSA tried to address this problem by asking HHS for an exemption from the relevant regulations for grantees using drug rebates, but the request was denied.[42]

Emerging Community Grants

The grant program for emerging communities defines such communities as metropolitan areas with cumulative total of at least 500 and fewer than 1,000 reported cases of AIDS during the most recent five calendar years. The metropolitan area continues as an emerging community until the metropolitan area fails for three consecutive fiscal years: (1) to have the required number of AIDS cases; and (2) to have a cumulative total of 750 or more living cases of AIDS as of December 31 of the most recent calendar year. The grant amount is determined by the amount set aside by the Secretary (authorized at $5 million) and by the proportion of the total number of living cases of HIV/AIDS in emerging communities in the state to the total number of living cases of HIV/AIDS in emerging communities in the United States.

ADAP

HRSA estimates that "about one in four HIV positive people in care in the U.S. receive their medications through state ADAPs."[43] ADAP funds are distributed via a formula based on each state's proportion of living HIV and AIDS cases.[44] P.L. 111-87 provides a continuation of the transition period for states that do not have a fully mature name-based HIV reporting system. Under the new law, these jurisdictions incur a 5% reduction in the number of non-AIDS HIV cases reported for the eligible area (to account for duplicate cases caused by code-based reporting) in making ADAP grant determinations for fiscal years prior to FY2012 and a 6% reduction for FY2012. Beginning with FY2013, only living name-based cases of HIV/AIDS would be used in making ADAP grant determinations. The same hold-harmless provision that applies to other Part A and Part B formula grants also applies to the ADAP formula grants.[45]

Five percent of the ADAP appropriation is set aside for ADAP supplemental grants. States are eligible for supplemental ADAP grants if they demonstrate a severe need to increase the availability of HIV/AIDS drugs. There is a state-match requirement ($1 state for every $4 federal) for ADAP supplemental grants, but this requirement can be waived under certain circumstances. The 2006 reauthorization established a formulary, that is, a list of HIV/AIDS therapeutics that all ADAPs must provide. The list is based on the clinical practice guidelines for use of HIV/AIDS drugs issued by HHS.[46]

According to the May 2010 National ADAP Monitoring Project, an annual report produced by the National Alliance of State and Territorial AIDS Directors, in FY2009 federal ADAP funds provide 49% of the national ADAP budget, state contributions provide 14%, and drug rebates provide another 31%; the remainder consists of funds from Part B Supplemental grants (3%), Part B Base grants (2%), Part A contributions (1%), and other state or federal funds (1%).[47] In previous years, many states have had to implement cost containment measures, such as waiting lists, because of insufficient ADAP funds.[48] According to the May 2010 National ADAP Monitoring Project Annual Report, as of April 2010 nine states had waiting lists with a combined total of 929 people.[49]

The May 2010 National ADAP Monitoring Project report states that ADAPs were situated in the eye of the "perfect storm" and that a number of factors have strained ADAP, such as "minimal increases in federal appropriations, significant state budget cuts, increased program demand due to unemployment, heightened national efforts on HIV testing and linkages into care, and new HIV Treatment Guidelines calling for earlier therapeutic treatments. These collective stressors are all contributing to a fiscal 'tipping point' for ADAPs from which recovery will be difficult."[50] ADAPs are reporting increased client demand due to changes in national HIV testing recommendations by the CDC and testing provisions put in place by the 2009 reauthorization of the Ryan White program. The goal of expanded testing is to increase the number of people who know their HIV status, and presumably many of these individuals are now receiving care through the Ryan White program.

In July 2010 HHS Secretary Kathleen Sebelius announced the reallocation of $25 million in funds from dozens of programs throughout HHS for ADAP.[51] The additional funds were targeted for states with ADAP waiting lists or other cost containment strategies.

PART C. EARLY INTERVENTION SERVICES

Part C "provides direct grants to 353 community and faith based primary health clinics and public health providers in 49 states, Puerto Rico, the District of Columbia and the U.S. Virgin Islands."[52] Part C grants provide medical services to underserved and uninsured people living with HIV/AIDS in rural and frontier communities. In April 2010, awards for Part C grants were announced.[53] Under current law, 75% of a Part C grant must be used for core medical services, and not less than 50% of a grant must be used for early intervention services. Part C grants are awarded to federally-qualified health centers, family planning clinics, hemophilia centers, rural health clinics, Indian Health Service facilities, and certain health facilities and community-based organizations that provide early intervention services to people infected with HIV/AIDS through intravenous drug use. Part C services include counseling, HIV testing, referrals, clinical and diagnostic services regarding HIV/AIDS, and drug treatments under ADAP.

PART D. GENERAL PROVISIONS

Part D provides grants to public and nonprofit entities for family-centered care for women, infants, children, and youth with HIV/AIDS. Such individuals are provided outpatient health care, case management, referrals, and other services to enable participation in the program including services designed to recruit and retain youth with HIV. Grantees must coordinate with programs promoting the reduction and elimination of risk of HIV/AIDS for youth.

The 2006 reauthorization required that, starting in FY2007, administrative expenses must be no more than 10% of the Part D grant, and GAO was directed to conduct an evaluation of Part D spending. GAO released its report in December 2008.[54] According to GAO, a majority of the Part D grantees reported that they have not made changes to client services in response to the administrative expense cap. However, a majority of Part D grantees reported that the cap has had a negative effect on their Part D program because clinical staff must now perform administrative tasks. Also, about half of grantees reported that not all of their Part D administrative expenses were covered by the 10% allowance. In FY2009, HRSA required that Part D grantees provide more detailed budget information.

P.L. 111-87 clarifies that Part D should be the payer of last resort when Part D clients have access to other forms of health care coverage, such as Medicaid and the Children's Health Insurance Program. The new law would also ensure that memoranda of understanding can be used by certain Part D providers to ensure clients have access to primary care.

PART E

Under prior law, Part E authorized grants for emergency response employees and established procedures for notifications of infectious diseases exposure; Part E was never funded. The 2006 reauthorization (P.L. 109-415) deleted all the old Part E sections and inserted into Part E several sections with some text changes from Part D (on coordination, audits, definitions, and a prohibition on promotion of intravenous drug use or sexual activity) and two new sections on public health emergencies and certain privacy protections.

P.L. 109-415 inadvertently deleted procedures for the notification of occupational infectious diseases exposure from Part E of Ryan White. This was a matter of some concern for the emergency response community and reinstatement of the relevant language was requested.[55] P.L. 111-87 reinserts the deleted language into a new Part G of Title XXVI of the PHS Act and includes a change from the original language that would permit the Secretary to suspend the requirements in a public health emergency.

PART F. DEMONSTRATION AND TRAINING

Part F provides support for the AIDS Dental Reimbursement (ADR) Program, the Community-Based Dental Partnership Program, the AIDS Education and Training Centers (AETCs), and the Special Projects of National Significance (SPNS) Program.[56] The ADR program reimburses dental schools for their treatment of HIV/AIDS patients. The AETC program provides specialized clinical education and consultation for health providers on HIV transmission, treatment, and prevention. In September 2010 HRSA announced awards for two new AETCs.[57]

The SPNS program awards grants to entities eligible for funding under Parts A, B, C, and D to (1) quickly respond to emerging needs of persons receiving assistance under this title, and (2) develop a standard electronic client information data system to improve grantee reporting of client-level data to the Secretary. The 2006 reauthorization provided new criteria for making SPNS grant awards that are focused on: obtaining client-level data to create a Severity of Need Index (SONI); creating and maintaining a safe, secure, and reliable qualified health information technology system; or newly emerging needs of persons receiving assistance under this title.

Under statute, the SPNS program is to be funded, up to $25 million, from amounts appropriated for Parts A, B, C, and D; this was not changed by reauthorization. However, beginning in FY2003, each Labor-HHS appropriations bill has provided $25 million for the SPNS program via a funding mechanism known as the "PHS evaluation tap."[58] The $25 million is divided, roughly proportionately, among Parts A, B, C, and D, which then make the individual SPNS grant awards.

P.L. 109-415 codified the Minority AIDS Initiative (MAI) as part of the Ryan White program under Part F of Title XXVI of the PHS Act.[59] Under P.L. 109-415, MAI provided funding for competitive grants under Parts A, B, C, D, and F that evaluate and address the disproportionate impact of HIV/AIDS on racial and ethnic minorities.

P.L. 111-87 directs HRSA to develop a formula for awarding MAI grants under Part A and Part B "that ensures that funding is provided based on the distribution of populations disproportionately impacted by HIV/AIDS."[60] The new law directs HRSA to synchronize the schedule of application submissions and funding of MAI grants with the schedule of the corresponding Ryan White Part (A, B, C, D, or F).

P.L. 111-87 requires GAO to provide a report for Congress within one year of enactment that describes MAI activities across HHS. The GAO report would "include a history of program activities, a description of activities conducted, people served and types of grantees funded." The GAO report would "collect and describe best practices in community outreach and capacity-building of community based organizations serving the communities that are disproportionately affected by HIV/AIDS." Within six months of publication of the GAO report, P.L. 111-87 would require that HHS submit to Congress a departmental plan for using MAI funds in all the relevant agencies to build capacity, taking into consideration the best practices described in the GAO report.

APPROPRIATIONS

FY2010

The Obama Administration's request for Ryan White programs in FY2010 was $2.267 billion; the amount appropriated in FY2009 was $2.213 billion (see Table 1). The House Appropriations Committee report (H.Rept. 111-220) on H.R. 3293, the Labor-HHS Appropriations bill for FY2010, states that the House bill would provide the same total amount for the Ryan White program as the request, but amounts for Parts A and D are increased and amounts for Parts C and F are decreased relative to the request amounts; Part B is the same as the request.

The Senate Appropriations Committee report (S.Rept. 111-66) on H.R. 3293 indicates that the Senate version of the bill would provide $2.248 billion, $19 million less than the amount provided by the House and the request. Most of the difference is in the amount provided for Part A: the Senate amount for Part A is $8 million less than the President's request and $16 million less than the House. In addressing the stop-loss issue (see "Stop-Loss Provisions"), the Senate report states, "The Committee notes that the FY2009 comparable level included a provision directing funds to particular metropolitan areas facing dramatic cuts as a result of the changes to the Ryan White formula. The Committee has not continued this provision in FY2010." An August 3, 2009, GAO analysis of the stop-loss provision in the House version of H.R. 3293 indicates that two EMAs and four TGAs would receive the funds set aside by the provision; 85% of the stop-loss funds would go to San Francisco, CA.[61] The amount for Part B in the Senate bill is the same as the House and the request.

The Ryan White program had been operating under two continuing resolutions (P.L. 111-68, P.L. 111-88), which funded the program at FY2009 levels through December 18, 2009. The Consolidated Appropriations Act, 2010 (P.L. 111-117), which became law on December 16, 2009, provided a total of $2.266 billion for the Ryan White program in FY2010. Amounts for the various parts of the Ryan White program can be found in Table 1.

In July 2010 HHS Secretary Kathleen Sebelius announced the reallocation of $25 million in funds from dozens of programs throughout HHS for ADAP.[62] The additional funds were targeted for states with ADAP waiting lists or other cost containment strategies.

FY2011

The Obama Administration's request for Ryan White programs in FY2011 is $2.305 billion, an increase of $39.513 million over the FY2010 appropriation. The request would provide increases for all Parts except Part A and Part D which would remain level (see Table 1).

The House Labor-HHS-Education Appropriations Subcommittee held a markup session in July 2010, but the full committee did not report a bill. The Senate Committee on Appropriations reported S. 3686 (S.Rept. 111-243) in August 2010, but the bill did not receive any further action. The Continuing Appropriations Act, 2011 (P.L. 111-242), as amended, provides temporary FY2011 funding through March 4, 2011, at the FY2010 rate of operations.

End Notes

[1] HRSA, *FY2011 Justification of Estimates for Appropriations Committees*, p. 212, http://www.hrsa.gov/about/budgetjustification/budgetjustification11.pdf.

[2] A provision at the end of P.L. 109-415 (Sec. 703) would have repealed the Ryan White program, Title XXVI of the PHS Act, as of the start of FY2010. The FY2010 Continuing Appropriations Resolution (Division B of P.L. 111-68), signed by President Obama on October 1, 2009, extended authority for the Ryan White program through October 31, 2009. P.L. 111-87 removed the sunset provision (section 703 of P.L. 109-415).

[3] For more information on PPACA in general, see CRS Report R40942, *Private Health Insurance Provisions in the Patient Protection and Affordable Care Act (PPACA)*, by Hinda Chaikind, Bernadette Fernandez, and Mark Newsom; CRS Report R41196, *Medicare Provisions in the Patient Protection and Affordable Care Act (PPACA): Summary and Timeline*, coordinated by Patricia A. Davis; and CRS Report R41210, *Medicaid and the State Children's Health Insurance Program (CHIP) Provisions in PPACA: Summary and Timeline*, coordinated by Julie Stone.

[4] HRSA FY2011 budget justification, p. 220, http://www.hrsa.gov/about/budgetjustification/budgetjustification11.pdf.

[5] The FY2010 Part A grant award announcement is at http://www.hhs.gov /news/press /2010pres/ 04/ 20100405a.html. Part A grant award amounts are listed at http:// newsroom.hrsa.gov /releases/2010/parta.htm.

[6] If an EMA no longer qualified as an EMA for FY2007, it was treated as a transitional grant area (TGA), even if it would not otherwise qualify as a TGA. Under the law prior to the 2006 reauthorization, a total of 51 EMAs received funding in FY2006. For FY2007 and FY2008, a total of 22 EMAs received funding; for FY2009, 24 EMAs received funding. Nassau-Suffolk, NY, and New Haven, CT, regained EMA status due to the results of a lawsuit filed by Nassau-Suffolk against HHS. Personal communication with HRSA Office of Legislation, and "County Executive Suozzi, Rep. Israel Declare Victory in Nassau-Suffolk Lawsuit to Save HIV/AIDS Funding," *US Fed News Service, including US State News*, April 28, 2008.

[7] A total of 29 areas that had been EMAs prior to the 2006 reauthorization received funding as TGAs starting in FY2007 and five metropolitan areas received funding as TGAs in FY2007 that were not previously eligible as an EMA: Indianapolis, IN; Baton Rouge, LA; Charlotte, NC; Memphis, TN; and Nashville, TN. For FY2007 and FY2008, a total of 34 TGAs received funding. For FY2009, 32 TGAs received funding; two former TGAs, New Haven, CT, and Nassau-Suffolk, NY, received an EMA grant rather than a TGA grant.

[8] HRSA identified six TGAs that might not have been eligible in FY2011 under P.L. 109-415 based on decreasing numbers of AIDS cases: Santa Rosa, CA; Vineland-Millville-Bridgeton, NJ; Ponce, PR; Middlesex-Somerset-Hunterdon, NJ; and Dutchess County, NY. "Section by Section Description of Ryan White HIV/AIDS Treatment Extension Act of 2009," p. 3, at http://energycommerce.house.gov/Press_111/ 20091013/Ryan_ White_ Section.pdf.

[9] If a TGA qualified as an EMA in a subsequent year, the amount reserved for TGA grants would decrease by the amount of the grant made to the former TGA in the preceding FY and an equal amount would be reserved for EMA grants. If an EMA failed to meet the eligibility criteria for three consecutive years and thus ceased to be an EMA, in the first subsequent year, any amount reserved for EMAs would be reduced by the amount of the formula grant received in the preceding fiscal year by the metropolitan area that was no longer an EMA. If the former EMA qualified as a TGA, the amount reserved for TGA grants would increase by the amount of the reduction in EMA reserved funds. If the former EMA did not qualify as a TGA, the amount by which EMA reserved funds decreased would be equal to $500,000 plus the amount of the formula grant received in the preceding fiscal year by the metropolitan area that was no longer an EMA; that money would be made available for Part B grants. Similarly, if a TGA failed to qualify as a TGA and did not qualify as an EMA, the amount reserved for TGA funds would be reduced by $500,000 plus the amount of the formula portion of the TGA grant for the former TGA in the preceding fiscal year, and those funds would be made available for Part B grants.

[10] The distribution under prior law (P.L. 106-345) was approximately fifty-fifty.

[11] Code-based reporting uses an alphanumeric code instead of a name.

[12] The number of living AIDS cases was estimated from the number of reported AIDS cases over a 10-year period with weighting factors to reflect that not all reported cases were still alive. Under the 2000 reauthorization (P.L. 106-345), statistics on HIV cases could have been used in the Ryan White grant formulas as early as FY2005 if the Secretary of HHS found that HIV incidence data were sufficiently accurate and reliable. In June 2004, the Secretary determined that HIV case reporting was incomplete and could not be used to distribute the grants.

[13] The 2000 reauthorization, P.L. 106-345, did not contain a transition period for states that were moving from code-based to name-based HIV reporting as recommended by the CDC. P.L. 109-415 provided a three-year transition period for qualifying areas. For purposes of the Part A formula, states without a sufficiently accurate and reliable name-based reporting system had a reduction of 5% in the number of non-AIDS HIV cases reported for an eligible area to account for duplicate cases. P.L. 109-415 identified 33 states and 2 territories that had a sufficiently accurate and reliable names-based reporting system as of December 31, 2005.

[14] California, Hawaii, Illinois, Maryland, Massachusetts, Oregon, Rhode Island and the District of Columbia did not have fully mature name-based HIV reporting systems. "Section by Section Description of Ryan White HIV/AIDS Treatment Extension Act of 2009," p. 2, at http:// energycommerce.house.gov /Press_ 111 /20091013 / Ryan_ White_Section.pdf. In addition, a September 18, 2009 GAO report identified three territories that have not begun collecting name-based HIV case counts.

[15] A hold-harmless provision protects grantees from large decreases in funding. The 1996, 2000 and 2006 reauthorizations also provided a hold harmless. In 2006 the hold harmless was extended for three years for EMAs that received a hold harmless amount in FY2006. For FY2007, an EMA that had received a hold harmless amount in FY2006 would receive not less than 95% of a grant amount equal to what the EMA would have gotten in FY2006 (including the hold harmless) if the FY2006 formula had distributed two-thirds of the FY2006 appropriation. For FY2008 and FY2009, under the language of P.L. 109-415 the EMA would receive not less than 100% of the grant amount for FY2007. The hold harmless does not apply to TGAs.

[16] U.S. Government Accountability Office, *Ryan White CARE Act: Effects of Certain Funding Provisions on GrantAwards*, GAO-09-894, September 18, 2009, http://www. gao.gov/new.items/d09894.pdf.

[17] In the 2006 reauthorization, the number of EMAs was reduced from 51 to 24, with the remainder being classified as TGAs. TGAs are not eligible for hold-harmless funding.

[18] Funding for FY2009 does not include amounts resulting from the stop-loss provision in the FY2009 appropriation act, P.L. 111-8. For an explanation of the stop-loss provision, see the "Stop-Loss Provisions" section of this report.

[19] GAO, *Ryan White CARE Act: Effects of Certain Funding Provisions on Grant Awards*, pp. 18-19.

[20] Ibid., p. 20.

[21] Ibid., p. 22.

[22] Ibid.

[23] Ibid., p. 23.

[24] The provision in P.L. 110-161 ensured that an area's total funding under Part A for FY2007 was not less than 86.6% of the amount of the area's total funding under Part A for FY2006. See the October 5, 2007 Government Accountability Office (GAO) report (GAO-08-137R), at http://www.gao.gov/new.items/d08137r.pdf. GAO analyzed the impact of a previously proposed hold harmless provision in an FY2008 Labor-HHS appropriations bill (H.R. 3043) that was not enacted. See also Shawn Zeller, "The AIDS Cash Clash," *CQ Weekly*, July 30, 2007, p. 2248.

[25] The provision in P.L. 111-8 ensured that an EMA's total funding under Part A for FY2008 was not less than 93.7% of the amount of the EMA's total funding under Part A for FY2006, and that a TGA's funding under Part A for FY2008 was not less than 88.7% of the amount of the TGA's total funding under Part A for FY2006. A March 6, 2009, GAO report (GAO-09-472R) analyzed the impact of the stop-loss provision in the FY2009 Omnibus Appropriations Act (H.R. 1105) as passed by the House.

[26] See http://newsroom.hrsa.gov/releases/2009/parta.htm.

[27] The House Appropriations Committee report on H.R. 3293, H.Rept. 111-220, stated "when allocating FY2010 supplemental funds under Part A ..., the Committee urges HRSA to provide additional increases to jurisdictions that have experienced cuts in their total awards relative to the amount awarded in FY2006." The Senate Appropriations Committee report (S.Rept. 111-66) on H.R. 3293 indicated that the Senate amount for Part A is $8 million less than the President's request and $16 million less than the House. The Senate report stated, "The Committee notes that the FY2009 comparable level included a provision directing funds to particular metropolitan areas facing dramatic cuts as a result of the changes to the Ryan White formula. The Committee has not continued this provision in FY2010."

[28] U.S. Government Accountability Office, *Ryan White CARE Act: Estimated Effect of Proposed Stop-Loss Provision in H.R. 3293 on Urban Areas*, GAO-09-947R, August 3, 2009, http://www.gao.gov/new.items/d09947r.pdf.

[29] FY2010 Part B grant award announcement is at http://www.hhs.gov/news /press/2010pres/04/20100405a.html. The Part B grant award amounts are listed at http://newsroom.hrsa.gov/releases/2010/partb.htm.

[30] The formula attempts to correct for a problem under a previous formula: specifically, states with EMAs received a larger amount of money, per case, than states without an EMA. U.S. Government Accountability Office, *Ryan*

White CARE Act: Factors that Impact HIV and AIDS Funding and Client Coverage, GAO-05-841T, June 2005, http://www.gao.gov/new.items/d05841t.pdf.

[31] The number of living AIDS cases was estimated from the number of reported AIDS cases over a 10-year period with weighting factors to reflect that not all reported cases were still alive. Under the 2000 reauthorization (P.L. 106-345), statistics on HIV cases would have been used in the Ryan White grant formulas as early as FY2005 if the Secretary of HHS found that HIV incidence data were sufficiently accurate and reliable. In June 2004, the Secretary determined that HIV case reporting was incomplete and could not be used to distribute the grants. Under P.L. 106-345 HIV case data would have been used for determining FY2007 grant amounts. However, P.L. 106-345 did not contain a transition period for states that were moving to name-based HIV reporting, as recommended by the CDC. P.L. 109-415 had a three-year transition period for qualifying areas.

[32] U.S. Government Accountability Office, *Ryan White CARE Act: Effects of Certain Funding Provisions on Grant Awards*, GAO-09-894, September 18, 2009, http://www.gao.gov/new.items/d09894.pdf.

[33] Ibid., p. 14. The seven grantees are as follows: CA, DC, IL, MD, MA, OR, RI. All but MD could have had HRSA use their name-based HIV case counts to determine formula funding but instead had HRSA use their code-based counts. MD's name-based HIV reporting system had not been determined to be operational and, therefore, did not have that option. The 5 grantees are as follows: HI, VT, the Federated States of Micronesia, Palau, and the Republic of the Marshall Islands. HI and VT transitioned to name-based reporting in 2008; the remaining 3 had not begun collecting name-based HIV case counts.

[34] Ibid., p. 14. According to the GAO report, eight grantees, CT, DE, KY, ME, MT, NH, PA, and WA, with systems less than four years old determined that their name-based HIV reporting systems were accurate and reliable such that case counts from these systems were used by HRSA to determine FY2009 funding.

[35] Ibid., p. 16.

[36] The Part B Supplemental has not been used by HRSA due to lack of funding (due to the requirements of the hold harmless provision). Personal communication with HRSA Office of Legislation, June 29, 2009, and Fact Sheet: The Ryan White Program, Henry J. Kaiser Family Foundation, February 2009, at http://www.kff.org/hivaids/upload/ 7582_05.pdf.

[37] A hold-harmless provision protects grantees from large decreases in funding. Under the P.L. 109-415 hold-harmless provision, for FY2007, a state could not receive less than 95% of the grant amount received in FY2006. For FY2008 and FY2009, a state could not receive less than 100% of the FY2007 grant amount.

[38] U.S. Government Accountability Office, *Ryan White CARE Act: Effects of Certain Funding Provisions on Grant Awards*, GAO-09-894, September 18, 2009, p. 24, http://www.gao.gov/ new.items /d09894.pdf. The 9 states were as follows: AZ, AR, CO, DE, ID, ME, NE, OH, and PA. The 7 territories were as follows: American Samoa, Commonwealth of the Northern Mariana Islands, the Federated States of Micronesia, Guam, Palau, the Republic of Marshall Islands, and the U.S. Virgin Islands. Part A grantees did not have unobligated balances over 2%.

[39] Ibid., p. 25.

[40] Ibid., p. 27.

[41] Ibid., p. 29.

[42] Ibid., pp. 30-31.

[43] HRSA FY2011 budget justification, p. 215, http://www.hrsa.gov/about/budgetjustification /budget justification11.pdf.

[44] ADAP operates in all 50 states, the District of Columbia, Puerto Rico, the U.S. Virgin Islands, Guam, American Samoa, the Commonwealth of the Northern Mariana Islands, and the Republic of the Marshall Islands.

[45] Grants for FY2010 would be an amount equal to 95% of funding in FY2009, funding in FY2011 and FY2012 would be an amount equal to 100% of FY2010, and funding in FY2013 would be an amount equal to 92.5% of FY2012.

[46] Guidelines are found at http://aidsinfo.nih.gov/Guidelines/Default.aspx? MenuItem =Guidelines.

[47] The National Alliance of State and Territorial AIDS Directors, National ADAP Monitoring Project Annual Report, May 2010, p. 8-9, at http://www.nastad.org/Docs/highlight/201053_2010%20National%20ADAP%20Monitoring%20Report.pdf.

[48] The George W. Bush Administration and Barack Obama Administration have provided supplemental ADAP grants in to help alleviate this problem. On September 18, 2007, the George W. Bush Administration announced supplemental ADAP grants totaling $39.5 million to 14 states (Alabama, Alaska, Georgia, Indiana, Iowa, Montana, North Carolina, Oklahoma, Oregon, South Carolina, Texas, Utah, Virginia, and Wisconsin), the Virgin Islands, and Puerto Rico; at http://archive. hrsa.gov /newsroom/releases/2007/ RyanWhitePartsBCD.htm. On June 23, 2004, the George W. Bush Administration announced what it

described as a one-time $20 million initiative for 10 states with ADAP waiting lists (Alabama, Alaska, Colorado, Idaho, Iowa, Kentucky, Montana, North Carolina, South Dakota, and West Virginia). In July 2010 HHS Secretary Kathleen Sebelius announced the reallocation of $25 million in funds from dozens of programs throughout HHS for ADAP. The additional funds were targeted for states with ADAP waiting lists or other cost containment strategies.

[49] The National Alliance of State and Territorial AIDS Directors, National ADAP Monitoring Project Annual Report, May 2010, p. 12, at http://www.nastad.org/Docs/highlight/ 201053_2010%20National %20ADAP% 20Monitoring%20Report.pdf.

[50] Ibid., p. 4.

[51] U.S. Department of Health and Human Services, "Statement from Secretary Sebelius on Reallocating $25 million for AIDS Drug Assistance," press release, July 9, 2010, http://www.hhs.gov/news/press/ 2010pres /07/20100709c.html.

[52] HRSA FY2011 budget justification, p. 231, http://www.hrsa.gov/about /budgetjustification /budget justification11.pdf.

[53] The FY2010 grant award announcement is at http://www.hhs.gov/news /press/2010pres/04/20100405a.html. A list of FY2010 Part C grant awards is at http://newsroom.hrsa.gov/releases/2010/partc.htm.

[54] U.S. Government Accountability Office, *Ryan White CARE Act: First-Year Experiences under the Part D Administrative Expense Cap*, GAO-09-140, December 19, 2008, http://www.gao.gov/products/GAO-09-140.

[55] Katherine West, "Ryan White Notification Law for Emergency Response Employees Deleted: 10 Reasons Why We Need it Back," *EMS Magazine*, October 2008, at http://www.emsresponder.com/print/EMS-Magazine/Ryan-WhiteNotificationLaw-for-Emergency-Response-Employees-Deleted—10-Reasons-Why-We-Need-It-Back/1$8394 ; James R. Cross, JD, "Ryan White Notification Law Repealed: The Deletion of Emergency Response Provisions Demands Attention," *Journal of Emergency Medical Services*, March 2008, p. 136-137; and National Association of State EMS Officials, "NASEMSO Issue Brief on the Repeal of Emergency-Response Provisions Contained in the Ryan White CARE Act," March 2008, at http://www.nasemsd. org/Advocacy /PositionsResolutions/documents/ RyanWhiteIssue Brief032508.pdf.

[56] Both the dental and the AETC programs were transferred legislatively from Title VII of the PHS Act.

[57] U.S. Department of Health and Human Services, "HHS Awards $3.5 Million to Expand HIV/AIDS Care Capacity for Minorities," press release, September 1, 2010, http://www.hrsa.gov/about/news/pressreleases/ 100901hhsawards35million toexpand hivaidscarecapacityforminorities.html.

[58] The tap, authorized under section 241 of the PHS Act, transfers money among PHS agencies for particular activities as specified by the appropriators.

[59] The MAI began in 1998 with the White House announcement of a series of initiatives targeting appropriated funds for HIV/AIDS prevention and treatment programs in minority communities. The Congressional Black Caucus worked with the Clinton Administration to formulate the approach. MAI activities are supported by the following agencies and offices in HHS: HRSA; CDC; National Institutes of Health; Substance Abuse and Mental Health Services Administration; Minority Communities Fund; Office of Minority Health; Office of Women's Health. GAO was required by P.L. 109-415 to provide a report on a variety of issues related to MAI: U.S. Government Accountability Office, *Ryan White CARE Act: Implementation of the New Minority AIDS Initiative Provisions*, GAO-09-315, March 27, 2009, http://www.gao.gov /new.items/d09315.pdf.

[60] Previously under P.L. 109-415 a competitive grant system was used to award Part A and Part B MAI grants.

[61] U.S. Government Accountability Office, *Ryan White CARE Act: Estimated Effect of Proposed Stop-Loss Provision in H.R. 3293 on Urban Areas*, GAO-09-947R, August 3, 2009, http://www.gao.gov/new.items/ d09947r.pdf.

[62] U.S. Department of Health and Human Services, "Statement from Secretary Sebelius on Reallocating $25 million for AIDS Drug Assistance," press release, July 9, 2010, http://www.hhs.gov/news/press/ 2010pres/ 07/20100709c.html.

In: Responding to HIV/AIDS
Editor: Lawrence T. Jensen

ISBN: 978-1-61324-618-4
© 2011 Nova Science Publishers, Inc.

Chapter 5

HOUSING FOR PERSONS LIVING WITH HIV/AIDS[*]

Libby Perl

SUMMARY

Since the beginning of the acquired immunodeficiency syndrome (AIDS) epidemic in the early 1980s, many individuals living with the disease have had difficulty finding affordable, stable housing. As individuals become ill, they may find themselves unable to work, while at the same time facing health care expenses that leave few resources to pay for housing. In addition, many of those persons living with AIDS struggled to afford housing even before being diagnosed with the disease. The financial vulnerability associated with AIDS, as well as the human immunodeficiency virus (HIV) that causes AIDS, results in a greater likelihood of homelessness among persons living with the disease. At the same time, those who are homeless may be more likely to engage in activities through which they could acquire or transmit HIV. Further, recent research has indicated that those individuals living with HIV who live in stable housing have better health outcomes than those who are homeless or unstably housed, and that they spend fewer days in hospitals and emergency rooms.

Congress recognized the housing needs of persons living with HIV/AIDS when it approved the Housing Opportunities for Persons with AIDS (HOPWA) program in 1990 as part of the Cranston-Gonzalez National Affordable Housing Act (P.L. 101-625). The HOPWA program, administered by the Department of Housing and Urban Development (HUD), funds short-term and permanent housing, together with supportive services, for individuals living with HIV/AIDS and their families. In addition, a small portion of funds appropriated through the Ryan White HIV/AIDS program, administered by the Department of Health and Human Services (HHS), may also be used to fund short-term housing for those living with HIV/AIDS.

In FY2010, Congress appropriated $335 million for HOPWA as part of the Consolidated Appropriations Act (P.L. 111-117). This is the most funding ever appropriated for the program, exceeding the FY2009 appropriation by $25 million. HOPWA funds are distributed to states and localities through both formula and competitive grants. HUD awards 90% of appropriated funds by formula to states and

---

[*] This is an edited, reformatted and augmented version of a Congressional Research Service publication, 7-5700 www.crs.gov. RL34318, dated January 24, 2011.

eligible metropolitan statistical areas (MSAs) based on population, reported cases of AIDS, and incidence of AIDS. The remaining 10% is distributed through a grant competition. Funds are used primarily for housing activities, although grant recipients must provide supportive services to those persons residing in HOPWA-funded housing.

INTRODUCTION

Acquired immunodeficiency syndrome (AIDS), a disease caused by the human immunodeficiency virus (HIV), weakens the immune system, leaving individuals with the disease susceptible to infections. As of 2007, AIDS had been diagnosed and reported in an estimated 465,441 individuals living in the 50 states, the District of Columbia, and the territories.[1] These estimates do not include those diagnosed with HIV where the disease has not yet progressed to AIDS or those who have not yet been diagnosed as HIV positive but are currently living with the disease. Currently there is no cure for HIV/AIDS, and in the early years of the AIDS epidemic, those persons infected with AIDS often died quickly. In recent years, however, medications have allowed persons living with HIV and AIDS to live longer and to remain in better health.

Despite improvements in health outcomes, affordable housing remains important to many who live with HIV/AIDS. This report describes recent research that shows how housing and health status are related and the effects of stable housing on patient health. It also describes the Housing Opportunities for Persons with AIDS (HOPWA) program, the only federal program that provides housing and services specifically for persons who are HIV positive or who have AIDS, together with their families. In addition, the report describes how a small portion of funds appropriated through the Ryan White HIV/AIDS program may be used by states and local jurisdictions to provide short-term housing assistance for persons living with HIV/AIDS.

HOUSING STATUS OF PERSONS LIVING WITH HIV/AIDS

The availability of adequate, affordable housing for persons living with HIV and AIDS has been an issue since AIDS was first identified in U.S. patients in the early 1980s. The inability to afford housing and the threat of homelessness confront many individuals living with HIV/AIDS. From the early years of the epidemic, those individuals who have been infected with HIV/AIDS face impoverishment as they become unable to work, experience high medical costs, or lose private health insurance coverage. The incidence of HIV/AIDS has also grown among low-income individuals who were economically vulnerable even before onset of the disease.[2]

Not surprisingly, researchers have found a co-occurrence between HIV/AIDS and homelessness. Homeless persons have a higher incidence of HIV/AIDS infection than the general population, while many individuals with HIV/AIDS are at risk of becoming homeless.[3] Research has found that rates of HIV among homeless people may be as much as three to nine times higher than among those living in stable housing.[4] Further, those who are HIV positive and homeless have been found to be more likely than those who are HIV positive and housed to engage in behaviors associated with the spread of HIV/AIDS. In one study, the use of injectable drugs, sharing needles, and exchanging sex for drugs or money were more likely among both homeless individuals and those who were unstably housed compared to those with stable housing.[5] (Those who were considered unstably housed lived in transitional housing, in jail, drug treatment or a halfway house, or were doubled up in someone else's home.[6]) When housing improved for individuals in the study, their odds of engaging in these behaviors were reduced. Another study found that homeless persons living with HIV/AIDS were almost twice as likely to engage in unprotected sex compared to those who had housing.[7] (Individuals were considered housed if they lived in a house or apartment alone or with others, a medical care facility, or a correctional institution.[8])

CREATION OF THE HOUSING OPPORTUNITIES FOR PERSONS WITH AIDS (HOPWA) PROGRAM

In 1988, Congress established the National Commission on AIDS as part of the Health Omnibus Extension Act (P.L. 100-607) to "promote the development of a national consensus on policy concerning acquired immune deficiency syndrome (AIDS); and to study and make recommendations for a consistent national policy concerning AIDS." In April 1990, in its second interim report to the President, the Commission recommended that Congress and the President provide "[f]ederal housing aid to address the multiple problems posed by HIV infection and AIDS."[9] About the same time that the Commission released its report, in March of 1990, the House Committee on Banking, Finance, and Urban Affairs held a hearing about the need for housing among persons living with HIV/AIDS. Witnesses as well as committee members discussed various barriers to housing for persons living with HIV/AIDS. Among the issues confronting those persons that were discussed at the hearing were poverty, homelessness, and discrimination[10] in attempting to secure housing.[11] Another issue discussed at the hearing was the eligibility for subsidized housing for persons living with the disease. A question raised during the hearing, but left unresolved, was whether persons living with HIV or AIDS met the definition of "handicap" in order to be eligible for the Section 202 Supportive Housing for the Elderly program (which also provided housing for persons with disabilities).[12] Another concern was that persons living with HIV/AIDS often had difficulty obtaining subsidized housing through mainstream HUD programs such as Public Housing and Section 8 due to the length of waiting lists; individuals often died while waiting for available units.[13]

In the 101st Congress, at least two bills were introduced that contained provisions to create a housing program specifically for persons living with AIDS. These proposed programs were called the AIDS Housing Opportunity Act (which was part of the Housing and Community Development Act of 1990, H.R. 1180) and the AIDS Opportunity Housing Act (H.R. 3423). The bills were similar, and both proposed to fund short-term and permanent housing, together with supportive services, for individuals living with AIDS and related diseases. The text from one of these bills, H.R. 1180, which included the AIDS Housing Opportunity Act, was incorporated into the Cranston-Gonzalez National Affordable Housing Act (S. 566) when it was debated and passed by the House on August 1, 1990. In conference with the Senate, the name of the housing program was changed to Housing Opportunities for Persons with AIDS (HOPWA). In addition, the several separate housing assistance programs that had been proposed in H.R. 1180—one for short-term housing, one for permanent housing supported through Section 8, and one for community residences—were consolidated into one formula grant program in which recipient communities could choose which activities to fund. The amended version of S. 566 was signed by the President on November 28, 1990, and became P.L. 101-625, the Cranston Gonzalez National Affordable Housing Act.

The HOPWA program is administered by the Department of Housing and Urban Development (HUD) and remains the only federal program solely dedicated to providing housing assistance to persons living with HIV/AIDS and their families.[14] The program addresses the need for reasonably priced housing for thousands of low-income individuals (those with incomes at or below 80% of the area median income). HOPWA was last reauthorized by the Housing and Community Development Act of 1992 (P.L. 102-550). Although authorization for HOPWA expired after FY1994, Congress continues to fund the program through annual appropriations.

DISTRIBUTION AND USE OF HOPWA FUNDS

Formula Grants

HOPWA program funding is distributed both by formula allocations and competitive grants. HUD awards 90% of appropriated funds by formula to states and eligible metropolitan statistical areas (MSAs) that meet the minimum AIDS case requirements according to data reported to the Centers for Disease Control and Prevention (CDC) in the previous year. (For the amounts distributed to eligible states and MSAs in recent years, see Appendix.) HOPWA formula funds are available through HUD's Consolidated Plan initiative. Jurisdictions applying for funds from four HUD formula grant programs, including HOPWA,[15] submit a single consolidated plan to HUD. The plan includes an assessment of community housing and development needs and a proposal that addresses those needs, using both federal funds and community resources. Communities that participate in the Consolidated Plan may receive HOPWA funds if they meet formula requirements. Formula funds are allocated in two ways:

- First, 75% of the total available formula funds, sometimes referred to by HUD as "base funding," is distributed to
    - the largest cities within metropolitan statistical areas (MSAs)[16] with populations of at least 500,000 and with 1,500 or more cumulative reported cases of AIDS (which includes those who have died); and
    - to states with at least 1,500 cases of AIDS in the areas outside of that state's eligible MSAs.[17]
- Second, 25% of total available formula funds—sometimes referred to by HUD as "bonus funding"—is distributed on the basis of AIDS incidence during the past three years.[18] Only the largest cities within MSAs that have populations of at least 500,000, with at least 1,500 reported cases of AIDS and that have a higher than

average per capita incidence of AIDS are eligible.[19] States are not eligible for bonus funding.

Although HOPWA funds are allocated to the largest city within an MSA, these recipient cities are required to allocate funds "in a manner that addresses the needs within the metropolitan statistical area in which the city is located."[20] While the distribution of balance of state funds is based on AIDS cases outside of eligible MSAs, states may use funds for projects in any area of the state, including those that received their own funds.[21] According to HUD guidance, states should serve clients in areas outside of eligible MSAs, but the state may operate anywhere in the state because it "may be coordinating the use of all resources in a way that address needs more appropriately throughout the state."[22] In FY2010, 92 MSAs (including the District of Columbia) received funds, while 40 states and Puerto Rico received funds for use in the areas outside of recipient MSAs.[23] HUD jurisdictions that receive HOPWA funds may administer housing and services programs themselves or may allocate all or a portion of the funds to subgrantee private nonprofit organizations. HOPWA formula funds remain available for obligation for two years.

As a result of language included in every HUD appropriations law since FY1999 (P.L. 105-276), states do not lose formula funds if their reported AIDS cases drop below 1,500, as long as they received funding in the previous fiscal year. States generally drop below 1,500 AIDS cases when a large metropolitan area becomes separately eligible for formula funds. These states are allocated a grant on the basis of the cumulative number of AIDS cases outside of their MSAs.[24]

Competitive Grants

The remaining 10% of HOPWA funding is available through competitive grants. Funds are distributed through a national competition to two groups of grantees: (1) states and local governments that propose to provide short-term, transitional, or permanent supportive housing in areas that are not eligible for formula allocations, and (2) government agencies or nonprofit entities that propose "special projects of national significance."[25] A project of national significance is one that uses an innovative service delivery model. In determining proposals that qualify, HUD must consider the innovativeness of the proposal and its potential replicability in other communities.[26] Competitive grants may not be used to provide supportive services alone; instead, services can only be provided in conjunction with housing activities, and funds for services cannot exceed 35% of a project's budget.[27]

The competitive grants are awarded through HUD's annual SuperNOFA (Notice of Funding Availability), which is generally published in the Federal Register in the early spring. Since FY2000 (P.L. 106-377), Congress has required HUD to renew expiring contracts for permanent supportive housing prior to awarding funds to new projects. In FY2009, the amount of funds required for project renewals meant that there were no funds available for new competitive grants.[28] HUD also anticipates that new competitive grants will not be awarded in FY2010 and FY2011.[29] Beginning in FY2006, competitive funds remain available for obligation for three years (from FY2002 through FY2005, competitive funds had been available only for two years). The extension makes the rules for HOPWA's competitive program consistent with those of other competitive programs advertised in HUD's SuperNOFA.

Eligibility for HOPWA-Funded Housing

In the HOPWA program, individuals are eligible for housing if they are either HIV positive or if they are diagnosed with AIDS.[30] In general, clients must also be low income, meaning that their income does not exceed 80% of the area median income.[31] HUD reports area median incomes for metropolitan areas and non-metropolitan counties on an annual basis.[32] Housing and some supportive services are available for family members of persons living with AIDS. When a person living in HOPWA-supported housing dies, his or her family members are given a grace period during which they may remain in the housing.[33] This period may not exceed one year, however. Individuals who are HIV positive or living with AIDS may also be eligible for other HUD-assisted housing for persons with disabilities. However, infection itself may not be sufficient to meet the definition of disability in these other programs. For example, in the case of housing developed prior to the mid-1990s under the Section 202 Supportive Housing for the Elderly program and those units developed under the Section 811 Supportive Housing for Persons with Disabilities program, an individual who is HIV positive or has AIDS must also meet the statutory definition of disability (in which HIV/AIDS status alone is not sufficient) to be eligible for housing.[34] The project-based Section 8 and Public Housing programs may also set aside units or entire developments for persons with disabilities. The definition of disability for these programs does "not exclude persons who have the disease of acquired immunodeficiency syndrome or any conditions arising from the etiologic agent" for AIDS.[35] However, the definition does not indicate whether the status of being HIV positive or having AIDS is alone sufficient to be considered disabled.

Eligible Uses of HOPWA Funds

HOPWA grantees may use funds for a wide range of housing, social services, program planning, and development costs. Supportive services must be provided together with housing. Formula grantees may also choose to provide supportive services not in conjunction with housing, although the focus of the HOPWA program is housing activities. Allowable activities include the following.

- The Development and Operation of Multi-Unit Community Residences, Including the Provision of Supportive Services for Persons Who Live in the Residences.[36] Funds may be used for the construction, rehabilitation, and acquisition of facilities, for payment of operating costs, and for technical assistance in developing the community residence.
- Short-Term Rental, Mortgage, and Utility Assistance to Persons Living with AIDS Who Are Homeless or at Risk of Homelessness.[37] Funds may be used to acquire and/or rehabilitate facilities that will be used to provide short-term housing, as well

as to make payments on behalf of tenants or homeowners, and to provide supportive services. Funds may not be used to construct short-term housing facilities.[38] Residents may not stay in short-term housing facilities more than 60 days in any 6-month period, and may not receive short-term rental, mortgage and utility assistance for more than 21 weeks in any 52 week period. These limits are subject to waiver by HUD, however, if a project sponsor is making an attempt to provide permanent supportive housing for residents and has been unable to do so. Funds may also be used to pay operating and administrative expenses.

- Project-Based or Tenant-Based Rental Assistance for Permanent Supportive Housing, Including Shared Housing Arrangements.[39] In general, tenants must pay approximately 30% of their income toward rent.[40] Grant recipients must ensure that residents receive supportive services, and funds may also be used for administrative costs in providing rental assistance.
- The New Construction or Acquisition and Rehabilitation of Property for Single-Room Occupancy Dwellings.[41]
- Supportive Services, Which Include Health Assessments, Counseling for Those with Addictions to Drugs and Alcohol, Nutritional Assistance, Assistance with Daily Living, Day Care, and Assistance in Applying for Other Government Benefits.[42]
- Housing Information Such as Counseling and Referral Services.[43] Assistance may include fair housing counseling for those experiencing discrimination.[44]

The majority of HOPWA funds are used to provide housing. According to HUD, in FY2008 and FY2009, 60% of HOPWA funding was used for housing assistance such as rent and facility operating costs. An additional 4% was used to help individuals find housing, and 3% for housing development.[45] Grantee performance reports indicate that clients who receive housing assistance through HOPWA are often at the lowest income levels; in its FY2011 Congressional Budget Justifications, HUD estimated that 83% of households served have extremely low incomes (at or below 30% of area median income) and 12% have very low incomes (at or below 50% of area median income).[46]

HOPWA PROGRAM FORMULA AND FUNDING

The HOPWA Formula

The HOPWA method for allocating formula funds has been an ongoing issue because the cumulative number of AIDS cases—including those who have died—is used to distribute funds. A 2006 Government Accountability Office (GAO) report found that the cumulative measure resulted in disproportionate funding per living AIDS case, depending on the jurisdiction. The GAO report looked at FY2004 HOPWA allocations and found that the amount of money grantees received per living AIDS case ranged from $387 per person to $1,290.[47] According to the report, if only living AIDS cases had been counted in that year, 92 of 117 grantees would have received more formula funding, while 25 would have received less.[48]

In each of President Bush's budgets from FY2007 through FY2009, the Administration proposed to change the way in which HOPWA funds are distributed. The FY2009 budget stated that "[w]hereas the current formula distributes formula grant resources by the cumulative number of AIDS cases, the revised formula will account for the present number of people living with AIDS, as well as differences in housing costs in the qualifying areas." The President's FY2007 and FY2008 budgets contained nearly identical language. HUD's budget justifications for FY2009 elaborated somewhat on the Administration's proposal to change the HOPWA distribution formula. HUD's explanation indicated that a new formula would use the number of persons living with AIDS, and that eventually, when consistent data on the number of persons living with HIV become available, that measure might also be used in determining the distribution of HOPWA funding.[49] In the FY2010 HUD budget justifications, HUD stated that it would review the formula and "make related recommendations at a future time."[50] The FY2011 HUD budget did not discuss the HOPWA formula.

Discussions regarding the HOPWA formula and its use of cumulative AIDS cases to distribute funds are not new. In 1997, GAO released a report regarding the performance of the HOPWA program in which it recommended that HUD look at recent changes to the formula used by the Ryan White CARE Act (now called the Ryan While HIV/AIDS program) to "determine what legislative revisions are needed to make the HOPWA formula more reflective of current AIDS cases ..."[51] (At the time of the GAO report, Congress had recently changed the CARE Act formula to use estimates of persons living with AIDS instead of cumulative AIDS cases.[52]) In response to the GAO report, the House Appropriations Committee included the GAO language in its report accompanying the FY1998 HUD Appropriations Act (P.L. 105-65) and directed HUD to make recommendations to Congress about its findings regarding an update to the formula.[53]

In response to the FY1998 Appropriations Act, HUD then issued a report to Congress in 1999 that proposed changes that could be made to the HOPWA formula.[54] The proposed formula in HUD's 1999 report would have used an estimate of persons living with AIDS (instead of all cumulative AIDS cases), together with housing costs, to distribute formula funds. It also would have included a protection for existing grantees. Those recommendations were not adopted by Congress.

No legislation to change the HOPWA formula has been introduced since the 109th Congress, when two bills (S. 2339 and H.R. 5009) would have changed the way that HOPWA formula funds are allocated by counting the number of "reported living cases of HIV disease" instead of cumulative AIDS cases. Neither bill was enacted.

HOPWA Funding

As a result of advances in medical science and in the care and treatment of persons living with HIV and AIDS, individuals are living longer with the disease.[55] As the number of those with AIDS grows, so do the jurisdictions that qualify for formula-based HOPWA funds. Since 1999, there has been a steady increase in the number of jurisdictions that meet the eligibility test to receive formula-based HOPWA funds. Funding for the HOPWA program has increased in almost every year since the program was created, with the exception of FY2005 through FY2007, when funding dropped from the FY2004 level of $295 million.

(See Table 1.) In FY2010, Congress appropriated $335 million as part of the Consolidated Appropriations Act (P.L. 111-117), the most ever appropriated for the program.

The number of households receiving HOPWA housing assistance (including short-term housing assistance, housing provided through community residences, or rental assistance in permanent housing) has declined in every year but one from FY2003 through FY2009. (See Table 1.)

Table 1. HOPWA Funding and Eligible Jurisdictions, FY2001-FY2011

Fiscal Year	Number of Qualifying Jurisdictions	Households Receiving Housing Assistance[a]	President's Request (dollars in thousands)	Appropriations (dollars in thousands)[b]
2001	105	72,117	260,000	257,432
2002	108	74,964	277,432	277,432
2003	111	78,467	292,000	290,102
2004	117	70,779	297,000	294,751
2005	121	67,012	294,800	281,728
2006	122	67,000	268,000	286,110
2007	123	67,850	300,100	286,110
2008	127	62,210	300,100	300,100
2009	131	58,367	300,100	310,000
2010	133	—	310,000	335,000
2011	134-136[c]	—	340,000	—

Source: Table prepared by the Congressional Research Service based on data from the Department of Housing and Urban Development budget justifications, P.L. 111-8, and P.L. 111-117 (number of qualifying jurisdictions and appropriation levels), FY2001 through FY2011 President's Budget Appendices (President's request), and FY2004, FY2006, FY2007, FY2008, and FY2009 HUD Performance and Accountability Reports (number of households assisted). For a breakdown of formula funding by jurisdiction, see the Appendix.

[a.] Housing assistance includes short-term assistance with rent, mortgage, or utilities; residence in short-term housing facilities; housing provided through community residences and single-room occupancy dwellings; and rental assistance for permanent supportive housing.

[b.] Includes rescissions.

[c.] In the FY2011 Congressional Budget Justifications, HUD estimated that 134-136 jurisdictions would qualify for HOPWA funds.

Between FY2003 and FY2009, the number of households served has dropped from 78,467 to 58,367.[56] These general reductions in households served could be due to a number of factors, including the growth in jurisdictions eligible for HOPWA grants (which have increased from 111 in FY2003 to 133 in FY2010), the amount of available funds, and housing costs.

HOUSING FUNDED THROUGH THE RYAN WHITE HIV/AIDS PROGRAM

In addition to funds for housing provided through HUD, funds appropriated to the Department of Health and Human Services (HHS) Ryan White HIV/AIDS program may be used to provide short-term housing assistance to persons living with HIV/AIDS. The Ryan White Comprehensive AIDS Resources Emergency Act (P.L. 101-381) established the Ryan White program in 1990. The program provides funds to states and metropolitan areas to help pay for health care and supportive services for persons living with HIV/AIDS (referred to as "support services" in the statute).[57] The statute governing the use of Ryan White funds does not specifically list housing as an eligible activity for which grantees may use funds. However, the statute provides that grantees may use Ryan White funds to provide support services for persons living with HIV and AIDS. These services are defined as those "that are needed for individuals with HIV/AIDS to achieve their medical outcomes ..."[58] In 1999, the HIV/AIDS Bureau of the Health Resources and Services Administration (HRSA) within HHS released policy guidance regarding the type of housing that Ryan White grantees could provide for their clients (Policy Notice 99-02).[59] According to the guidance, grantees may use funds for housing referral services and for emergency or short-term housing. Ryan White funds must be the payer of last resort, meaning that other sources of funds for housing must be exhausted before using Ryan White funds.

Initially, the policy regarding use of Ryan White funds for housing did not require that specific time limits be placed on short-term housing. In its report regarding the new guidance, HRSA stated: "Although we are restricting the policy to transitional/temporary housing, we don't define 'transitional/temporary.' Because we don't know yet what the recent changes in medical treatment of HIV/AIDS mean to the evolution of the epidemic, it is foolish to adopt any definition of 'short-term.'"[60] However, when the Ryan White program was reauthorized in 2006, the new law limited the amount of grants to states and urban areas that could be used for supportive services to no more than 25% by requiring that at least 75% of funds be used for "core medical services."[61] Previously the law did not limit the amount of funds that could be used for supportive services.

In December 2006, in response to the "more restrictive funding limits established for support services in the 2006 reauthorization," HHS issued a proposed policy notice to limit the amount of time that any client could spend in Ryan White-funded transitional housing to 24 months in a lifetime, effective retroactively.[62] This would have meant that those individuals who had already exhausted the 24-month time period would not be able to receive housing benefits. After receiving over 200 comments regarding the policy of the 24-month lifetime limit and released a final policy notice on February 27, 2008 (Amendment proposal, HHS eventually removed the provision requiring retroactive application #1 to Policy Notice 99-02).[63] The policy took effect on March 27, 2008. However, as the 24-month deadline approached, in February 2010 HRSA released another notice announcing that it was rescinding Amendment #1 to Policy Notice 99-02, and that grantees would not be required to enforce the previous 24-month limit on housing services.[64] HRSA also noted that it would be "undertaking a comprehensive review of the Housing Policy."[65]

In 2007, HRSA reported that 476 Ryan White-funded service organizations provided housing services for individuals living with HIV/AIDS.[66] In 2006, an estimated 42,178 persons living with AIDS received some sort of housing service. Note that this estimate includes duplicated services, so an individual who received both housing referral services and spent time in emergency housing may be counted more than once.[67]

THE RELATIONSHIP BETWEEN STABLE HOUSING AND HEALTH OUTCOMES

As mentioned earlier in this report, HIV/AIDS status is associated with homelessness: those persons who are homeless are more likely to be HIV positive than those who are housed. In addition, recent research has found that the health outcomes of homeless individuals living with HIV/AIDS may be improved with stable housing. In response to evidence from recent studies, the Administration's National HIV/AIDS Strategy, published in 2010, acknowledged that "access to housing is an important precursor to getting many people into a stable treatment regimen. Individuals living with HIV who lack stable housing are more likely to delay HIV care, have poorer access to regular care, are less likely to receive optimal antiretroviral therapy, and are less likely to adhere to therapy."[68] The National HIV/AIDS Strategy included pursuing the goal of housing as one of the ways to increase access to care and improve health outcomes for individuals living with HIV and AIDS.[69]

This section of the report gives a short overview of several studies that have examined how access to stable housing influences health outcomes for those living with HIV and AIDS.

Community Health Advisory and Information Network (Chain) Project Data

The CHAIN Project is a longitudinal study, begun in 1994, of a sample of individuals who are living with HIV/AIDS in New York City and the northern suburbs. In 2007, researchers released a study that used the CHAIN data to examine the effects of stable housing on health care for individuals living with HIV and AIDS.[70]

The study looked at those who were unstably housed—meaning that they were either living in some form of transitional housing; in a jail, drug treatment facility, or halfway house; in a hospice; or temporarily living in someone else's home—or who were homeless, meaning that they were living in a shelter or place not meant for human habitation. Researchers measured the likelihood of six scenarios involving the receipt or continuity of both medical care in general and appropriate HIV medical care. In general, individuals who were unstably housed were less likely to enter into and retain both medical care and appropriate HIV care.[71]

However, the likelihood of obtaining and retaining medical care increased if individuals received some form of housing assistance.[72] In addition, receipt of mental health services and social services case management had a statistically significant relationship to individuals entering into and retaining medical care.

Housing and Health Study

In the Housing and Health Study, HUD, together with the CDC, provided HIV positive individuals who were homeless or at severe risk of homelessness with HOPWA-funded rental housing. (The study considered individuals to be at severe risk of homelessness if they frequently moved from one temporary housing situation to another.) Those individuals in the comparison group received services, including assistance with finding housing, but did not receive HOPWAfunded housing.[73] Despite the differences in rental assistance provided between the treatment and comparison groups, both groups had a statistically significant increase in stable housing.[74] After 18 months, 82% of HOPWA-assisted renters and 52% of individuals in the comparison group were living in their own housing. Perhaps due to the fact that the comparison group also had some success in achieving and maintaining housing, both groups saw statistically significant improvements in health outcomes. After 18 months, both groups had fewer emergency room visits, fewer hospitalizations, reduced opportunistic infections (those infections that occur due to weakened immune systems), and reduced use of medical care generally. Self-reported depression and perceived stress saw improvement as well.

Chicago Housing for Health Partnership Study

The Chicago Housing for Health Partnership study identified homeless individuals with chronic illnesses, including HIV, for participation. Among those who participated in the study, 36% were HIV positive. The treatment group received housing funded through either HOPWA or HUD's Supportive Housing Program for homeless individuals, while the comparison, or usual care group, received available supportive services but no separate assistance with rent. The study found that, after 12 months, the group receiving housing assistance had higher rates of intact immunity compared to the comparison group and were more likely to have undetectable viral loads.[75] There was no statistically significant difference between CD4 counts for the treatment and usual care group. (Very generally, CD4 counts are a measure of immune system strength.) At the conclusion of the study, the treatment group was found to have spent fewer days in emergency rooms and hospitals during the 18 month period in which the researchers followed participants. Specifically, compared to those in the usual care group, those in the treatment group showed 29% reduction in hospitalizations, a 29% reduction in the number of days spent in the hospital, and a 24% reduction in visits to the emergency room.[76]

APPENDIX. RECENT HOPWA FORMULA ALLOCATIONS

Table A-1. HOPWA Formula Allocations, FY2004-FY2010

MSA, State, or Territory	FY2004	FY2005	FY2006	FY2007	FY2008	FY2009	FY2010
Alabama State Program	1,139,000	1,117,000	1,145,000	1,163,000	1,241,000	1,299,792	1,403,821
Birmingham	520,000	497,000	511,000	516,000	538,000	554,848	593,523
Arkansas State Program	752,000	723,000	707,000	720,000	766,000	797,682	531,915
Little Rock	—	—	—	—	—	—	317,437
Arizona State Program	164,000	164,000	173,000	180,000	191,000	198,919	219,282
Phoenix	1,434,000	1,391,000	1,433,000	1,456,000	1,541,000	1,608,397	1,769,291
Tucson	402,000	390,000	389,000	390,000	411,000	420,497	453,391
California State Program	3,042,000	2,869,000	2,929,000	2,926,000	2,746,000	2,557,875	2,746,244
Bakersfield(a)	—	—	—	—	323,000	472,334	635,917
Fresno(a)	—	—	—	—	—	315,824	346,048
Los Angeles	10,476,000	11,848,000	10,310,000	10,393,000	10,437,000	10,764,091	12,384,800
Oakland	2,006,000	1,879,000	1,905,000	1,896,000	1,952,000	2,038,921	2,208,481
Riverside	1,772,000	1,683,000	1,684,000	1,689,000	1,751,000	1,850,429	1,990,870
Sacramento	844,000	795,000	786,000	784,000	818,000	844,003	906,991
San Diego	2,683,000	2,527,000	2,549,000	2,551,000	2,646,000	2,731,528	2,935,661
San Francisco	8,562,000	8,466,000	8,070,000	8,189,000	8,193,000	9,233,417	9,977,748
San Jose	792,000	736,000	738,000	739,000	767,000	796,679	871,489
Santa Ana	1,436,000	1,342,000	1,359,000	1,345,000	1,402,000	1,458,807	1,568,178
Colorado State Program	366,000	354,000	364,000	363,000	379,000	392,424	425,407
Denver	1,424,000	1,342,000	1,359,000	1,361,000	1,414,000	1,452,390	1,572,773
Connecticut State Program	251,000	242,000	253,000	252,000	263,000	268,902	286,319
Bridgeport	779,000	717,000	737,000	739,000	771,000	854,931	846,219
Hartford	1,023,000	1,285,000	1,108,000	1,098,000	1,140,000	1,084,029	1,153,422
New Haven	1,232,000	1,624,000	1,178,000	1,075,000	946,000	963,113	1,021,853
Washington, DC	11,802,000	10,535,000	11,370,000	11,118,000	11,541,000	12,213,518	14,118,841

Table A-1. (Continued).

MSA, State, or Territory	FY2004	FY2005	FY2006	FY2007	FY2008	FY2009	FY2010
Delaware State Program	164,000	162,000	166,000	167,000	179,000	186,286	202,783
Wilmington(b)	798,000	703,000	679,000	552,000	604,000	651,902	771,469
Florida State Program	4,063,000	3,581,000	3,312,000	3,316,000	3,191,000	3,012,662	3,655,741
Cape Coral(c)	—	—	336,000	332,000	350,000	368,963	402,434
Deltona	—	—	—	—	—	312,215	0
Fort Lauderdale	6,240,000	6,106,000	6,637,000	6,878,000	7,351,000	7,545,922	8,646,967
Jacksonville	1,564,000	1,624,000	1,587,000	1,630,000	1,988,000	2,265,720	2,510,630
Lakeland(c)	—	378,000	445,000	418,000	509,000	491,383	545,040
Miami	10,715,000	10,351,000	11,189,000	11,689,000	12,370,000	12,599,526	12,935,584
Orlando	3,189,000	2,871,000	2,906,000	2,895,000	3,234,000	3,533,132	3,347,552
Palm Bay(c)	—	—	—	—	311,000	317,829	341,871
Sarasota/Bradenton	397,000	548,000	390,000	391,000	409,000	421,099	460,283
Tampa	2,389,000	3,049,000	2,542,000	2,772,000	3,193,000	3,449,810	3,721,763
West Palm Beach	3,836,000	3,426,000	3,595,000	3,235,000	3,271,000	3,200,060	3,466,709
Georgia State Program	1,515,000	1,527,000	1,576,000	1,621,000	1,744,000	1,860,455	2,025,746
Atlanta	4,899,000	6,592,000	5,290,000	6,801,000	7,034,000	8,788,464	9,224,086
Augusta	373,000	418,000	376,000	394,000	385,000	398,640	429,792
Hawaii State Program	181,000	169,000	162,000	160,000	164,000	168,039	181,691
Honolulu	452,000	428,000	429,000	419,000	433,000	444,761	473,440
Iowa State Program	347,000	329,000	330,000	336,000	354,000	367,359	400,137
Illinois State Program	864,000	827,000	875,000	875,000	916,000	945,467	1,014,962
Chicago	8,338,000	5,379,000	5,561,000	5,572,000	5,819,000	5,993,040	6,426,836
Indiana State Program	836,000	806,000	818,000	822,000	863,000	892,730	971,314
Indianapolis	759,000	738,000	751,000	752,000	782,000	806,705	878,589
Kansas State Program	363,000	349,000	331,000	332,000	346,000	357,333	384,683
Kentucky State Program	423,000	407,000	410,000	408,000	431,000	452,782	493,906
Louisville	462,000	443,000	447,000	453,000	476,000	502,511	554,887
Louisiana State Program	940,000	932,000	951,000	975,000	1,034,000	1,090,045	1,203,335
Baton Rouge	1,813,000	1,659,000	1,572,000	1,409,000	1,433,000	1,797,197	2,225,972
New Orleans	2,992,000	3,398,000	2,997,000	2,914,000	2,769,000	3,089,672	3,385,486

MSA, State, or Territory	FY2004	FY2005	FY2006	FY2007	FY2008	FY2009	FY2010
Massachusetts State Program	525,000	178,000	168,000	166,000	173,000	180,471	194,639
Boston	1,829,000	1,721,000	1,719,000	1,690,000	1,747,000	1,779,243	1,889,165
Lowell	659,000	623,000	627,000	622,000	644,000	658,318	702,955
Lynn	—	316,000	317,000	312,000	326,000	331,866	355,028
Springfield	461,000	433,000	424,000	418,000	426,000	445,162	481,793
Worcester	369,000	348,000	354,000	349,000	368,000	377,385	408,282
Maryland State Program	345,000	335,000	348,000	345,000	357,000	362,346	401,808
Baltimore	7,936,000	7,754,000	7,649,000	8,038,000	8,195,000	8,657,224	10,043,043
Frederick(d)	535,000	518,000	524,000	539,000	575,000	603,776	977,937
Michigan State Program	911,000	862,000	877,000	893,000	941,000	980,158	1,056,103
Detroit	1,979,000	1,554,000	1,597,000	1,640,000	1,979,000	2,066,997	1,944,506
Warren	405,000	392,000	397,000	409,000	437,000	456,391	498,501
Minnesota State Program	110,000	105,000	112,000	114,000	119,000	124,525	137,625
Minneapolis	839,000	797,000	829,000	833,000	873,000	903,558	977,370
Missouri State Program	496,000	475,000	455,000	450,000	473,000	492,485	526,694
Kansas City	978,000	924,000	918,000	918,000	955,000	1,016,453	1,108,522
St. Louis	1,217,000	1,158,000	1,150,000	1,140,000	1,227,000	1,264,901	1,362,053
Mississippi State Program	756,000	749,000	778,000	783,000	833,000	858,039	948,759
Jackson	724,000	998,000	868,000	899,000	885,000	881,503	970,233
North Carolina Program	2,082,000	2,010,000	2,097,000	2,154,000	2,272,000	2,387,029	2,685,680
Charlotte	571,000	565,000	597,000	626,000	671,000	714,063	793,382
Wake County	352,000	337,000	366,000	382,000	434,000	459,800	721,566
Nebraska State Program	—	—	—	—	306,000	317,829	344,586
New Jersey State Program(b)	1,106,000	1,050,000	1,064,000	1,056,000	1,079,000	1,109,696	1,180,213
Camden	657,000	628,000	620,000	610,000	642,000	655,912	713,814

Table A-1. (Continued).

MSA, State, or Territory	FY2004	FY2005	FY2006	FY2007	FY2008	FY2009	FY2010
Jersey City	—	2,240,000	2,545,000	2,443,000	2,534,087	2,358,602	2,926,790
Newark	5,182,000	5,014,000	5,246,000	4,924,000	5,167,000	4,913,428	6,620,013
Paterson	—	1,265,000	1,282,000	1,250,000	1,286,736	1,301,766	1,404,206
Woodbridge	1,462,000	1,366,000	1,375,000	1,351,000	1,390,000	1,408,877	1,516,177
New Mexico State Program	533,000	503,000	514,000	514,000	532,000	552,442	272,536
Albuquerque	—	—	—	—	—	—	320,778
Nevada State Program	238,000	219,000	219,000	219,000	228,000	236,818	254,785
Las Vegas	916,000	886,000	882,000	897,000	952,000	1,002,015	1,098,706
New York State Program	1,776,000	1,702,000	1,797,000	1,809,000	1,897,000	1,938,459	2,139,773
Albany	429,000	415,000	436,000	439,000	462,000	471,430	508,525
Buffalo	472,000	456,000	480,000	480,000	507,000	521,962	565,329
Islip	1,660,000	1,565,000	1,617,000	1,608,000	1,675,000	1,711,266	1,848,859
New York City	60,355,000	47,056,000	56,610,000	54,723,000	56,811,177	52,654,359	54,718,998
Poughkeepsie	604,000	577,000	679,000	812,000	947,000	655,310	702,119
Rochester	597,000	575,000	599,000	605,000	640,000	658,519	709,220
Ohio State Program	1,041,000	1,024,000	1,037,000	1,051,000	1,108,000	1,157,420	1,249,280
Cincinnati	550,000	517,000	518,000	530,000	562,000	584,124	643,644
Cleveland	854,000	822,000	826,000	840,000	870,000	895,337	960,454
Columbus	584,000	584,000	596,000	608,000	641,000	667,342	735,952
Oklahoma State Program	518,000	494,000	498,000	506,000	226,000	230,000	243,925
Oklahoma City	466,000	441,000	435,000	437,000	459,000	483,261	513,746
Tulsa	—	—	—	—	307,000	324,647	342,706
Oregon State Program	—	321,000	319,000	317,000	335,000	350,114	374,867
Portland	1,006,000	949,000	947,000	943,000	988,000	1,016,854	1,088,055
Pennsylvania State Program	1,540,000	1,511,000	1,548,000	1,527,000	1,670,000	1,755,180	1,615,167
Allentown	—	—	—	—	—	—	317,228

MSA, State, or Territory	FY2004	FY2005	FY2006	FY2007	FY2008	FY2009	FY2010
Philadelphia	7,632,000	7,336,000	7,083,000	6,650,000	7,052,000	8,716,376	8,786,271
Pittsburgh	626,000	620,000	623,000	619,000	649,000	676,967	731,148
Puerto Rico State Program	1,748,000	1,636,000	1,633,000	1,616,000	1,679,000	1,709,461	1,825,260
San Juan	7,140,000	5,324,000	5,874,000	5,632,000	6,144,000	6,266,967	6,430,001
Providence	807,000	764,000	776,000	773,000	801,000	820,541	874,203
South Carolina State Program	1,387,000	1,356,000	1,387,000	1,403,000	1,491,000	1,563,881	1,708,727
Charleston	418,000	390,000	397,000	401,000	419,000	437,943	477,408
Columbia	1,270,000	1,160,000	1,041,000	1,034,000	1,138,000	1,404,470	1,566,258
Tennessee State Program	739,000	718,000	747,000	756,000	796,000	830,568	911,377
Memphis	2,134,000	1,462,000	1,882,000	1,879,000	2,115,000	2,019,277	1,701,201
Nashville	737,000	840,000	737,000	757,000	795,000	829,966	903,441
Texas State Program	2,736,000	2,634,000	2,691,000	2,733,000	2,841,000	2,625,853	2,818,502
Austin	988,000	931,000	940,000	947,000	987,000	1,029,086	1,103,927
Dallas	3,192,000	3,867,000	3,141,000	3,134,000	3,332,000	3,642,608	3,722,637
El Paso	—	—	—	—	—	327,655	355,028
Fort Worth	835,000	805,000	813,000	819,000	863,000	892,529	950,848
Houston	5,068,000	9,669,000	6,039,000	6,579,000	6,038,000	7,315,504	7,793,944
San Antonio	1,027,000	960,000	971,000	972,000	1,025,000	1,064,378	1,151,125
Utah State Program	120,000	111,000	112,000	111,000	115,000	117,707	126,975
Salt Lake City	386,000	354,000	353,000	346,000	357,000	363,348	387,189
Virginia State Program	640,000	612,000	618,000	615,000	634,000	667,943	703,999
Richmond	692,000	658,000	665,000	660,000	690,000	702,433	774,169
Virginia Beach	1,022,000	958,000	941,000	937,000	968,000	1,002,215	1,079,493
Washington State Program	652,000	619,000	620,000	622,000	651,000	671,553	728,016
Seattle	1,688,000	1,611,000	1,615,000	1,604,000	1,663,000	1,705,852	1,821,710

Table A-1. (Continued).

MSA, State, or Territory	FY2004	FY2005	FY2006	FY2007	FY2008	FY2009	FY2010
Wisconsin State Program	405,000	383,000	389,000	391,000	407,000	422,102	455,271
Milwaukee	512,000	487,000	497,000	492,000	515,000	531,988	574,936
West Virginia State Program	—	—	—	—	—	309,608	336,232
—Subtotal formula grants	263,039,000	251,323,000	256,162,000	256,162,000	267,417,000	276,089,000	298,485,000
—Subtotal competitive grants	29,227,000	27,925,000	28,463,000	28,463,000	29,713,000	30,676,000	33,165,000
—Subtotal technical asst.	2,485,000	2,480,000	1,485,000	1,485,000	1,485,000	1,485,000	3,350,000
Total HOPWA	294,751,000	281,728,000	286,110,000	286,110,000	300,100,000	310,000,000	335,000,000

Source: U.S. Department of Housing and Urban Development, Office of Community Planning and Development. Program Formula Allocations, http://www.hud.gov/offices/cpd/about/budget/budget10/index.cfm, and the Office of Community Planning and Development Appropriations Budget page, http://www.hud.gov/offices/cpd/about/budget/index.cfm.

a) The State of California administers the grant for the Bakersfield and Fresno MSAs (See FY2011 HUD Congressional Budget Justifications, p. Z-12).
b) According to directions in HUD Appropriations Acts, funds awarded to the Wilmington MSA are transferred to the State of New Jersey to administer the HOPWA program for the one New Jersey county that is in the Wilmington MSA (Salem county).
c) The State of Florida administers the grants for the Cape Coral, Lakeland, and Palm Bay MSAs.
d) The State of Maryland administers the grant for the Bethesda-Frederick-Gaithersburg MSA.

End Notes

[1] Note that this represents persons living with AIDS, not a cumulative total. U.S. Department of Health and Human Services, Centers for Disease Control and Prevention, *HIV Surveillance Report 2008*, vol. 20, Atlanta, Georgia, 2010, p. 83, table 16b, http://www.cdc.gov/hiv/surveillance/resources/reports/2008report/pdf/2008 SurveillanceReport.

[2] John M. Karon, Patricia L. Fleming, Richard W. Steketee, and Kevin M. DeCock, "HIV in the United States at the Turn of the Century: An Epidemic in Transition," *American Journal of Public Health* 91, no. 7 (July 2001): 1064-1065.
See also, Paul Denning and Elizabeth DiNenno, *Communities in Crisis: Is There a Generalized HIV Epidemic in Impoverished Urban Areas of the United States?*, Centers for Disease Control and Prevention, August 2010, http://www.cdc.gov/hiv /topics /surveillance/ resources/other/pdf/poverty_poster.pdf.

[3] See, for example, D.P. Culhane, E. Gollub, R. Kuhn, and M. Shpaner, "The Co-Occurrence of AIDS and Homelessness: Results from the Integration of Administrative Databases for AIDS Surveillance and Public Shelter Utilization in Philadelphia," *Journal of Epidemiology and Community Health* 55, no. 7 (2001): 515-520. Marjorie Robertson, et al., "HIV Seroprevalence Among Homeless and Marginally Housed Adults in San Francisco," *American Journal of Public Health* 94, no. 7 (2004): 1207-1217. Angela A. Aidala and Gunjeong Lee, *Housing Services and Housing Stability Among Persons Living with HIV/AIDS*, Joseph L. Mailman School of Public Health, May 30, 2000, http://www.nyhiv.org/pdfs/chain/ CHAIN%20Housing% 20 Stability%2032.pdf

[4] Daniel P. Kidder, Richard J. Wolitski, and Scott Royal, et al., "Access to Housing as a Structural Intervention for Homeless and Unstably Housed People Living with HIV: Rational, Methods, and Implementation of the Housing and Health Study," *AIDS and Behavior*, vol. 11, no. 6 (November 2007, supplement), pp. 149-150.

[5] Angela Aidala, Jay E. Cross, Ron Stall, David Harre, and Esther Sumartojo, "Housing Status and HIV Risk Behaviors: Implications for Prevention and Policy," *AIDS and Behavior* 9, no. 3 (2005): 251-265.

[6] Ibid., p. 254.

[7] Daniel P. Kidder, Richard J. Wolitski, and Sherri L. Pals, et al., "Housing Status and HIV Risk Behaviors Among Homeless and Housed Persons with HIV," *Journal of Acquired Immune Deficiency Syndromes*, vol. 49, no. 4 (December 1, 2008), pp. 453-454.

[8] Ibid., p. 452.

[9] The second interim report was released on April 24, 1990. Its recommendations were reprinted in National Commission on Acquired Immune Deficiency Syndrome, *Annual Report to the President and Congress*, August 1990, pp. 106-109.

[10] Individuals living with HIV/AIDS have experienced housing discrimination even though they are protected as persons with a "handicap" under the Fair Housing Act (FHA). 42 U.S.C. §§ 3601-3631. A number of court cases have established that the definition of "handicap" protects persons who are HIV positive and persons with AIDS. See, for example, *Baxter* v. *City of Belleville, Ill.*, 720 F.Supp. 720, 729-730 (S.D.Ill.1989), and *Support Ministries for Persons With AIDS, Inc.* v. *Village of Waterford, N.Y.*, 808 F.Supp. 120, 129-133 (N.D.N.Y. 1992).

[11] Hearing before the House Committee on Banking, Finance, and Urban Affairs, Subcommittee on Housing and Community Development, "Housing Needs of Persons with Acquired Immune Deficiency Syndrome," March 21, 1990, (hereafter Hearing on Housing Needs). See also, Statement of Representative James A. McDermott, 135 Cong. Rec. 23641, October 5, 1989.

[12] Hearing on Housing Needs, pp. 25-30. See footnote 11.

[13] U.S. Congress, House Committee on Banking, Finance, and Urban Affairs, *Housing and Community Development Act of 1990*, report to accompany H.R. 1180, 101st Cong., 2nd sess., June 21, 1990, H.Rept. 101-559.

[14] The law is codified at 42 U.S.C. §§ 12901-12912, with regulations at 24 C.F.R. Parts 574.3-574.655.

[15] The others are the Community Development Block Grant, the Emergency Shelter Grants, and HOME.

[16] MSAs are defined as having at least one "urbanized" area of 50,000 or more and "adjacent territory that has a high degree of social and economic integration with the core as measured by commuting ties." See Office of Management and the Budget Bulletin 10-02, "Update of Statistical Area Definitions and Guidance on Their Uses," December 1, 2009, Appendix, p. 2, http://www.whitehouse.gov/omb/assets/bulletins/b10-02.pdf.

[17] 42 U.S.C. § 12903(c)(1)(A).

[18] AIDS incidence is measured as the number of new AIDS cases during a given time period.

[19] 42 U.S.C. § 12903(c)(1)(B).

[20] 42 U.S.C. § 12903(f).

[21] 24 C.F.R. § 574.3.

[22] U.S. Department of Housing and Urban Development, *2010 HOPWA Formula Operating Instructions*, April 1, 2010, p. 2, http://www.hudhre.info/documents/ 2010 Operating_ Formula.pdf.

[23] U.S. Department of Housing and Urban Development, Office of Community Planning and Development, Formula Allocations for FY2010, http://www.hud.gov/offices /cpd/about/budget/ budget10/index.cfm.

[24] The states that have retained funding under this provision are Arizona, Connecticut, Delaware, Hawaii, Massachusetts, Minnesota, Nevada, Oklahoma, and Utah. See U.S. Department of Housing and Urban Development, *Congressional Justifications for FY2011*, p. Z-12, http://hud.gov/offices/cfo/reports/2011 /cjs/hofpwAIDS2011.pdf (hereinafter, *FY2011 Congressional Budget Justifications*).

[25] 42 U.S.C. § 12903(c)(3).

[26] Ibid.

[27] See, for example, U.S. Department of Housing and Urban Development, "FY2008 Notice of Funding Availability Housing Opportunities for Persons with AIDS," 73 *Federal Register* 27266, May 12, 2008.

[28] See HUD's website, http://www.hud.gov/offices/adm/grants/nofa09/grphopwa.cfm.

[29] *FY2011 Congressional Budget Justifications*, p. Z-13.

[30] The HOPWA statute defines an eligible person as one "with acquired immunodeficiency syndrome or a related disease." 42 U.S.C. § 12902(12). The regulations have further specified that "acquired immunodeficiency syndrome or related diseases means the disease of acquired immunodeficiency syndrome or any conditions arising from the etiologic agent for acquired immunodeficiency syndrome, including infection with the human immunodeficiency virus (HIV)." 24 C.F.R. § 574.3.

[31] 42 U.S.C. § 12908 and § 12909. The statutory provisions regarding short-term housing and community residences do not require individuals to be low income, although to be eligible for short-term housing a person must be homeless or at risk of homelessness. See 42 U.S.C. § 12907 and § 12910.

[32] U.S. Department of Housing and Urban Development, Office of Policy Development and Research, *Fiscal Year 2010 HUD Income Limits Briefing Material*, May 13, 2010, p. 1, http://www.huduser.org/portal /datasets/il/il10/ IncomeLimitsBriefingMaterial_FY10.pdf. Tables showing area median incomes in recent years are available at http://www.huduser.org/datasets/il.html.

[33] 24 C.F.R. § 574.310(e).

[34] For more information about housing for persons with disabilities and the definitions of disability under these programs, see CRS Report RL34728, *Section 811 and Other HUD Housing Programs for Persons with Disabilities*, by Libby Perl.

[35] 42 U.S.C. § 1437a(b)(3).

[36] 42 U.S.C. § 12910.

[37] 42 U.S.C. § 12907.

[38] HOWPA funds may only be used for construction of community residences and single-room occupancy dwellings. See 24 C.F.R. § 574.300(b)(4).

[39] 42 U.S.C. § 12908.

[40] See 24 C.F.R. § 574.310(d).

[41] 42 U.S.C. § 12909.

[42] 24 C.F.R. § 574.300(b)(7).

[43] 42 U.S.C. § 12906.

[44] 24 C.F.R. § 574.300(b)(1).

[45] *FY2011 Congressional Budget Justifications*, p. Z-4.

[46] Ibid, p. Z-3.

[47] U.S. Government Accountability Office, *Changes Needed to Improve the Distribution of Ryan White CARE Act and Housing Funds*, GAO-06-332, February 2006, p. 23, http://www.gao.gov/new.items/d06332.pdf.

[48] Ibid., p. 24.

[49] U.S. Department of Housing and Urban Development, *Congressional Justifications for FY2009*, p. Q-2, http://www.hud.gov/offices/cfo/reports/2009/cjs/cpd1.pdf.

[50] *FY2010 Congressional Budget Justifications*, p. X-13.

[51] U.S. Government Accountability Office, *HUD's Program for Persons with AIDS*, GAO/RCED-97-62, March 1997, p. 27, http://www.gao.gov/archive/1997/rc97062.pdf.

[52] Ryan White CARE Act Amendments of 1996, P.L. 104-146. In 2006, when the Ryan White HIV/AIDS program was reauthorized as part of the Ryan White HIV/AIDS Treatment Modernization Act of 2006 (P.L. 109-415), the formula began to incorporate living HIV cases in addition to living AIDS cases.

[53] See U.S. Congress, House Committee on Appropriations, Subcommittee on VA, HUD, and Independent Agencies, *Departments of Veterans Affairs and Housing and Urban Development and Independent Agencies Appropriations Bill*, report to accompany H.R. 2158, 105th Cong., 1st sess., July 11, 1997, H.Rept. 105-175, pp. 33-34.

[54] U.S. Department of Housing and Urban Development, *1999 Report on the Performance of the Housing Opportunities for Persons with AIDS Program*, October 6, 1999 (hereafter *1999 HUD Report*).

[55] For example, researchers who analyzed data from 25 states found that from 1996 to 2005, average life expectancy after HIV diagnosis increased from 10.5 to 22.5 years. See Kathleen McDavid Harrison, Ruiguang Song, and Xinjian Zhang, "Life Expectancy after HIV Diagnosis Based on National HIV Surveillance Data from 25 States, United States," *Journal of Acquired Immune Deficiency Syndromes*, vol. 53, no. 1 (January 2010), pp. 124-130.

[56] HUD provides estimates of the numbers of households served in its annual Performance and Accountability Reports. The most recent is the *FY2009 Performance and Accountability Report*, November 16, 2009, p. 349, http://www.hud.gov/offices/cfo/reports/hudfy2009par.pdf.

[57] For more information about the Ryan White program, see CRS Report RL33279, *The Ryan White HIV/AIDS Program*, by Judith A. Johnson.

[58] 42 U.S.C. § 300ff-14(d)(1) and § 300ff-22(c)(1). At the time that HHS established its housing policy, the statute stated that funds could be used "for the purpose of delivering or enhancing HIV-related outpatient and ambulatory health and support services, including case management and comprehensive treatment services ..." The statute was amended to read as stated in the text of this report as part of the Ryan White HIV/AIDS Treatment Modernization Act of 2006, P.L. 109-415.

[59] Policy Notice 99-02 is reproduced in U.S. Department of Health and Human Services, Health Resources and Services Administration, *Housing is Health Care: A Guide to Implementing the HIV/AIDS Bureau (HAB) Ryan White CARE Act Housing Policy*, 2001, p. 3, ftp://ftp.hrsa.gov/hab/housingmanualjune.pdf (hereinafter, *Housing is Health Care*).

[60] *Housing is Health Care*, p. 7. See footnote 59.

[61] The program was reauthorized in the Ryan White HIV/AIDS Treatment Modernization Act of 2006 (P.L. 109-415). See Section 105.

[62] U.S. Department of Health and Human Services, "HIV/AIDS Bureau Policy Notice 99-02," 71 *Federal Register* 70781, December 6, 2006.

[63] U.S. Department of Health and Human Services, "HIV/AIDS Bureau Policy Notice 99-02 Amendment #1," 73 *Federal Register* 10260-10261, February 26, 2008.

[64] U.S. Department of Health and Human Services, Health Resources and Services Administration, "HIV/AIDS Bureau: Policy Notice 99-02 Amendment #1," 75 *Federal Register* 6672-6673, February 10, 2010.

[65] Ibid.

[66] Information provided to CRS by HRSA on December 4, 2008.

[67] U.S. Department of Health and Human Services, Health Resources and Services Administration, *Ryan White HIV/AIDS Program Annual Data Summary*, 2006, p. P11.

[68] *National HIV/AIDS Strategy for the United States*, July 13, 2010, p. 28, http://www.whitehouse.gov/sites/default/files/uploads/NHAS.pdf.

[69] Ibid., pp. 27-28.

[70] Angela A. Aidala, Gunjeong Lee, and David M. Abramson, et al., "Housing Need, Housing Assistance, and Connection to HIV Medical Care," *Aids and Behavior*, vol. 11, no. 6 (November 2007, supplement), pp. S101-S115.

[71] The statistical significance of the likelihood varied among the models used. See Table 3, pp. S110-S111 for significance.

[72] Findings were statistically significant in all but one of six models—continuity of appropriate HIV medical care.

[73] The methodology of the study is described in Daniel P. Kidder, Richard J. Wolitski, and Scott Royal, et al., "Access to Housing as a Structural Intervention for Homeless and Unstably Housing People Living with HIV: Rationale, Methods, and Implementation of the Housing and Health Study," *AIDS and Behavior*, vol. 11, no. 6 (November 2007, supplement), pp. 149-161.

[74] Richard J. Wolitski, Daniel P. Kidder, and Sherri L. Pals, et al., "Randomized Trial of the Effects of Housing Assistance on the Health and Risk Behaviors of Homeless and Unstably Housing People Living with HIV," *AIDS and Behavior*, vol. 14, no. 3 (2010), pp. 493-503.

[75] David Buchanan, Romina Kee, and Laura S. Sadowski, et al., "The Health Impact of Supportive Housing for HIVPositive Homeless Patients: A Randomized Controlled Trial," *American Journal of Public Health*, vol. 99, no. S3 (November 2009), pp. S675-S680.

[76] Laura S. Sadowski, Romina A. Kee, and Tyler J. VanderWeele, et al., "Effects of a Housing and Case Management Program on Emergency Department Visits and Hospitalizations Among Chronically Ill Homeless Adults," *Journal of the American Medical Association*, vol. 301, no. 17 (May 6, 2009), pp. 1775-1776.

In: Responding to HIV/AIDS
Editor: Lawrence T. Jensen

ISBN 978-1-61324-618-4
©2011 Nova Science Publishers, Inc.

Chapter 6

FEDERAL AND STATE EFFORTS TO IDENTIFY INFECTED INDIVIDUALS AND CONNECT THEM TO CARE[*]

The United States Government Accountability Office

ABBREVIATIONS

AETC	AIDS Education and Training Centers
AIDS	acquired immunodeficiency syndrome
CARE Act	Ryan White Comprehensive AIDS Resources Emergency Act of 1990
CDC	Centers for Disease Control and Prevention
HAART	highly active antiretroviral therapy
HHS	Department of Health and Human Services
HIV	human immunodeficiency virus
HMO	health maintenance organization
HRSA	Health Resources and Services Administration
NASTAD	National Alliance of State and Territorial AIDS Directors
NHIS	National Health Interview Survey
STD	sexually transmitted disease

WHY GAO DID THIS STUDY

Of the estimated 1.1 million Americans living with HIV, not all are aware of their HIV-positive status. Timely testing of HIV-positive individuals is important to improve health outcomes and to slow the disease's transmission. It is also important that individuals have access to HIV care after being diagnosed, but not all diagnosed individuals are receiving such care.

---

[*] This is an edited, reformatted and augmented version of The United States Government Accountability Office publication 09-985, dated September, 2009.

The Centers for Disease Control and Prevention (CDC) provides grants to state and local health departments for HIV prevention and collects data on HIV. In 2006, CDC recommended routine HIV testing for all individuals ages 13- 64. The Health Resources and Services Administration (HRSA) provides grants to states and localities for HIV care and services.

GAO was asked to examine issues related to identifying individuals with HIV and connecting them to care. This report examines: 1) CDC and HRSA's coordination on HIV activities and steps they have taken to encourage routine HIV testing; 2) implementation of routine HIV testing by select state and local health departments; 3) available information on CDC funding for HIV testing; and 4) available data on the number of HIV-positive individuals not receiving care for HIV. GAO reviewed reports and agency documents and analyzed CDC, HRSA, and national survey data. GAO interviewed federal officials, officials from nine state and five local health departments chosen by geographic location and number of HIV cases, and others knowledgeable about HIV.

WHAT GAO FOUND

The Secretary of Health and Human Services (HHS) is required to ensure that HHS agencies, including CDC and HRSA, coordinate HIV programs to enhance the continuity of prevention and care services. CDC and HRSA have coordinated to assist health care professionals who provide HIV-related services. For example, in 2007 and 2008, CDC provided funding to HRSA to expand consultation services at the National HIV/AIDS Clinicians' Consultation Center. Both CDC and HRSA have taken steps to encourage routine HIV testing—that is, testing all individuals in a health care setting without regard to risk. For example, CDC has funded initiatives on routine HIV testing and HRSA has provided for training as part of these initiatives.

Officials from over half of the 14 selected state and local health departments in GAO's review reported implementing routine HIV testing in their jurisdictions. However, according to officials we interviewed, those that implemented it generally did so at a limited number of sites. Officials from most of the selected health departments and other sources knowledgeable about HIV have identified barriers that exist to implementing routine HIV testing, including lack of funding and legal barriers.

CDC officials estimated that approximately 30 percent of the agency's annual HIV prevention funding is spent on HIV testing. For example, according to CDC officials, in fiscal 2008, this would make the total amount spent on HIV testing about $200 million out of the $652.8 million CDC allocated for domestic HIV prevention to its Division of HIV/AIDS Prevention. However, CDC officials said that they could not provide the exact amount the Division spends on HIV testing, because they do not routinely aggregate how much all grantees spend on a given activity, including HIV testing.

CDC estimated that 232,700 individuals with HIV were undiagnosed—that is, unaware that they were HIV positive—in 2006, and were therefore not receiving care for HIV. CDC has not estimated the total number of diagnosed HIV-positive individuals not receiving care, but has estimated that 32.4 percent, or approximately 12,000, of HIV-positive individuals diagnosed in 2003 did not receive care for HIV within a year of diagnosis. State-level estimates of the number of undiagnosed and diagnosed HIV-positive individuals not receiving care for HIV are not available from CDC. HRSA collects states' estimates of the number of diagnosed individuals not receiving care, but data are not consistently collected or reported by states, and therefore estimates are not available for comparison across all states.

HHS provided technical comments on a draft of this report, which GAO incorporated as appropriate.

September 23, 2009
The Honorable Michael B. Enzi
Ranking Member
Committee on Health, Education, Labor, and Pensions United States Senate
The Honorable Richard Burr United States Senate
The Honorable Tom A. Coburn United States Senate
The Honorable Lisa Murkowski United States Senate

It has been more than 28 years since the first cases of acquired immunodeficiency syndrome (AIDS) in the United States were reported in June 1981. Since that time, approximately 1.7 million Americans have been infected with human immunodeficiency virus (HIV), including more than 580,000 who have died.[1] The most recent data available from the Department of Health and Human Services' (HHS) Centers for Disease Control and Prevention (CDC) estimates that there were 1.1 million people living with HIV in the United States at the end of 2006, and that 56,300 new HIV infections occurred that year.[2]

Not all of those living with HIV are aware of their HIV-positive status. Timely testing of individuals who are HIV positive but have not yet been diagnosed is important both in improving health outcomes for those individuals and in slowing transmission of the disease. Research has shown that the earlier individuals are treated for HIV the better their prognosis becomes. In addition, many individuals who know that they are HIV positive adopt behaviors that reduce their risk of spreading the disease, while those who are unaware of their status are more likely to pass HIV on to others. According to CDC, it has been estimated that the majority of new HIV infections are transmitted from individuals who are unaware of their status.

Testing for HIV can occur in health care settings,[3] such as public health clinics, private doctors' offices, health maintenance organizations (HMO), and emergency rooms, or in non-health care settings, such as community-based organizations.[4] According to data from the 2007 National Health Interview Survey (NHIS), less than 40 percent of adults in the United States reported having ever been tested for HIV.[5] Further, CDC estimates that in 2006, 36 percent of those who were diagnosed with HIV were not tested until late in the course of their disease, meaning that they were diagnosed with AIDS within 1 year of receiving an HIV-positive result. A number of studies have shown that late testing can occur after HIV-positive individuals have made numerous visits to health care settings, indicating missed opportunities to test for HIV.

HIV testing is the first step to connecting HIV-positive individuals to the care that they need. Connecting HIV-positive individuals to care can occur through, for example, assistance in scheduling appointments and by providing transportation to and from appointments. It is also important to ensure that individuals have access to and remain in care after they have been diagnosed. New advances in HIV treatments have reduced mortality rates and have the potential to extend the lives of individuals diagnosed with HIV. However, not all diagnosed HIV-positive individuals are accessing care options.

CDC provides funding to state and local health departments for HIV prevention, including counseling, testing, and referral services, through cooperative agreements, grants, and contracts.[6] CDC also provides funding to community-based organizations and a smaller amount to national professional organizations such as the National Medical Association. In addition to providing funding, CDC conducts research, surveillance, and epidemiologic studies on HIV.[7] CDC has also issued a series of recommendations related to HIV testing in health care settings, the most recent of which were released in 2006.[8] A major component of the 2006 recommendations is for all health care settings to test all individuals for HIV without regard to risk—a practice called routine HIV testing.[9] This represents a significant change from prior CDC guidance, which generally recommended that health care settings target testing to groups at high risk of contracting HIV or to high-prevalence areas.[10] Additionally, CDC has identified the requirement for separate written informed consent or pretest counseling as barriers to routine HIV testing.[11] While the 2006 recommendations suggest these practices not be required for HIV testing, there is some disagreement over whether this would take away important protections. States and localities are not required to adopt CDC's recommendations, and state HIV testing laws vary. For example, according to a study on state HIV testing laws, some states' laws require separate written informed consent for HIV testing and others do not.[12]

While CDC is the federal agency primarily responsible for HIV prevention, HHS' Health Resources and Services Administration (HRSA) is the agency responsible for administering grant programs authorized by the Ryan White Comprehensive AIDS Resources Emergency Act of 1990 (CARE Act) and subsequent legislation that provide funding to states, localities, and others for HIV-related services. The CARE Act was enacted to address the needs of jurisdictions, health care providers, and people with HIV and their family members.[13] Each year, assistance to over 530,000 mostly low-income, underinsured, or uninsured individuals living with HIV is provided through CARE Act programs. The 2006 reauthorization of CARE Act programs, like the 2000 reauthorization, required states to submit an estimate of the size and demographics of the population with HIV within the state and a determination of those who have HIV but are not receiving HIV-related services. HRSA characterizes this as an unmet need estimate, that is, the number of individuals in a state who know their HIV-positive status but who are not receiving care for HIV.[14] In addition to administering CARE Act programs, HRSA provides training to health care providers and community service workers who work with people with HIV and evaluates best-practice models of health care delivery.

Given their respective roles in funding HIV prevention and care, CDC and HRSA have coordinated on HIV activities in the past. Additionally, the CARE Act requires the Secretary of HHS to ensure that HHS agencies, including CDC and HRSA, coordinate HIV programs to enhance the continuity of prevention and care services for individuals with HIV or those at risk of the disease.[15]

As Congress prepares to reauthorize CARE Act programs, you asked us to examine various issues related to identifying and caring for individuals with HIV. In this report, we examine: (1) the actions taken by CDC and HRSA since 2006 to coordinate on HIV-related activities, and steps the agencies have taken to encourage implementation of routine HIV testing; (2) the extent to which select state and local health departments have implemented routine HIV testing in their jurisdictions and what barriers exist to its implementation; (3) available information on how much of CDC's HIV prevention funding is spent on HIV testing;[16] (4) national data on the types of settings where HIV tests are conducted and the types of settings where HIV-positive results occur; (5) available data on national and state estimates of the number of undiagnosed and diagnosed HIV-positive individuals who are not receiving care for HIV; and (6) what barriers exist to care for HIV and what initiatives are being implemented to connect diagnosed HIV-positive individuals to such care. In this report, we also provide information on transitioning prisoners with HIV to care upon their release. This information is provided in appendix I.[17]

To examine the actions taken by CDC and HRSA to coordinate on HIV-related activities, and steps the agencies have taken to encourage implementation of routine HIV testing, we reviewed reports that describe programs administered by the two agencies. We also reviewed meeting minutes from the CDC/HRSA Advisory Committee on HIV and Sexually Transmitted Diseases (STD) Prevention to identify HIV activities coordinated by CDC and HRSA. In addition, we interviewed officials at CDC and HRSA as well as a judgmental sample of officials from 14 state and local health departments knowledgeable about these topics.[18] We selected health departments based on their geographic location and the number of HIV cases in their jurisdiction. Our sample is not generalizable to all state and local health departments.

To examine the extent to which select state and local health departments have implemented routine HIV testing in their jurisdictions and what barriers exist to its implementation, we interviewed our sample of officials from state and local health departments as well as officials from the Henry J. Kaiser Family Foundation, the National Alliance of State and Territorial AIDS Directors (NASTAD), and other organizations that work on HIV-related issues, including an organization that contracts with state and local health departments to coordinate HIV-related issues and an association for HIV providers. We also reviewed medical journal articles and reports by the Henry J. Kaiser Family Foundation and NASTAD on the implementation of routine testing. We did not conduct a state-by-state review of all laws related to HIV testing or independently verify information related to state laws.

To examine available information on how much of CDC's HIV prevention funding is spent on HIV testing, we reviewed CDC budget information and interviewed officials at CDC.

To examine national data on the types of settings where HIV tests are conducted, we examined NHIS data from 2007 on the number of HIV tests conducted by setting type. We performed data reliability checks by testing for missing data and outliers and compared our results to published data on this topic and determined that these data were sufficiently reliable for our purposes. To examine available data on the types of settings where HIV-positive results occur, we obtained and reviewed 2007 CDC surveillance data on the number of HIV-positive results by facility of diagnosis. We reviewed related documentation and interviewed agency officials and determined these data were sufficiently reliable for our purposes.

To examine available data on national and state estimates of the number of undiagnosed and diagnosed HIV-positive individuals who are not receiving care for HIV, we reviewed CDC surveillance data and the unmet need estimates reported by CARE Act grantees to HRSA. We also obtained and reviewed information from CDC and HRSA on how these estimates are calculated. We reviewed related documentation and interviewed agency officials to determine if national- and state-level data were reliable for our purposes. We determined that national data on undiagnosed HIV-positive individuals not receiving care were sufficiently reliable for our purposes. We also determined that national data on the number of diagnosed HIV-positive individuals not receiving care were reliable, but not comprehensive. Finally, we determined that state-level data on the number of diagnosed HIV-positive individuals not receiving care are not consistently collected or reported across states, and therefore were not reliable for our purposes.

To examine what barriers exist to care for HIV and what initiatives are being implemented to connect diagnosed HIV-positive individuals to such care, we interviewed officials at CDC and HRSA and our sample of officials from state and local health departments.

We conducted this performance audit from April 2009 through September 2009 in accordance with generally accepted government auditing standards. Those standards require that we plan and perform the audit to obtain sufficient, appropriate evidence to provide a reasonable basis for our findings and conclusions based on our audit objectives. We believe that the evidence obtained provides a reasonable basis for our findings and conclusions based on our audit objectives.

BACKGROUND

According to 2007 NHIS data, fewer than 40 percent of adults in the United States reported ever having been tested for HIV. In a recent survey by the Henry J. Kaiser Family Foundation, the primary reason people gave for not being tested is that they do not think they are at risk.[19] The second most common reason was that their doctor never recommended HIV testing. While 38 percent of adults said that they had talked to their doctor about HIV, only 17 percent said that their doctor had suggested an HIV test. According to this survey, African Americans and Latinos were more likely than adults overall to have had such a conversation with their doctor and for the doctor to have suggested testing. Sixty-seven percent of African Americans and 45 percent of Latinos said that they had talked to their doctor about HIV and 29 percent of African Americans and 28 percent of Latinos said that their doctor had suggested an HIV test.

Technological advances have increased the benefits associated with HIV testing as well as with regular care and treatment for HIV. First, advances in testing methods, such as rapid HIV tests, have made testing more feasible in a variety of different settings and increased the likelihood that individuals will receive their results. Rapid tests differ from conventional HIV tests in that results are ready sometime from immediately after the test is performed to 20 minutes after the test is performed, which means that individuals can get tested and receive their results in the same visit.[20] Second, the advent of highly active antiretroviral therapy (HAART) has transformed HIV from a fatal disease to a treatable condition.[21] For example, a 25-year-old individual who is in care for HIV can expect to live only 12 years less than a 25-year-old individual who does not have HIV.

In addition, studies have found that people generally reduce risky behaviors once they learn of their HIV-positive status. According to one study, people who are unaware that they are HIV positive are 3.5 times more likely to transmit the disease to their partners than people who know their status.[22] At the same time, research has shown that individuals are often unaware of their status until late in the course of the disease despite visits to health care settings. For example, one study looked at HIV case reporting in a state over a 4-year period. The study found that of people who were diagnosed with HIV late in the course of the disease, 73 percent made at least one visit to a health care setting prior to their first reported positive HIV test, and the median number of prior visits was four.[23]

FUNDING FOR HIV TESTING

Funding for HIV testing can come from insurance reimbursement by private insurers as well as Medicaid and Medicare, although these payers do not cover HIV testing under all circumstances.[24] Funding for HIV testing can also come from other government sources, such as CDC, CARE Act programs, or state and local funding. A study by CDC and the Henry J. Kaiser Family Foundation that looked at the insurance coverage of individuals at the time of their HIV diagnosis from 1994-2000 found that 22 percent were covered by Medicaid, 19 percent were covered by other public-sector programs, and 27 percent were uninsured.

The cost of an HIV test varies based on a number of factors, including the type of test performed, the test result, and the amount of counseling that is associated with the test. For example, from a payer's perspective, the costs of a rapid HIV test are higher for someone who is HIV positive than for someone who is not, primarily because rapid testing requires an initial rapid test and a confirmatory test when the result is positive with counseling conducted after both tests. Additionally, eliminating pretest counseling can lower the cost of HIV testing by about $10, regardless of the type of test. According to the most recent data available from CDC, in 2006, the cost of an HIV test could range from $10.16 to $86.84 depending on these and other factors.

CDC HIV TESTING RECOMMENDATIONS

CDC issued its first recommendations for HIV testing in health care settings in 1987. These recommendations focused on individuals engaged in high-risk behaviors and specifically recommended that people who were seeking treatment for STDs be tested for HIV on a routine basis. Throughout the 1990s and 2000s CDC updated these recommendations periodically to reflect new information about HIV. For example, in 2001, CDC modified its recommendations for pregnant women to emphasize that HIV testing should be a routine part of prenatal care and that the testing process should be simplified to eliminate barriers to testing, such as requiring pretest counseling.[25] CDC's 2001 recommendations also recommended that HIV testing be conducted routinely in all health care settings with a high prevalence of HIV; in low-prevalence settings it was recommended that HIV testing be conducted based on an assessment of risk. In 2003, CDC introduced a new initiative called "Advancing HIV Prevention: New Strategies for a Changing Epidemic." The initiative had a number of strategies, including two that specifically applied to health care settings: (1) making HIV testing a routine part of medical care; and (2) further reducing perinatal transmission of HIV by universally testing all pregnant women and by using HIV rapid tests during labor and delivery or postpartum if the mother had not been tested previously.

Elements of the Advancing HIV Prevention initiative were incorporated into CDC's revised HIV testing recommendations for heath care settings in 2006.[26] The 2006 recommendations represent a major shift from prior recommendations for health care settings in that they no longer base HIV testing guidelines on risk factors. Rather, they recommend that routine HIV testing be conducted for all patients ages 13 through 64 in all health care settings on an opt-out basis.[27] CDC also recommends that persons at high risk of HIV be tested annually; that general consent for medical care encompass consent for HIV testing (i.e., separate written consent is not necessary); and that pretest information, but not pretest counseling be required.[28]

CDC HIV AND AIDS SURVEILLANCE

According to CDC, tracking the prevalence of HIV is necessary to help prevent the spread of the disease. CDC's surveillance system consists of case counts submitted by states on the number of HIV and AIDS diagnoses, the number of deaths among persons with HIV, the number of persons living with HIV or AIDS, and the estimated number of new HIV infections. HIV laboratory tests, specifically CD4 or viral load tests, can be used to determine the stage of the disease, measure unmet health care needs among HIV-infected persons, and evaluate HIV testing and screening activities.[29]

Current CDC estimates related to HIV are not based on data from all states because not all states have been reporting such data by name long enough to be included in CDC's estimates. While all states collect AIDS case counts through name-based systems, prior to 2008 states collected HIV data in one of two different formats, either by name or by code.[30] CDC does not accept code-based case counts for counting HIV cases because CDC does not consider them to be accurate and reliable, primarily because they include duplicate case counts. In order for CDC to use HIV case counts from a state for CDC's estimated diagnoses of HIV infection, the name-based system must be mature, meaning that the state has been reporting HIV name-based data to CDC for 4 full calendar years. CDC requires this time period to allow for the stabilization of data collection and for adjustment of the data in order to monitor trends. In its most recent surveillance report, CDC used the name-based HIV case counts from 34 states and 5 territories and associated jurisdictions in its national estimates.[31] Name-based HIV reporting had been in place in these jurisdictions since the end of 2003 or earlier.

THE CARE ACT

Under the CARE Act, approximately $2.2 billion in grants were made to states, localities, and others in fiscal year 2009. Part A of the CARE Act provides for grants to selected metropolitan areas that have been disproportionately affected by the HIV epidemic to provide care for HIV-positive individuals. Part B provides for grants to states and territories and associated jurisdictions to improve quality, availability, and organization of HIV services. Part A and Part B base grants are determined by formula based on the number of individuals living with HIV and AIDS in the grantee's jurisdiction.[32] For the living HIV/AIDS case counts HRSA used to determine fiscal year 2009 Part A and Part B base grants, see appendices II and III. Part C provides for grants to public and private nonprofit entities to provide early intervention services, such as HIV testing and ambulatory care.[33] Part F provides for grants for demonstration and evaluation of innovative models of HIV care delivery for hard-to-reach populations, training of health care providers, and for Minority AIDS Initiative grants.[34]

Since the 2006 reauthorization of CARE Act programs, HRSA has placed an emphasis on states' unmet need, which is the number of individuals in a state's jurisdiction who know they are HIV positive but who are not receiving care for HIV. According to the framework used by HRSA, addressing unmet need is a three-step process. First, states are required to produce an unmet need estimate, which is submitted to HRSA on the state's annual Part B grant application.[35] To calculate the unmet need, the state must determine the total number of individuals who are aware of their HIV positive status in their jurisdiction, and then subtract the number of individuals who are receiving care for HIV.[36] Second, the state must assess the service needs and barriers to care for individuals who are not receiving care for HIV, including finding out who they are and where they live. Third, the state must address unmet need by connecting these individuals to care.

CDC AND HRSA HAVE COORDINATED ON HIV ACTIVITIES TO ASSIST HEALTH CARE PROFESSIONALS, AND BOTH AGENCIES HAVE TAKEN STEPS TO ENCOURAGE ROUTINE HIV TESTING

CDC and HRSA have coordinated on activities to assist health care professionals who provide HIV-related services. HRSA has encouraged routine HIV testing by providing for training for health care providers, as part of CDC-funded initiatives. CDC has taken other steps to encourage routine HIV testing by funding special initiatives that focus on certain populations.

CDC AND HRSA HAVE COORDINATED ACTIVITIES TO ASSIST HEALTH CARE PROFESSIONALS WHO PROVIDE HIV-RELATED SERVICES

Since 2006, CDC and HRSA have coordinated activities to assist health care professionals who provide HIV-related services. In 2007, CDC and HRSA initiated a clinic-based research study to develop, implement, and test the efficiency and effectiveness of an intervention designed to increase client appointment attendance among patients at risk of missing scheduled appointments in HIV clinics, "Increasing Retention in Care among Patients Being Treated for HIV Infection." An interagency agreement outlined the responsibilities of CDC and HRSA with respect to the study.[37] For example, under the agreement, CDC is responsible for maintaining data gathered from the study and HRSA is responsible for presenting their findings at national and international conferences. Each agency provided $1.3 million for the study in fiscal year 2009 and will continue to provide funds for the study until its final year of operation in 2011.

In coordination with a federal interagency work group, CDC and HRSA have also participated in the development and publication of a document for case managers who work with individuals with HIV.[38] The document, "Recommendations for Case Management Collaboration and Coordination in Federally Funded HIV/AIDS Programs," outlines best practices for, and six recommended components of, HIV case management for federally funded HIV case management agencies.[39] The document also describes how case management is practiced in different settings and methods for strengthening linkages among case management programs.[40] CDC and HRSA were the lead authors of the document and shared staff time and production expenses. The agencies published the document in February 2009.

CDC also provided HRSA with funding to expand HIV consultation services offered to health care professionals at the National HIV/AIDS Clinicians' Consultation Center. The National HIV/AIDS Clinicians' Consultation Center is a component of the HRSA-administered AIDS Education and Training Centers (AETC) program.[41] The Consultation Center operates hotline systems to provide consultation to health care professionals, including the PEPline and Perinatal Hotline. Health care professionals access the PEPline to receive information on post-exposure management for health care professionals exposed to blood-borne pathogens and the Perinatal Hotline for information on treatment and care for HIV-diagnosed pregnant women and their infants. CDC provided HRSA with $169,000 to support the PEPline and Perinatal Hotline in fiscal year 2007 and $90,000 to support the PEPline in fiscal year 2008. In addition, CDC provided HRSA with $180,000 during fiscal years 2007 and 2008 for the enhancement of existing consultation services at the Consultation Center for health care professionals who expand HIV testing and need assistance in managing a resulting increase in patients who are HIV positive.

In addition, CDC and HRSA have coordinated to prevent duplication of HIV training provided to health care professionals. The CDC-funded National Network of STD/HIV Prevention Training Centers, HRSA-funded AETCs, and other federal training centers, participate in the Federal Training Centers Collaboration to ensure that HIV training opportunities are not duplicated among the centers.[42] The agencies hold biennial national meetings to increase training coordination of STD/HIV prevention and treatment, family planning/reproductive health, and substance abuse prevention to maximize the use of training resources.[43]

In addition to coordinating on HIV activities that assist health care professionals, CDC and HRSA have participated in the CDC/HRSA Advisory Committee on HIV and STD Prevention and Treatment. The Advisory Committee was established by the Secretary of HHS in November 2002 to assess HRSA and CDC objectives, strategies, policies, and priorities for HIV and STD prevention and care and serves as a forum to discuss coordination of HIV activities. The committee meets twice a year and is comprised of 18 individuals who are nominated by the HHS Secretary to serve 2- to 4-year terms and are knowledgeable in such public health fields as epidemiology, infectious diseases, drug abuse, behavioral science, health care delivery and financing, state health programs, clinical care, preventive health, and clinical research. The members assess the activities administered by HRSA and CDC, including HIV testing initiatives and training programs, and make recommendations for improving coordination between the two agencies to senior department officials, including the HHS Secretary. Officials from CDC and HRSA regularly attend the meetings to present current HIV initiatives administered by their agencies.

Officials from 6 of the 14 state and local health departments we interviewed said that CDC and HRSA coordination on HIV activities could be improved. For example, officials from 3 of these health departments attributed the lack of coordination to differing guidelines CDC and HRSA use for their grantees. Officials from 1 health department stated that although they have the same desired outcome, CDC and HRSA do not always coordinate on activities that they fund. They noted that the two agencies have inconsistent policies for HIV-related activities, such as confidentiality guidelines and policies for data sharing. Officials from another health department stated that the two agencies could improve coordination on HIV testing and guidelines for funding HIV testing initiatives.

HRSA HAS ENCOURAGED ROUTINE HIV TESTING BY PROVIDING FOR TRAINING FOR HEALTH CARE PROVIDERS AS PART OF CDC-FUNDED INITIATIVES

Since the release of CDC's 2006 routine HIV testing recommendations, HRSA has encouraged routine HIV testing by providing for training for health care providers, as part of CDC-funded initiatives. CDC and HRSA developed interagency agreements through which CDC provided $1.75 million in 2007 and $1.72 million in 2008 to HRSA-funded AETCs to develop curricula, training, and technical assistance for health care providers interested in implementing CDC's 2006 routine HIV testing recommendations.[44] As of June 2008, AETCs had conducted over 2,500 training sessions to more than 40,000 health care providers on the recommendations.

HRSA provided for training during CDC-funded strategic planning workshops on routine HIV testing for hospital staff. CDC officials said that in 2007, the agency allocated over $900,000 for workshops in eight regions across the country on implementing routine HIV testing in emergency departments. CDC reported that 748 attendees from 165 hospitals participated in these workshops. HRSA-funded AETCs from each of the eight regions provided information on services they offer hospitals as they prepare to implement routine HIV testing, and also served as facilitators during the development of hospital-specific strategic plans.

In addition, HRSA provided for training as part of a CDC-funded pilot project to integrate routine HIV testing into primary care at community health centers. HRSA officials said that their primary role in this project, called "Routine HIV Screening within Primary Care in Six Southeastern Community Health Centers," was to provide for training on routine HIV testing and to ensure that HIV-positive individuals were connected to care, and that CDC provided all funding for the project. CDC officials told us that the first phase of the project funded routine HIV testing in two sites in Mississippi, two sites in South Carolina, and two sites in North Carolina. The CDC officials said that in 2008 four sites in Ohio were added and that these sites are receiving funding through CDC's Expanded HIV Testing initiative. CDC officials said that they plan to start a second phase of the project with additional testing sites.

CDC HAS TAKEN OTHER STEPS TO ENCOURAGE ROUTINE HIV TESTING

CDC has taken other steps to encourage routine HIV testing by funding special initiatives that focus on certain populations. In 2007, CDC initiated a 3-year project for state and local health departments called the "Expanded and Integrated Human Immunodeficiency Virus (HIV) Testing for Populations Disproportionately Affected by HIV, Primarily African Americans" initiative or the Expanded HIV Testing initiative. In the first year of the initiative, CDC awarded just under $35 million to 23 state and local health departments that had an estimated 140 or more AIDS cases diagnosed among African Americans in 2005. Individual awards were proportionately based on the number of cases, with amounts to each jurisdiction ranging from about $700,000 to over $5 million. Funding after the first year of the initiative was to be awarded to departments on a noncompetitive basis assuming availability of funds and satisfactory performance.[45] Funding for the second year of the initiative was just over $36 million and included funding for 2 additional health departments, bringing the total number of funded departments to 25.

CDC asked health departments participating in the Expanded HIV Testing initiative to develop innovative pilot programs to expand testing opportunities for populations disproportionately affected by HIV— primarily African Americans—who are unaware of their status. CDC required health departments to spend all funding on HIV testing and related activities, including the purchase of HIV rapid tests and connecting HIV-positive individuals to care. CDC strongly encouraged applicants to focus at least 80 percent of their pilot program activities on health care settings, including settings to which CDC had not previously awarded funding for HIV testing, such as emergency rooms, inpatient medical units, and urgent care clinics. Additionally, CDC required that programs in health care settings follow the agency's 2006 routine HIV testing recommendations to the extent permitted by law. Programs in non-health care settings were to have a demonstrated history of at least a 2 percent rate of HIV-positive test results.

The 2006 reauthorization of CARE Act programs included a provision for the Early Diagnosis Grant program under which CDC would make HIV prevention funding for each of fiscal years 2007 through 2009 available to states that had implemented policies related to routine HIV testing for certain populations.[46] These policies were (1) voluntary opt-out testing of all pregnant women and universal testing of newborns or (2) voluntary opt-out testing of patients at STD clinics and substance abuse treatment centers.[47] CDC's fiscal year 2007 appropriation prohibited it from using funding for Early Diagnosis grants. In fiscal year 2008, CDC's appropriation provided up to $30 million for the grants. CDC officials told us that in 2008, the agency awarded $4.5 million to the six states that had implemented at least one of the two specified policies as of December 31, 2007. In fiscal year 2009, CDC's appropriation provided up to $15 million for grants to states newly eligible for the program.[48] CDC officials said that in 2009, one state received funding for implementing voluntary opt-out testing at STD clinics and substance abuse treatment centers.[49] CDC officials also told us that they provided HRSA with information on how the Early Diagnosis Grant program would be implemented, but have not coordinated with the agency on administration of the program.

MOST SELECTED STATE AND LOCAL HEALTH DEPARTMENTS REPORTED NOT WIDELY IMPLEMENTING ROUTINE HIV TESTING IN THEIR JURISDICTIONS AND BARRIERS EXIST TO ITS IMPLEMENTATION

Officials from just over half of the state and local health departments we interviewed said that their departments had implemented routine HIV testing in their jurisdictions, but that they generally did so in a limited number of sites. Officials from most of the health departments we interviewed and other sources knowledgeable about HIV have identified barriers to routine HIV testing, including lack of funding.

OVER HALF OF THE SELECTED STATE AND LOCAL HEALTH DEPARTMENTS REPORTED IMPLEMENTING ROUTINE HIV TESTING IN THEIR JURISDICTIONS, BUT GENERALLY DID SO IN A LIMITED NUMBER OF SITES

Officials from 9 of the 14 state and local health departments we interviewed said that their departments had implemented routine HIV testing, but 7 said that they did so in a limited number of sites. Specifically, officials from 5 of the state health departments we interviewed said that their departments had implemented routine HIV testing in anywhere from one to nine sites and officials from 2 of the local health departments said that their departments had implemented it in two and four sites, respectively. Officials from all but 1 of these 7 departments said that their departments used funding from CDC's Expanded HIV Testing initiative to implement routine HIV testing.[50] CDC's goal for its Expanded HIV Testing initiative is to test 1.5 million individuals for HIV in areas disproportionately affected by the disease and identify 20,000 HIV-infected persons who are unaware of their status per year. During the first year of the initiative,[51] health departments that received funding under the CDC initiative reported conducting just under 450,000 HIV tests and identifying approximately 4,000 new HIV-positive results.[52]

The two other health departments that had implemented routine HIV testing—one state health department and one local health department located in a large city—had been able to implement routine HIV testing more broadly. These departments had implemented routine HIV testing prior to receiving funding through the Expanded HIV testing initiative, and used the additional funding to expand the number of sites where it was implemented. For example, the local health department had started an initiative to achieve universal knowledge of HIV status among residents in an area of the city highly affected by HIV. The department used funding from the Expanded HIV Testing initiative and other funding sources to implement routine HIV testing in this area and other sites throughout thecity, including 20 emergency rooms. An official from the state health department said that while the department had already funded routine HIV testing in some settings, for example STD clinics and community health centers, funding from the Expanded HIV Testing initiative allowed them to fund routine HIV testing in other types of settings, for example emergency rooms.

Officials from five health departments we interviewed said that their departments had not implemented routine HIV testing in their jurisdictions, including three state health departments and two local health departments. None of these health departments received funding through CDC's Expanded HIV Testing initiative, and officials from two of the state health departments specifically cited this as a reason why they had not implemented routine HIV testing. Officials from all of the departments that had not implemented routine HIV testing said that their departments do routinely test certain populations for HIV, including pregnant women, injection drug users, and partners of individuals diagnosed with HIV.

OFFICIALS FROM SELECTED STATE AND LOCAL HEALTH DEPARTMENTS AND OTHER SOURCES HAVE IDENTIFIED BARRIERS THAT EXIST TO IMPLEMENTING ROUTINE HIV TESTING

Officials from 11 of the 14 state and local health departments we interviewed and other sources knowledgeable about HIV have identified barriers that exist to implementing routine HIV testing. Officials from 5 of the 11 health departments cited lack of funding as a barrier to routine HIV testing. For example, an official from 1 state health department told us that health care providers have said that they would do routine HIV testing if they could identify who would pay for the cost of the tests. The need for funding was corroborated by officials from an organization that contracts with state and local health departments to coordinate HIV-related care and services. These officials told us that they had often seen routine HIV testing end when funding streams dried up and noted that there has been little implementation of CDC's 2006 routine HIV testing recommendations in their area outside of STD clinics and programs funded through the Expanded HIV Testing initiative.

Officials from state and local health departments we interviewed and other sources also cited lack of insurance reimbursement as a barrier to routine HIV testing. When identifying lack of funding as a barrier to routine HIV testing, officials from two state health departments we interviewed explained that there is a general lack of insurance reimbursement for this purpose. Other organizations we interviewed and CDC also raised the lack of insurance reimbursement for routine HIV testing as a barrier. For example, one provider group that we spoke with said that many providers are hesitant to offer HIV tests without knowing whether they will be reimbursed for it. In a recent presentation, CDC reported that out of 11 insurance companies, as of May 2009, all covered targeted HIV testing,[53] but only 6 reimbursed for routine HIV testing.[54] CDC also reported that as of this same date only one state required that insurers reimburse for HIV tests regardless of whether testing is related to the primary diagnosis.[55] CDC noted that legislation similar to this state's has been introduced, but not passed, in two other states as well as at the federal level.

Medicare does not currently reimburse for routine HIV testing, though the Centers for Medicare & Medicaid Services initiated a national coverage analysis as the first step in determining whether Medicare should reimburse for this service.[56] While federal law allows routine HIV testing as a covered service under Medicaid, individual states decide whether or not they will reimburse for routine HIV testing. According to one study, reimbursement for routine HIV testing has not been widely adopted by state Medicaid programs.[57] Many insurers, including Medicare and Medicaid, base their reimbursement policies on the recommendations of the U.S. Preventive Services Task Force, which is the leading independent panel of private-sector experts in prevention and primary care.[58] While the Task Force has recommended that clinicians conduct routine HIV testing when individuals are at increased risk of HIV infection and for all pregnantwomen, it has not made a recommendation for routine HIV testing when individuals are not at increased risk, saying that the benefit in this case is too small relative to the potential harms.[59]

In addition, officials from three state health departments we interviewed discussed legal barriers to implementing routine testing. For example, officials from one department said that implementation of routine HIV testing would require a change in state law to eliminate the requirement for pretest counseling and written informed consent. Similarly, officials from another department said that while their department had been able to conduct routine testing through the Expanded HIV Testing initiative, expanding it further might require changing state law to no longer require written informed consent for HIV testing. The officials explained that while the initiative did have a written informed consent form, the department had been able to greatly reduce the information included on the form in this instance. The department is currently in the process of looking for ways to further expand HIV testing without having to obtain changes to state law. According to a study published in the Annals of Internal Medicine, as of September 2008, 35 states' laws did not present a barrier to implementing routine HIV testing, though the 3 states discussed above were identified as having legal barriers.[60]

Officials from 3 of the state and local health departments we interviewed discussed operational barriers to integrating routine HIV testing with the policies and practices already in place in health care settings. For example, an official from a state health department said that the department tries to work past operational barriers to routine HIV testing, but if after 6 months the barriers prove too great in one site the department moves implementation of routine HIV testing to another site. An official from another state health department noted that in hospital settings it can take a long time to obtain approval for new protocols associated with routine HIV testing. NASTAD conducted a survey of the 25 state and local health departments that received funding through the Expanded HIV Testing initiative and found that health departments reported some barriers in implementing routine HIV testing, including obtaining buy-in from staff in health care settings and providing adequate training, education, and technical assistance to this staff. Other barriers mentioned by officials from health departments we interviewed included health care providers not being comfortable testing everyone for HIV and the ability of providers to provide care for the increased number of people who might be diagnosed through expanded HIV testing.

CDC OFFICIALS ESTIMATED THAT ABOUT 30 PERCENT OF THE AGENCY'S ANNUAL HIV PREVENTION FUNDING IS SPENT ON HIV TESTING

CDC officials estimated that approximately 30 percent of the agency's annual HIV prevention funding is spent on HIV testing. For example, according to CDC officials, in fiscal year 2008 this would make the total amount spent on HIV testing about $200 million out of the $652.8 million CDC allocated for domestic HIV prevention to its Division of HIV/AIDS Prevention.61 Of the $200 million CDC officials estimated was spent on testing, CDC did report that, in fiscal year 2008, $51.1 million was spent on special HIV testing initiatives, such as the Expanded HIV testing initiative and the Early Diagnosis Grant program.[62]

CDC officials said that, outside of special testing initiatives, they could not provide the exact amount CDC spent on HIV testing. CDC's Division of HIV/AIDS Prevention spends the majority of its domestic HIV prevention budget in connection with cooperative agreements, grants, and contracts to state and local health departments and other funded entities. CDC officials explained that grantees submit reports to CDC on the activities they fund at the middle and end of the year. The officials said that while project officers check to see that these reports are consistent with how grantees planned to spend their funding, CDC does not routinely aggregate how much all grantees spent on a given activity, including HIV testing. In addition, outside of the Expanded HIV Testing initiative, CDC does not maintain data on how funds for HIV testing are distributed to different settings within jurisdictions. For example, this would mean that CDC does not have data on how much money a state health department spends on testing in emergency rooms, versus how much money it spends on testing in community-based organizations.

NATIONAL DATA SUGGEST THAT MOST HIV TESTS AND NEARLY HALF OF HIV-POSITIVE RESULTS OCCUR IN A PRIVATE DOCTOR'S OFFICE, HMO, OR HOSPITAL SETTING, BUT THE DATA ON SETTINGS WHERE PEOPLE TEST POSITIVE HAVE LIMITATIONS

According to data from NHIS, nearly 70 percent of all HIV tests in the United States were conducted in a private doctor's office, HMO, or hospital setting in 2007. Specifically, 50 percent of all HIV tests were conducted in a private doctor's office or HMO and nearly 20 percent of all HIV tests were conducted in a hospital setting, including emergency departments. The remaining tests were conducted in a variety of settings, including public clinics and HIV counseling and testing sites. Less than 1 percent of all HIV tests were conducted in a correctional facility, STD clinic, or a drug treatment facility. These data are similar to earlier data from NHIS. In 2002, NHIS found that 44 percent of all HIV tests were conducted in a private doctor's office or HMO and 22 percent of all HIV tests were conducted in a hospital setting.

Analysis of CDC surveillance data on the settings in which HIV-positive individuals are diagnosed suggests that approximately 40 percent of all HIV-positive results in the United States occurred in a private doctor's office, HMO, or hospital setting in 2007,[63] the most recent year for which data were available.[64] These data also suggest that hospital inpatient settings account for a disproportionate number of HIV-positive results discovered late in the course of the disease. In 2007, hospital inpatient settings accounted for 16 percent of all HIV-positive results. Among HIV cases diagnosed in 2006, these same settings accounted for 31 percent of HIV-positive results that occurred within 1 year of an AIDS diagnosis.

While CDC surveillance data can provide some indication of the types of settings where the greatest percentage of HIV-positive results occur, data limitations did not permit a more detailed analysis of HIV-positive results by setting type. Specifically, information on facility of diagnosis was missing or unknown for nearly one out of every four HIV cases reported through the surveillance system in 2007.[65] CDC officials told us that in the past the agency used data from the Supplement to HIV/AIDS Surveillance project to examine the types of settings where individuals test positive for HIV, but this project ended in 2004.[66] CDC reported that in place of the Supplement to HIV/AIDS Surveillance project, the agency has implemented the Medical Monitoring Project.[67] However, data from the Medical Monitoring Project were not available at the time of our analysis.[68]

A NATIONAL ESTIMATE OF THE NUMBER OF UNDIAGNOSED HIV- POSITIVE INDIVIDUALS IS AVAILABLE, BUT AN ESTIMATE IS NOT AVAILABLE FOR THE TOTAL NUMBER OF DIAGNOSED INDIVIDUALS NOT RECEIVING CARE NATIONALLY AND NEITHER ESTIMATE IS AVAILABLE AT THE STATE LEVEL

CDC has calculated a national estimate of more than 200,000 undiagnosed HIV-positive individuals—that is, individuals who were unaware they are HIV positive and were therefore not receiving care for HIV. CDC estimated that 232,700 individuals, or 21 percent of the 1.1 million people living with HIV at the end of 2006, were unaware that they were HIV positive.[69]

CDC does not have a national estimate of the total number of diagnosed individuals not receiving care, but CDC has calculated a national estimate of more than 12,000 diagnosed HIV-positive individuals who did not receive care within a year after they were diagnosed with HIV in 2003. CDC reported that the estimated proportion of individuals with HIV who did not receive care within a year of diagnosis—which CDC measures by the number of HIV-positive individuals who did not have a reported CD4 or viral load test within this time—was 32.4 percent, or 12,285 of the 37,880 individuals who were diagnosed with HIV in 2003.[70] Since this estimate is based on the number of HIV-positive individuals who did not receive care within a year of diagnosis, this estimate does not include all individuals diagnosed with HIV who are not receiving care. For example, an individual may receive care within a year of diagnosis, but subsequently drop out of care 2 years later. Or an individual may receive care 2 years after diagnosis. In these examples, the individuals' change in status as receiving care or not receiving care is not included in CDC's estimate of the proportion of diagnosed individuals not receiving care.

Although CDC has published these estimates, the agency has noted limitations to the data used to calculate the number of diagnosed HIV-positive individuals not receiving care for

HIV. First, not all states require laboratories to report all CD4 and viral load test results; without this information being reported, CDC's estimates may overstate the number of individuals who did not enter into care within 1 year of HIV diagnosis.[71] Additionally, in the past, CDC only required jurisdictions to report an individual's first CD4 or viral load test, which did not allow CDC to provide an estimate of all HIV-positive individuals who are not receiving care for HIV after the first year. CDC is currently disseminating updated data collection software which will permit the collection and reporting of all results collected by states. However, CDC officials told us that this software is still going through quality control checks.

While CDC calculates national estimates of the number of undiagnosed HIV-positive individuals not receiving care for HIV and the number of diagnosed HIV-positive individuals who did not receive care within a year of diagnosis, the agency does not calculate these estimates at the state level. CDC officials said that these estimates are not available at the state level because not all states have mature name-based HIV reporting systems.[72] CDC officials said that the agency is determining what it will need to estimate the number of undiagnosed individuals at the state level once all states have mature HIV reporting systems. CDC officials also said that once the new data collection software to collect CD4 and viral load test results from states is ready, data on all diagnosed HIV-positive individuals not receiving care may be available at the state level for those states with mature name-based HIV reporting systems with laboratory reporting requirements.[73]

HRSA also collects states' estimates of the number of diagnosed HIV-positive individuals not receiving care for HIV, but data are not consistently collected or reported by states, and therefore estimates are not available for comparison across all states. States report their estimates of the number of diagnosed HIV-positive individuals who are not receiving care as unmet need estimates to HRSA as a part of the states' CARE Act Part B grant applications. However, these estimates have limitations and are not comparable across states. One limitation is that not all states require laboratory reporting of CD4 and viral load results for all individuals who receive the tests. States use reported CD4 and viral load test results to calculate their unmet need, and, according to HRSA, without data for all individuals who receive CD4 or viral load tests, a state may overestimate its unmet need. Another limitation is that the estimates submitted in the states' fiscal year 2009 grant applications were calculated using differing time periods. For example, New Hampshire calculated its unmet need estimate using HIV cases collected as of December 31, 2004, while Colorado calculated its estimate using data collected as of June 30, 2008. Additionally, not all states have access to information on the number of individuals receiving care through private insurance; therefore, these individuals are counted as part of the state's unmet need.

OFFICIALS WE INTERVIEWED IDENTIFIED BARRIERS TO CARE THAT EXIST FOR HIV, BUT AGENCIES HAVE IMPLEMENTED INITIATIVES TO CONNECT HIV-POSITIVE INDIVIDUALS TO CAR

According to officials we interviewed, several barriers exist that could prevent HIV-positive individuals from receiving care. HRSA officials told us that structural barriers within the health care system, such as no or limited availability of services, inconvenient service locations and clinic hours, and long wait times for appointments can influence whether an individual is receiving care for HIV. Other barriers identified by HRSA officials are the quality of communication between the patient and provider, lack of or inadequate insurance, financial barriers, mental illness, and substance abuse. HRSA officials also noted that personal beliefs, attitudes, and cultural barriers such as racism, sexism, homophobia, and stigma can also have an impact on an individual's decision to seek care. Officials from two states and one local health department we spoke with stated that transportation was a barrier, while officials from two state health departments stated that lack of housing was a barrier for access to care. Unstable housing can prevent individuals with HIV from accessing health care and adhering to complex HIV treatments because they must attend to the more immediate need of obtaining shelter.[74]

Agencies have implemented initiatives to connect diagnosed individuals to care for HIV. For example, part of CDC's Expanded HIV Testing initiative focused on connecting individuals diagnosed with HIV to care. In the first year of the initiative, 84 percent of newly diagnosed patients received their HIV test results and 80 percent of those newly diagnosed were connected to care. CDC has also funded two studies that evaluated a case management intervention to connect HIV-positive individuals to care for HIV. In these studies, case management was conducted in state and local health departments and community-based organizations and included up to five visits with a case manager over a 3-month period. In one of these studies, 78 percent of individuals who participated in case management were still in care 6 months later.

HRSA has developed two initiatives as Special Projects of National Significance.[75] The first initiative, "Enhancing Access to and Retention in Quality HIV Care for Women of Color," was developed to implement and evaluate the effectiveness of focused interventions designed to improve timely entry and retention into quality HIV care for women of color. The second initiative, the "Targeted HIV Outreach and Intervention Model Development" initiative, was a 5-year, 10-site project implemented to bring underserved HIV-positive individuals into care for HIV. According to HRSA, results of the initiative indicated that individuals are less likely to have a gap of 4 months or more of care when they have had nine or more contacts with an outreach program within the first 3 months of these programs.

In collaboration with AIDS Action, an advocacy organization formed to develop policies for individuals with HIV, HRSA has also funded the "Connecting to Care" initiative. AIDS Action and HRSA developed the initiative to highlight successful methodologies to help connect or reconnect individuals living with HIV to appropriate and ongoing medical care. The methodologies were identified from cities across the country and are being utilized in different settings. The initiative includes two publications with 42 interventions that have been reported to be successful in connecting HIV-positive individuals to care. The publications provide a description, logistics, strengths and difficulties, and outcomes of each intervention and focus specifically on homeless individuals, Native Americans, immigrant women, low-income individuals in urban and rural areas, and currently or formerly incarcerated individuals. AIDS Action has held training workshops that provided technical assistance to explain the interventions, including how to apply the best practices from successful programs.

HRSA provides grants under Part C of the CARE Act to public and private nonprofit entities to provide early intervention services to HIV-positive individuals on an outpatient basis that can help connect people to care. Part C grantees are required to provide HIV medical care services that can include outpatient care, HIV counseling, testing, and referral, medical evaluation and clinical care, and referrals to other health services. These programs also provide services to improve the likelihood that undiagnosed individuals will be identified and connected to care, such as outreach services to individuals who are at risk of contracting HIV, patient education materials, translation services, patient transportation to medical services, and outreach to educate individuals on the benefits of early intervention.

HRSA and CDC are currently collaborating on a clinic-based research study, "Increasing Retention in Care among Patients Being Treated for HIV Infection." The study is designed to develop, implement, and test the efficacy of an intervention intended to increase appointment attendance among individuals at risk of missing scheduled appointments in HIV clinics.

In addition to CDC and HRSA initiatives, officials we interviewed told us that state and local health departments have implemented their own initiatives to connect HIV-positive individuals to care. Officials from six states and five local health departments we spoke with stated that their departments use case management to assist HIV-positive individuals through the process of making appointments and to help address other needs of the individuals. For example, officials from one of these health departments explained that some case managers sign up qualified individuals for an AIDS Drug Assistance Program and others assist with locating housing or with substance abuse issues, which can also be barriers to staying in care. Case managers make sure individuals are staying in care by finding patients who have missed appointments or who providers have been unable to contact. In addition, officials from one state and four local health departments we spoke with told us that their departments use mental health professionals and officials from one state and three local health departments told us that their departments use substance abuse professionals to connect individuals to care, since individuals who need these services are at a high risk of dropping out of care. Officials from two health departments said that their departments use counseling and officials from one health department said that partner counseling is conducted when an individual is diagnosed with HIV. HHS provided technical comments on a draft of the report, which we incorporated as appropriate.

APPENDIX I. INFORMATION ON TRANSITIONING PRISONERS WITH HIV TO CARE UPON THEIR RELEASE

U.S. federal prisons have become a principal screening and treatment venue for thousands of individuals who are at high risk for human immunodeficiency virus (HIV) or who have HIV.[1] According to a 2008 report by the Bureau of Justice Statistics, the overall rate of estimated confirmed acquired immune deficiency syndrome (AIDS) cases among the prison population (.46 percent) was more than 2.5 times the rate of the general U.S. population at the end of calendar year 2006.[2] The Bureau of Justice Statistics also reported that 1.6 percent of male inmates and 2.4 percent of female inmates in state and federal prisons were known to be HIV positive. To ensure that infected individuals are aware of their HIV-positive status and to ensure that they receive care while in prison, 21 states tested all inmates for HIV at admission or at some point during their incarceration. Forty-seven states and all federal prisons tested inmates if they had HIV-related symptoms or if they requested an HIV test.

The Ryan White Comprehensive AIDS Resources Emergency Act of 1990 (CARE Act) was enacted to address the needs of jurisdictions, health care providers, and people with HIV and their family members.[3] CARE Act programs have been reauthorized three times (1996, 2000, and 2006) and are scheduled to be reauthorized again in 2009.[4] The CARE Act Amendments of 2000 required the Health Resources and Services Administration (HRSA) to consult with the Department of Justice and others to develop a plan for the medical case management and provision of support services to individuals with HIV when they are released from the custody of federal and state prisons. The plan was to be submitted to Congress no later than 2 years after the date of enactment of the CARE Act Amendments of 2000.

You asked us to review the implementation status of the plan and to determine the extent of any continued coordination between HRSA and the Department of Justice to transition prisoners with HIV to CARE Act programs. However, HRSA officials told us that they did not create this plan or coordinate with the Department of Justice to create this plan. Additionally, the requirement for this plan was eliminated by the 2006 Ryan White Treatment Modernization Act. We are therefore providing information related to other steps that HRSA has taken to address the provision of HIV prevention and care for incarcerated persons with HIV transitioning back to the community and into CARE Act funded programs. Additionally, we provide information on steps taken by the Centers for Disease Control and Prevention (CDC) and states to address this issue.[5]

To provide information related to the steps that CDC and HRSA have taken to address the provision of HIV prevention and care for incarcerated persons, we interviewed CDC and HRSA officials. We also interviewed officials from nine state health departments about their programs for incarcerated persons with HIV transitioning back to the community and into CARE Act-funded programs, and the limitations of these programs.[6] From these nine state health departments, officials from eight states provided responses about their programs. The remaining state did not have a transition program in place. Our sample is not generalizable to all state and local health departments.

BACKGROUND

The U.S. prison system has been the focus of many studies on HIV testing for prisoners and care for those with HIV while in prison and upon their release. Studies have been conducted to determine the number of individuals who are accessing HIV testing and treatment for the first time upon their incarceration. Studies have also been conducted to evaluate how infected prisoners fare in their HIV treatment upon release from prison, as inmates often encounter social and economic changes including the need to secure employment and housing, establish connections with family, and manage mental health and substance abuse disorders. For example, one recent study of the Texas state prison system published in the Journal of the American Medical Association discussed an evaluation of the proportion of infected individuals who filled a highly active antiretroviral therapy (HAART) prescription within 10, 30, and 60 days after their release from prison, respectively.[7] The study found that 90 percent of recently released inmates did not fill a prescription for HAART therapy soon enough to avoid a treatment interruption (10 days) and more than 80 percent did not fill a prescription within 30 days of release. Only 30 percent of those released filled a prescription within 60 days. Individuals on parole and those who received assistance in completing a Texas AIDS Drug Assistance Program application were more likely to fill a prescription within 30 and 60 days.[8] Because those who discontinue HAART are at increased risk of developing a higher viral burden (resulting in greater infectiousness and higher levels of drug resistance), it is important for public health that HIV-positive prisoners continue their HAART treatment upon release from prison. CDC, HRSA, and several states we interviewed have implemented programs to aid in the transition of HIV-positive persons from prison to the community with emphasis on their continued care and treatment.

CDC, HRSA, AND STATES HAVE TAKEN STEPS TO ADDRESS THE PROVISION OF HIV PREVENTION AND CARE FOR PRISONERS WITH HIV UPON THEIR RELEASE

CDC and HRSA have funded demonstration projects to address HIV prevention and care for prisoners with HIV upon their release from incarceration. Selected state health departments and their respective state departments of corrections have coordinated to help HIV-positive prisoners in their transition back to the community.

CDC AND HRSA HAVE FUNDED DEMONSTRATION PROJECTS TO ADDRESS HIV PREVENTION AND CARE FOR PRISONERS WITH HIV AND PROVIDED GUIDANCE TO STATES REGARDING HIV-RELATED PROGRAMS

CDC and HRSA have funded various projects to address the provision of HIV prevention and care for prisoners with HIV upon their release from incarceration. CDC and HRSA have also provided guidance to states regarding HIV-related programs. The list below describes the projects and guidance.

- CDC and HRSA jointly funded a national corrections demonstration project in seven states (California, Florida, Georgia, Illinois, Massachusetts, New Jersey, and New York). This demonstration project was funded from 1999 to 2004. The goal of the demonstration project was to increase access to health care and improve the health status of incarcerated and at-risk populations disproportionately affected by the HIV epidemic. The "HIV/AIDS Intervention, Prevention, and Community of Care Demonstration Project for Incarcerated Individuals within Correctional Settings and the Community" involved jail, prison, and juvenile detention settings. The project targeted inmates with HIV, but also those with hepatitis B and hepatitis C, tuberculosis, substance abuse, and sexually transmitted diseases (STD). According to

a HRSA report, the project was able to enhance existing programs in facilities, and develop new programs both within facilities and outside of them.[9] Many states integrated lessons learned through the project at varying levels throughout their state.
- CDC funded Project START to develop an HIV, STD, and hepatitis prevention program for young men aged 18-29 who were leaving prison in 2001. The goal of this project was to test the effectiveness of the Project START interventions in reducing sexually risky behaviors for prisoners transitioning back to the community. State prisons in California, Mississippi, Rhode Island, and Wisconsin were selected. A study describing the Project START interventions indicated a multi-session community re-entry intervention can lead to a reduction in sexually risky behavior in recently released prisoners.[10]
- CDC funded a demonstration project at multiple sites in four states (Florida, Louisiana, New York, and Wisconsin) where prisoners in short-term jail facilities were offered routine rapid initial testing and appropriate referral to care, treatment, and prevention services within the facility or outside of it. From December 2003 through June 2004, more than 5,000 persons had been tested for HIV, and according to a CDC report, 108 (2.1 percent) had received confirmed positive results.[11]
- CDC officials told us that CDC is currently completing three pilot studies which began in September 2006. These studies were conducted to develop interventions for HIV-positive persons being released from several prisons or halfway houses in three states: California (prisons), Connecticut (prisons), and Pennsylvania (halfway houses).
- CDC officials explained that CDC has established a Corrections Workgroup within the National Center for HIV/AIDS, Viral Hepatitis, STD, and Tuberculosis Prevention. In March of 2009, the workgroup hosted a Corrections and Public Health Consultation: "Expanding the Reach of Prevention." This forum provided an opportunity for subject matter experts in the fields of corrections and academia as well as representatives from health departments and community-based organizations to develop effective prevention strategies for their correctional systems.
- According to a Special Projects of National Significance program update, HRSA's "Enhancing Linkages to HIV Primary Care and Services in Jail Settings" initiative seeks to develop innovative methods for providing care and treatment to HIV-positive inmates who are reentering the community.[12] This 4-year project, which began in September 2007, is different from the "HIV/AIDS Intervention, Prevention, and Co mmunity of Care Demonstration Project for Incarcerated Individuals within Correctional Settings and in the Community" in that it focuses entirely on jails. HRSA defines jails as locally operated facilities whose inmates are typically sentenced for 1 year or less or are awaiting trial or sentencing following trial. Under the initiative, HRSA has awarded grants to 10 demonstration projects in the following areas: Atlanta, Georgia; Chester, Pennsylvania; Chicago, Illinois; Cleveland, Ohio; Columbia, South Carolina; New Haven, Connecticut; New York, New York; Philadelphia, Pennsylvania; Providence, Rhode Island; and Springfield, Massachusetts.

Besides funding demonstration projects and creating workgroups, HRSA and CDC have issued guidance to states. HRSA issued guidance in September 2007 explaining allowable expenditures under CARE Act programs for incarcerated persons.[13] The guidance states that expenditures under the CARE Act are only allowable to help prisoners achieve immediate connections to community-based care and treatment services upon release from custody, where no other services exist for these prisoners, or where these services are not the responsibility of the correctional system. The guidance provides for the use of funds for transitional social services including medical case management and social support services. CARE Act grantees can provide these transitional primary services by delivering the services directly or through the use of contracts. Grantees must also develop a mechanism to report to HRSA on the use of funds to provide transitional social services in correctional settings. In 2009, CDC issued HIV Testing Implementation Guidance for Correctional Settings.[14] This guidance recommended routine opt-out HIV testing for correctional settings and made suggestions for how HIV services should be provided and how prisoners should be linked to services.[15] The guidance also addressed challenges that may arise for prison administrators and health care providers who wish to implement the guidelines in their correctional facilities.

SELECTED STATE HEALTH DEPARTMENTS HAVE COORDINATED WITH THEIR RESPECTIVE STATE DEPARTMENTS OF CORRECTIONS ON HIV-POSITIVE PRISONER TRANSITION PROGRAMS

Of the eight state health departments in our review that had HIV transition programs in place, several have implemented programs that coordinate with the state's department of corrections to provide prisoners with support services to help them in their transition back to the community. We provide examples of three of these programs below.

- Officials from one state health department said that their department uses CARE Act and state funding to provide a prerelease program that uses the state's department of corrections prerelease planners to make sure that prisoners with HIV are linked to care. Prisoners meet with their prerelease planner 60-90 days prior to release, and the planner links them to care services, has them sign up for the AIDS Drug Assistance Program and Medicaid, and follows up with them after their release to ensure that they remain in care. Additionally, the department of corrections provides 30 days of medications to prisoners upon release. The state department of health has been working with the department of corrections to help them transition HIV-positive prisoners for the past 10 years.
- According to officials from another state health department, their department uses state funds to provide transitional case management for HIV prisoners who are transitioning back into the community. Specialized medical case managers meet and counsel prisoners with HIV who are within 6 months of being released. Within 90 days of release, the prisoner and the medical case manager may meet several times to arrange housing, complete a Medicaid application, obtain referrals to HIV specialists and to the AIDS Drug Assistance Program, and provide the prisoner with assistance in obtaining a state identification card. Case managers will also work with the

prisoner for 3 months after release so that the prisoner is stable in the community. After 90 days, the person can be transferred into another case management program or they can drop out. The client is kept on the AIDS Drug Assistance Program if they are not disabled.

According to officials from a third state health department, their department uses "Project Bridge," a nationally recognized program to transition prisoners back into the community and into CARE Act programs. The Project Bridge program provides transition services to prisoners. Ninety-seven percent of the Project Bridge participants receive medical care during the first month of their release from prison. The state attributes the success of this program to the productive relationship between the state health department and the department of corrections. Project Bridge participants are involved in discharge planning with case managers starting 6 months before their discharge. Participants then receive intense case management for approximately 18-24 months after their release. During this period they are connected with medical and social services. According to state officials, the program has also been effective in decreasing recidivism rates.

Officials we interviewed from state health departments described several limitations to their departments' programs. One state health department official explained that their department does not have the staff to coordinate services for all of the state's 110 jails. Officials from two other state health departments explained that state budget cuts are threatening the continuation of their departments' prisoner transition programs. One state health department official explained that finding the transitioning HIV-positive prisoner housing in the community is often very difficult. The lack of available housing has impacted their HIV care because they are so focused on finding housing that they are unable to focus on taking their medication or going to medical appointments. One state health department official explained that their department's prisoners with HIV are sometimes not interested in being connected to care in the community. Another state health department official explained that the lack of funding for prisoner transition programs is a limitation of their program.

APPENDIX II. PART A GRANTEES' LIVING HIV/AIDS CASES USED BY HRSA TO DETERMINE FISCAL YEAR 2009 CARE ACT BASE GRANTS

Part A Grantee	HIV	AIDS	Total
Atlanta, Ga.	6,260	11,571	17,831
Austin, Tex.	1,630	2,458	4,088
Baltimore, Md.	11,901	9,488	21,389

(Continued).

Part A Grantee	HIV	AIDS	Total
Baton Rouge, La.	1,867	1,888	3,755
Bergen-Passaic, N.J.	1,858	2,190	4,048
Boston, Mass.	6,270	7,748	14,018

Part A Grantee	HIV	AIDS	Total
Caguas, P.R.	483	761	1,244
Charlotte-Gastonia, N.C.-S.C.	3,216	1,809	5,025
Chicago, Ill.	13,166	13,945	27,111
Cleveland, Ohio	2,020	2,158	4,178
Dallas, Tex.	6,589	8,346	14,935
Denver, Colo.	4,721	3,232	7,953
Detroit, Mich.	3,944	4,635	8,579
Dutchess County, N.Y.	452	803	1,255
Fort Lauderdale, Fla.	6,730	7,724	14,454
Fort Worth, Tex.	1,681	2,238	3,919
Hartford, Conn.	1,085	2,565	3,650
Houston, Tex.	8,047	10,809	18,856
Indianapolis, Ind.	1,825	1,990	3,815
Jacksonville, Fla.	2,169	2,970	5,139
Jersey City, N.J.	2,166	2,528	4,694
Kansas City, Mo.	1,953	2,390	4,343
Las Vegas, Nev.	2,968	2,763	5,731
Los Angeles, Calif.	15,106	22,431	37,537
Memphis, Tenn.	3,421	2,688	6,109
Miami, Fla.	10,877	12,988	23,865
Middlesex-Somerset-Hunterdon, N.J.	1,212	1,442	2,654
Minneapolis-St. Paul, Minn.	2,964	2,173	5,137
Nashville, Tenn.	2,036	2,215	4,251
Nassau-Suffolk, N.Y.	1,877	3,621	5,498
New Haven, Conn.	1,813	4,200	6,013
New Orleans, La.	3,397	4,006	7,403
New York, N.Y.	35,856	59,700	95,556
Newark, N.J.	6,237	6,669	12,906
Norfolk, Va.	3,329	2,353	5,682
Oakland, Calif.	2,431	4,173	6,604
Orange County, Calif.	2,370	3,662	6,032
Orlando, Fla.	3,953	4,550	8,503
Philadelphia, Pa.	9,070	13,596	22,666
Phoenix, Ariz.	4,528	3,775	8,303
Ponce, P.R.	627	1,371	1,998
Portland, Ore.	1,508	2,339	3,847
Riverside-San Bernardino, Calif.	3,167	4,686	7,853
Sacramento, Calif.	970	1,699	2,669
San Antonio, Tex.	1,711	2,568	4,279
San Diego, Calif.	5,161	6,403	11,564
San Francisco, Calif.	6,641	10,532	17,173

Part A Grantee	HIV	AIDS	Total
San Jose, Calif.	1,102	1,816	2,918
San Juan, P.R.	4,029	7,023	11,052
Santa Rosa, Calif.	415	844	1,259
Seattle, Wash.	3,099	3,914	7,013
St. Louis, Mo.	2,897	3,099	5,996
Tampa-St. Petersburg, Fla.	3,975	5,264	9,239
Vineland-Millville-Bridgeton, N.J.	375	461	836
Washington, D.C.	12,678	16,350	29,028
West Palm Beach, Fla.	2,881	4,513	7,394
Total	254,714	334,133	588,847

Source: HRSA.

Note: Fourteen Part A grantees—Baltimore, Md.; Boston, Mass.; Chicago, Ill.; Los Angeles, Calif.; Oakland, Calif.; Orange County, Calif.; Portland, Ore.; Riverside-San Bernardino, Calif.; Sacramento, Calif.; San Diego, Calif.; San Francisco, Calif.; San Jose, Calif.; Santa Rosa, Calif.; and Washington, D.C.—submitted code-based HIV case counts to HRSA for the fiscal year 2009 funding formula and were assessed a 5 percent reduction in their HIV case counts in accordance with the CARE Act. For more information, see GAO-09-894, 8-10.

APPENDIX III. PART B GRANTEES' LIVING HIV/AIDS CASES USED BY HRSA TO DETERMINE FISCAL YEAR 2009 CARE ACT BASE GRANTS

Part B Grantee	HIV	AIDS	Total
Alabama	5,702	4,164	9,866
Alaska	278	340	618
Arizona	5,949	5,180	11,129
Arkansas	2,388	2,296	4,684
California	41,730	63,187	104,917
Colorado	5,974	4,313	10,287
Connecticut	3,215	7,403	10,618
Delaware	1,259	1,813	3,072
District of Columbia	6,575	8,559	15,134
Florida	38,303	49,055	87,358
Georgia	10,883	17,447	28,330
Hawaii	845	1,251	2,096
Idaho	356	311	667

(Continued).

Part B Grantee	HIV	AIDS	Total
Illinois	15,447	16,513	31,960
Indiana	3,953	4,218	8,171

Part B Grantee	HIV	AIDS	Total
Iowa	637	912	1,549
Kansas	1,260	1,369	2,629
Kentucky	1,635	2,788	4,423
Louisiana	7,663	8,522	16,185
Maine	421	534	955
Maryland	15,793	15,029	30,822
Massachusetts	7,258	8,651	15,909
Michigan	6,177	6,900	13,077
Minnesota	3,370	2,457	5,827
Mississippi	4,575	3,570	8,145
Missouri	5,061	5,751	10,812
Montana	120	205	325
Nebraska	680	784	1,464
Nevada	3,447	3,214	6,661
New Hampshire	480	587	1,067
New Jersey	15,851	17,564	33,415
New Mexico	934	1,330	2,264
New York	44,973	73,879	118,852
North Carolina	12,812	8,718	21,530
North Dakota	83	78	161
Ohio	8,274	7,380	15,654
Oklahoma	2,259	2,333	4,592
Oregon	1,746	2,938	4,684
Pennsylvania	12,401	18,647	31,048
Puerto Rico	6,519	11,335	17,854
Rhode Island	985	1,346	2,331
South Carolina	6,591	7,604	14,195
South Dakota	209	144	353
Tennessee	7,032	6,822	13,854
Texas	25,894	34,734	60,628
Utah	932	1,206	2,138
Vermont	206	236	442
Virginia	10,092	8,573	18,665
Washington	4,420	5,734	10,154
West Virginia	662	786	1,448
Wisconsin	2,418	2,283	4,701
Wyoming	98	109	207
American Samoa	2	1	3
Commonwealth of the Northern Mariana Islands	3	3	6
Federated States of Micronesia	8	0	8

Part B Grantee	HIV	AIDS	Total
Guam	55	35	90
Palau	0	0	0
Republic of the Marshall Islands	0	1	1
U.S. Virgin Islands	235	335	570
Total	367,128	461,477	828,605

Source: HRSA.

Note: Ten Part B grantees—California, the District of Columbia, Hawaii, Illinois, Maryland, Massachusetts, Oregon, Rhode Island, Vermont, and the Federated States of Micronesia—submitted code-based HIV case counts to HRSA for the fiscal year 2009 funding formula and were assessed a 5 percent reduction in their HIV case counts in accordance with the CARE Act. For more information, see GAO-09-894, 8-10.

End Notes

[1] HIV is the virus that causes AIDS. In this report, except where noted, we use the term HIV to refer to HIV disease, inclusive of cases that have and have not progressed to AIDS. When we use the term AIDS alone it refers exclusively to HIV disease that has progressed to AIDS.

[2] CDC estimates HIV case counts based on information it receives from states, the District of Columbia, and the U.S. territories and associated jurisdictions.

[3] For the purposes of this report, we use the term setting to refer to a type of facility, for example, emergency rooms. Settings can include multiple sites. We use the term site to refer to an individual facility, for example, a specific hospital's emergency room.

[4] Community-based organizations are organizations that provide social services at the local level. 5NHIS, which has been conducted since 1957, collects information on a broad range of health topics through personal household interviews. Information on HIV testing has been included in the NHIS since 1997. The survey is one of the major data collection programs of the National Center for Health Statistics, which is part of CDC.

[6] A cooperative agreement is a mechanism used to provide financial support when substantial interaction is expected between a federal agency and a state, local government, or other funded entity. In this report, except where noted, we use the term state to include all 50 states, the District of Columbia, and the U.S. territories and associated jurisdictions.

[7] Surveillance is an ongoing, systematic collection, analysis, interpretation, and dissemination of data regarding a health-related event. CDC's HIV surveillance system observes, records, and disseminates reports about cases of HIV and AIDS.

[8] CDC has also issued HIV testing recommendations for non-heath care settings, such as community-based organizations. CDC is currently working on revising these recommendations, which were last updated in 2001. For more information on the 2001 recommendations, see CDC, "Revised guidelines for HIV counseling, testing, and referral," *Morbidity and Mortality Weekly Report*, Vol. 50, No. RR-19 (2001).

[9] These CDC recommendations apply to adults and adolescents ages 13-64 and specify that routine HIV testing should be done on an opt-out basis. Opt-out testing is a type of routine testing where a patient is notified that testing will be performed unless the patient elects to decline testing and consent is inferred unless the patient declines.

[10] CDC defines high prevalence of HIV as greater than 1 percent. However, CDC now recommends conducting routine HIV testing unless the prevalence of undiagnosed HIV infection has been shown to be less than 0.1 percent.

[11] According to CDC, informed consent is a process of communication between a patient and a health care provider through which an informed patient can choose whether to undergo HIV testing or decline to do so. CDC defines counseling as a process of assessing risk, recognizing specific behaviors that increase the risk of acquiring or transmitting HIV, and developing a plan to reduce risks.

[12] For more information on this study see, A. Mahajan, et al., "Consistency of State Statutes with the Centers for Disease Control and Prevention HIV Testing Recommendations for Health Care Settings," *Annals of Internal Medicine*, Vol. 150, No. 4 (2009). In addition, the National HIV/AIDS Clinicians' Consultation Center

[13] continuously revises and releases an online Compendium of State HIV Testing Laws. See http://www.nccc.ucsf.edu/StateLaws/Index.html.

[13] Pub. L. No. 101-381, 104 Stat. 576 (codified as amended at 42 U.S.C. §§ 300ff through 300ff-121). The 1990 CARE Act added title XXVI to the Public Health Service Act. Unless otherwise indicated, references to the CARE Act are to the current title XXVI.

[14] Pub. L. No. 106-345, § 205(a)(2), 114 Stat. 1319, 1332 (codified at 42 U.S.C. § 300ff-27(b)(2)-(3)(A)).

[15] See 42 U.S.C. § 300ff-81.

[16] Federal funding for HIV testing can come from sources other than HIV prevention funding, such as Medicaid reimbursement. Medicaid is a joint federal-state health care financing program for certain categories of low-income individuals. However, for this report, we focus exclusively on how much of CDC's HIV prevention funding is spent on testing. We focus on CDC because the agency spent more than 85 percent of the nearly $900 million that the federal government spent on domestic HIV prevention in fiscal year 2008.

[17] For additional information on the implementation of the CARE Act see GAO, *Ryan White CARE Act: Effects of Certain Funding Provisions on Grant Awards*, GAO-09-894 (Washington, D.C.: Sept. 18, 2009).

[18] We interviewed officials from nine state health departments and five local health departments. We interviewed officials from the following state health departments: California, Florida, Hawaii, Indiana, Missouri, North Carolina, Pennsylvania, Rhode Island, and Washington. We interviewed officials from the following local health departments: Harris County, Tex.; Maricopa County, Ariz.; Memphis, Tenn.; New York, N.Y.; and Sacramento County, Calif.

[19] The Henry J. Kaiser Family Foundation, *Survey Brief: Views and Experiences with HIV Testing in the U.S.* (Menlo Park, CA: June 2009).

[20] Rapid tests also do not require any special equipment and thus can be performed outside of health care settings. Rapid test results require further testing to confirm a positive test result.

[21] HAART means any combination of three or more antiretroviral drugs. While HAART has greatly improved survival rates of individuals living with HIV, there is currently no cure for the disease.

[22] G. Marks, N. Crepaz, and R.S. Janssen, "Estimating Sexual Transmission of HIV from Persons Aware and Unaware that they are Infected with the Virus in the USA," *AIDS*, Vol. 20, No. 10 (2006).

[23] CDC, "Missed Opportunities for Earlier Diagnosis of HIV Infection—South Carolina, 1997–2005," *Morbidity and Mortality Weekly Report*, Vol. 55, No. 47 (2006).

[24] Medicare is the federal health care financing program for elderly and certain disabled individuals. Medicaid is a joint federal-state health care financing program for certain categories of low-income individuals.

[25] According to CDC, many health care providers have since adopted these recommendations leading to increased prenatal screening and a 95 percent decline in perinatally acquired AIDS cases.

[26] CDC, "Revised Recommendations for HIV Testing of Adults, Adolescents, and Pregnant Women in Health-Care Settings," *Morbidity and Mortality Weekly Report*, Vol. 55, No. RR-14 (September 2006). In this report we refer to these recommendations as CDC's 2006 routine HIV testing recommendations.

[27] CDC specified that if routine testing yields a prevalence of undiagnosed HIV infection of less than 0.1 percent in a health care setting, routine testing is no longer necessary.

[28] The 2006 recommendations also included updated recommendations regarding HIV testing for pregnant women. However, for the purposes of this report we focus on HIV testing for the general population.

[29] CD4 cells help the body fight infection and are susceptible to attack by the HIV virus. A CD4 test is used to determine the number of CD4 cells in the blood to assess the functioning of the immune system. An HIV-positive individual will have a lower CD4 cell count than an individual without HIV. A viral load test measures the amount of HIV in the blood.

[30] In name-based systems, cases are collected by name, while in a code-based system cases are collected using a code identifier. Even though all states collect AIDS cases by name, some states had to transition their reporting systems for cases of HIV that have not progressed to AIDS from code to name. Due to the differences in reporting and CDC's use of these data, when we refer to name-based HIV reporting systems or the data collected through those systems, we are referring to cases of HIV that have not progressed to AIDS.

[31] The 34 states and 5 territories and associated jurisdictions that had mature name-based HIV reporting systems were: Alabama, Alaska, Arizona, Arkansas, Colorado, Florida, Georgia, Idaho, Indiana, Iowa, Kansas, Louisiana, Michigan, Minnesota, Mississippi, Missouri, Nebraska, Nevada, New Jersey, New Mexico, New York, North Carolina, North Dakota, Ohio, Oklahoma, South Carolina, South Dakota, Tennessee, Texas, Utah, Virginia, West Virginia, Wisconsin, Wyoming, American Samoa, the Commonwealth of the Northern Mariana Islands, the Commonwealth of Puerto Rico, Guam, and the U.S. Virgin Islands. See CDC, *HIV/AIDS Surveillance Report, 2007*, Vol. 19 (2009).

[32] Most other Part A and Part B grants are distributed competitively. For more information on Part A and Part B grants, see GAO-09-894, 2-4.
[33] The CARE Act also allows Part A and B grantees some flexibility to use funding for HIV testing through early intervention services.
[34] There is also a Part D, which provides for grants to private nonprofit and public entities for family-centered comprehensive care to children, youth, and women and their families, and a Part E, which does not provide for funding for HIV services, but rather includes provisions to address various administrative functions.
[35] For purposes of this report, we look only at the unmet need estimates of states that are reported in their CARE Act Part B grant applications.
[36] According to HRSA's unmet need framework, an individual diagnosed with HIV is considered to be in care if there is evidence that the individual has received a viral load test, CD4 count, or provision of antiretroviral therapy within a 12-month time frame. Reported CD4 or viral load tests can be used to determine if an individual has entered into care because these tests are monitored routinely in the clinical setting.
[37] Interagency Agreement Numbers: HAB0700301 (HRSA) and ST07-012.01(CDC), *Retaining HIV Positive Patients in Medical Care* (August 2008).
[38] The interagency work group included HRSA's HIV/AIDS Bureau; CDC's Division on HIV/AIDS Prevention; Centers for Medicare & Medicaid Services; the Substance Abuse and Mental Health Services Administration's Center for Mental Health Services; the National Institutes of Health's National Institute on Drug Abuse; the Department of Housing and Urban Development's Housing Opportunities for Persons with AIDS; and the National Association of Social Workers.
[39] HHS, *Recommendations for Case Management Collaboration and Coordination in Federally Funded HIV Programs* (Washington, D.C.: August 2008). http://www.cdcnpin.org/scripts/features/CaseManagement.pdf.
[40] In the context of HIV, case management is a process through which programs facilitate access to care, stable housing, and support services for individuals with HIV and their families.
[41] HRSA funds AETCs under Part F of the CARE Act. Specifically, HRSA provides grants to a network of 11 regional AETCs that conduct training programs for health care providers treating individuals with HIV. HRSA oversees AETCs by conducting a number of activities, including reviewing grantee progress reports, conducting site visits at AETC locations, and scheduling meetings to discuss AETCs activities.
[42] In addition to the National Network of STD/HIV Prevention Training Centers and AETCs, other organizations that participate in the Federal Training Centers Collaboration include the Regional Training Centers for Family Planning, Addiction Technology Transfer Centers, Viral Hepatitis Education and Training Projects, and Tuberculosis Regional Training and Medical Consultation Centers.
[43] The participating agencies held meetings in 2002, 2004, 2006, and 2008.
[44] Interagency Agreement Numbers: HAB0600521 (HRSA) and 07FED705251(CDC), *Training and Technical Assistance to Support the Adoption of CDC's Recommendation for HIV Testing in Health-Care Settings* (August 2007) and Interagency Agreement Numbers: HAB0700403 (HRSA) and 07FED705251-1(CDC), *Training and Technical Assistance to Support the Adoption of CDC's Recommendation for HIV Testing in Health-Care Settings* (August 2008).
[45] CDC plans to hold a new competition for the Expanded HIV Testing initiative after the first 3-year funding cycle. CDC also plans to expand the initiative to better meet the needs of the Latino population and gay and bisexual men.
[46] Pub. L. No. 109-415, § 209, 120 Stat. 2767, 2802-03 (codified at 42 U.S.C. § 300ff-33).
[47] Opt-out testing is a type of routine testing where a patient is notified that testing will be performed unless the patient elects to decline testing and consent is inferred unless the patient declines.
[48] Appropriations in 2008 and 2009 limited the amount that could be made available to any one state to $1 million.
[49] States that received funding for implementing a policy in 2008 could not receive funding for that same policy in 2009. For example, if a state received funding for implementing voluntary opt-out testing of patients at STD clinics and substance abuse treatment centers in 2008 it could not receive funding for having implemented this policy in 2009.
[50] Officials from one health department said that they funded routine HIV testing through the Early Intervention Services portion of their CARE Act Part A grant.
[51] Under the Expanded HIV Testing initiative, CDC provided funding to 23 health departments in the first year of the initiative and 2 of these departments did not report data to CDC. Two additional health departments received funding in the second year of the initiative.
[52] Though the initiative did not reach its goal in the first year, this could be related to the time it takes states and local areas to start up routine HIV testing. NASTAD officials we interviewed said that it takes time for states and local areas to build the capacity to conduct routine HIV testing, but that once the infrastructure is in place

testing can increase quickly. According to CDC, the number of tests conducted during the second half of the first year of the Expanded HIV Testing initiative was more than four times the number conducted during the first half.

[53] HIV testing is targeted when it is based on an assessment of risk.

[54] CDC, *Update on HIV Testing* (presentation given at the CDC-HRSA Advisory Committee meeting, Atlanta, GA: May 2009).

[55] Requiring insurers to reimburse for HIV testing regardless of primary diagnosis means that plans have to cover HIV testing for individuals who are asymptomatic and for whom exposure to infection is uncertain. It also requires plans to cover testing done by an emergency or urgent care service provider, even if the testing is unrelated to the reason for the visit.

[56] As a result of this analysis, on September 9, 2009, the Centers for Medicare & Medicaid Services issued a proposal to cover routine HIV testing for certain populations.

[57] L. Cheever, et al., "Ensuring Access to Treatment for HIV Infection," *Clinical Infectious Diseases*, Vol. 45, No. 4 (2007).

[58] The U.S. Preventive Services Task Force was first convened by the U.S. Public Health Service in 1984. Since 1998, the Task Force has been sponsored by HHS' Agency for Healthcare Research and Quality. According to the Agency for Health Care Research and Quality, the Task Force conducts rigorous, impartial assessments of the scientific evidence for the effectiveness of a broad range of clinical preventive services, including screening, counseling, and preventive medications. Its recommendations are considered the "gold standard" for clinical preventive services.

[59] The U.S. Preventive Services Task Force defines increased risk for HIV infection as reporting one or more individual risk factors or receiving health care in a high-prevalence or high-risk clinical setting.

[60] For more information on this study, see A. Mahajan, et al., "Consistency of State Statutes with the Centers for Disease Control and Prevention HIV Testing Recommendations for Health Care Settings," *Annals of Internal Medicine*, Vol. 150, No. 4 (2009).

[61] According to CDC officials, in fiscal year 2008 CDC allocated approximately $79 million in domestic HIV prevention funding to other divisions in the agency, including the Division of Adolescent and School Health, the Division of STD Prevention, the Division of Reproductive Health, and the Division of TB Elimination. For the purposes of this report, we focus on the Division of HIV/AIDS Prevention because it received nearly 90 percent of CDC's HIV prevention funding.

[62] Other federal agencies have also provided funding for special HIV testing initiatives. For example, HHS' Office of Population Affairs provided $10 million to 77 projects in 34 states to expand HIV testing in family planning projects over 2 years. The Substance Abuse and Mental Health Services Administration has committed $60 million from 2007-2012 to expand routine HIV testing in 22 states.

[63] CDC officials noted that the settings where HIV diagnoses are reported can sometimes differ from the settings where individuals test positive for HIV. Specifically, they said that in the 2007 surveillance data, individuals who tested positive for HIV in the emergency room were included in the HIV diagnoses reported for hospital inpatient settings.

[64] CDC surveillance data on the settings in which HIV-positive individuals were diagnosed in 2007 are from the 34 states that had mature name-based HIV reporting systems that year.

[65] CDC surveillance data also exclude states that do not have mature name-based HIV reporting systems. In 2007, 16 states and the District of Columbia did not have a mature name-based HIV reporting system, including some large states such as California and Massachusetts. In addition, name-based data do not include individuals taking an anonymous HIV test. As of April 2008, 41 states and 4 territories and ssociated jurisdictions offered anonymous testing.

[66] The Supplement to HIV/AIDS Surveillance project was a collaborative effort between CDC and 19 state and local areas that conducted cross-sectional interviews with individuals with HIV from 1990 to 2004.

[67] The Medical Monitoring Project is conducted in 23 participating project areas that are estimated to include over 80 percent of the total HIV cases in the United States.

[68] Data from the first year of CDC's Expanded HIV Testing initiative can also provide information on the types of settings where HIV-positive results occur. For example, these data suggest that HIV testing in emergency rooms may yield a disproportionate number of positive results per HIV test conducted. However, data from this initiative are not generalizable, because the types of settings funded through the initiative are not representative of the types of settings where HIV testing is conducted in the United States.

[69] CDC uses a statistical method to calculate these estimates. For more information on this method, see CDC, "HIV Prevalence Estimates—United States," *2006, Morbidity and Mortality Weekly Report*, Vol. 57, No. 39 (2008).

[70] These estimates are based on the 33 states with mature confidential name-based HIV reporting used in CDC's 2005 surveillance report. These states have had name-based HIV reporting systems in place since at least 2000. See CDC, "Reported CD4+ T-lymphocyte results for adults and adolescents with HIV/AIDS—33 states, 2005," *HIV/AIDS Surveillance Supplemental Report*, Vol. 11, No. 2 (2005).

[71] According to CDC, not all states require laboratories to report CD4 and viral load results at all levels. Individuals whose tests are not reported are included in the number of HIVpositive individuals not receiving care for HIV because CDC has no indication that theses individuals are in care. As of December 2008, 26 states, the District of Columbia, and Puerto Rico required laboratory reporting of all CD4 and viral load test results.

[72] Even though all states are collecting AIDS cases by name, some states are transitioning their reporting systems for cases of HIV that have not progressed to AIDS from code- to name-based. Due to the differences in reporting and CDC's use of these data, when we refer to name-based HIV reporting systems or the data collected through those systems, we are referring to cases of HIV that have not progressed to AIDS. Although all states and territories and associates jurisdictions, with the exception of the Federated States of Micronesia, Palau, and the Republic of the Marshall Islands, have switched to a name-based HIV reporting system, not all systems are mature. Systems are required to be mature in order to be used in CDC's surveillance estimates. All systems in which name-based HIV counts are being collected will be mature by 2012 and case counts will be available in 2014.

[73] CDC officials noted that underreporting of CD4 and viral load test results may continue to occur under the new data collection software, and additional study may be required to provide estimates of the number of diagnosed HIV-positive individuals not receiving care at the state level.

[74] See GAO, *Ryan White CARE Act: Implementation of the New Minority AIDS Initiative Provisions*, GAO-09-315 (Washington, D.C.: March 2009), 43-47.

[75] Special Projects of National Significance grants are authorized by Part F of the CARE Act. These grants fund programs to quickly respond to emerging needs and programs to develop a standard electronic data system.

End Notes for Appendix I

[1] HIV is the virus that causes acquired immune deficiency syndrome (AIDS). In this report, except where noted, we use the term HIV to refer to HIV disease, inclusive of cases that have and have not progressed to AIDS. When we use the term AIDS alone it refers exclusively to HIV disease that has progressed to AIDS.

[2] Calendar year 2006 data were the most recent data available at the time of this report. U.S. Department of Justice, Bureau of Justice Statistics, *HIV in Prisons, 2006* (Washington, D.C.: 2008). http://www.ojp.usdoj.gov/bjs/pub/html1/hivp/2006/hivp06.htm.

[3] Pub. L. No. 101-381, 104 Stat. 576 (codified as amended at 42 U.S.C. §§ 300ff through 300ff-121). The 1990 CARE Act added title XXVI to the Public Health Service Act. Unless otherwise indicated, references to the CARE Act are to the current title XXVI.

[4] CARE Act programs were previously reauthorized by the Ryan White CARE Act Amendments of 1996 (Pub. L. No. 104-146, 110 Stat. 1346), the Ryan White CARE Act Amendments of 2000 (Pub. L. No. 106-345, 114 Stat. 1319), and the Ryan White HIV/AIDS Treatment and Modernization Act of 2006 (Pub. L. No. 109-415, 120 Stat. 2767).

[5] CDC provides funding to state and local health departments for HIV prevention, including counseling, testing, and referral services, primarily through cooperative agreements and grants.

[6] We interviewed officials from the following state health departments: California, Florida, Hawaii, Indiana, Missouri, North Carolina, Pennsylvania, Rhode Island, and Washington.

[7] Highly active antiretroviral therapy (HAART) means any combination of three or more antiretroviral drugs. While HAART has greatly improved survival rates of individuals living with HIV/AIDS, there is currently no cure for the disease.

[8] J. Bailargeon, et al., "Accessing Antiretroviral Therapy Following Release from Prison," *Journal of the American Medical Association*, Vol. 301, No. 8 (2009).

[9] Department of Health and Human Services, Health Services and Resources Administration, *Opening Doors: The HRSA-CDC Corrections Demonstration Project for People Living with HIV/AIDS* (Washington, D.C.: 2007). http://hab.hrsa.gov/tools/openingdoors/index.htm.

[10] R. J. Wolitski, et al., "Relative Efficacy of a Multisession Sexual Risk–Reduction Intervention for Young Men Released from Prisons in 4 States," *American Journal of Public Health*, Vol. 96, No. 10 (2006).

[11] CDC, *Demonstration Projects for State and Local Health Departments: Routine Rapid HIV Testing of Inmates in Short-Stay Correctional Facilities* (Atlanta, GA: 2004). http://www.cdc.gov/hiv/topics/prev_prog/ahp/resources/factsheets/Correctional_Facilities.htm.

[12] Department of Health and Human Services, Health Resources and Services Administration HIV/AIDS Bureau, *What's Going on @ SPNS. Enhancing Linkages: Opening Doors for Jail Inmates* (Washington, D.C.: 2008). http://hab.hrsa.gov/special/products2g.htm.

[13] Department of Health and Human Services, Health Resources and Services Administration HIV/AIDS Bureau, *Policy Notice 07-04: The Use of Ryan White HIV/AIDS Program Funds for Transitional Social Support and Primary Care Services for Incarcerated Persons* (Washington, D.C.: 2007). http://hab.hrsa.gov/law/0704.htm.

[14] CDC, *HIV Testing Implementation Guidance for Correctional Settings* (Atlanta, GA: 2009). http://www.cdc.gov/hiv/topics/testing/resources/guidelines/correctionalsettings/index.htm.

[15] Opt-out testing is when a patient is notified that testing is a routine part of medical care and will be performed unless the patient declines.

INDEX

A

Abraham, 44, 114
abuse, 26, 110, 122, 137, 194, 202
accountability, 16, 36, 38, 48, 77, 127, 132
acculturation, 121, 138
acquired immunodeficiency syndrome, viii, 161, 166, 180, 183, 185
adolescents, 7, 24, 44, 82, 94, 96, 97, 124, 211, 215
adults, 11, 24, 33, 34, 44, 45, 90, 94, 96, 97, 110, 137, 142, 144, 185, 188, 211, 215
advocacy, 35, 51, 84, 85, 201
affirming, 35, 70
African Americans, 15, 22, 26, 32, 33, 42, 43, 68, 69, 138, 188, 194
African-American, 43, 84, 90, 99, 115, 116, 117, 118, 124
age, 2, 3, 4, 7, 20, 21, 22, 25, 27, 42, 49, 61, 77, 80, 82, 90, 108, 113, 115, 128, 136
agencies, 2, 5, 16, 19, 25, 27, 28, 35, 36, 37, 38, 48, 49, 50, 51, 52, 55, 57, 58, 59, 60, 62, 63, 64, 65, 67, 69, 70, 72, 73, 74, 75, 76, 77, 78, 80, 89, 123, 127, 128, 129, 132, 134, 154, 159, 165, 184, 186, 187, 192, 193, 213, 214
Alaska, 15, 16, 31, 43, 47, 58, 88, 90, 119, 138, 158, 209, 212
Alaska Natives, 15, 43, 58, 138
American Samoa, 88, 158, 210, 212
Americans with Disabilities Act, 34, 84, 129
antiretroviral therapy, 17, 18, 19, 25, 28, 32, 33, 41, 43, 44, 45, 98, 110, 114, 118, 124, 137, 171, 183, 213, 215
appointments, 100, 101, 102, 108, 125, 129, 185, 191, 201, 202, 207
appropriations, 142, 143, 147, 152, 154, 155, 157, 164, 165, 168, 178

assessment, 28, 76, 164, 189, 214
at-risk populations, 96, 204
awareness, 20, 82, 90

B

ban, 34, 97, 98
barriers, 23, 24, 27, 28, 90, 96, 100, 103, 105, 110, 112, 113, 118, 124, 125, 127, 130, 136, 137, 144, 148, 149, 163, 184, 186, 187, 188, 189, 191, 195, 196, 197, 200, 202
base, 3, 83, 146, 149, 151, 164, 190, 191, 197
basic needs, 4, 21, 23, 27, 28, 51, 62
behaviors, 3, 9, 13, 18, 19, 20, 24, 26, 33, 34, 42, 44, 45, 54, 93, 94, 120, 121, 132, 139, 163, 185, 188, 189, 205, 211
benchmarks, 11, 58
benefits, 20, 26, 28, 93, 104, 105, 124, 142, 144, 188, 202
bisexual men, 3, 6, 12, 13, 15, 16, 29, 30, 31, 32, 33, 41, 42, 53, 56, 67, 68, 69, 78, 82, 114, 121, 138, 139, 213
blacks, 12, 15, 29, 30, 31, 53, 67, 119, 123
blood, 8, 32, 41, 123, 192, 212
brothers, 90, 109
budget cuts, 152, 207
businesses, 1, 2, 7, 8, 10, 33, 35, 50, 61, 70, 72, 104

C

campaigns, 16, 20, 61, 95, 125
cancer, 3, 11, 27, 118
Census, 138, 144
Centers for Medicare & Medicaid Services (CMS), 37
challenges, vii, 2, 4, 6, 9, 21, 22, 23, 28, 36, 37, 39, 40, 57, 62, 67, 73, 75, 76, 80, 83, 93, 99,

103, 104, 105, 112, 117, 118, 120, 122, 130, 206
Chicago, 110, 172, 174, 205, 208, 209
children, 3, 11, 20, 93, 120, 141, 153, 213
chronic illness, 27, 124, 172
cities, 13, 82, 83, 105, 125, 141, 144, 164, 165, 201
citizens, vii, 2, 81
City, 28, 41, 83, 84, 105, 106, 115, 117, 118, 124, 129, 171, 175, 176, 177, 179, 208
civil rights, 34, 35, 68, 77, 129
clients, 21, 23, 52, 57, 60, 62, 63, 100, 102, 105, 106, 107, 112, 153, 165, 166, 167, 170
clinical practice standards, 17, 28, 76
clinical trials, 122, 132
collaboration, 5, 25, 28, 36, 38, 50, 51, 62, 63, 64, 72, 73, 76, 80, 128, 201
color, iv, 6, 82, 89, 112, 115, 116, 117, 118, 121, 201
Commonwealth of the Northern Mariana Islands, 158, 210, 212
communication, 93, 106, 129, 139, 156, 158, 201, 211
competition, 162, 165, 213
complications, 21, 23, 24, 27, 108, 111
conference, 85, 143, 163
confidentiality, 62, 193
Congress, iv, 2, 16, 36, 56, 74, 98, 129, 135, 141, 143, 148, 150, 154, 161, 163, 164, 165, 168, 169, 179, 181, 186, 203
consensus, 95, 163
consent, 186, 190, 197, 211, 213
Consolidated Appropriations Act, 142, 147, 155, 161, 169
construction, 166, 180
consumer protection, 4, 22
consumers, 80, 119, 125
cooperation, 34, 35, 70
cooperative agreements, 38, 186, 198, 215
coordination, 5, 24, 26, 35, 36, 38, 50, 51, 55, 62, 67, 72, 73, 76, 77, 78, 83, 100, 108, 109, 128, 129, 132, 153, 184, 192, 193, 203
correlation, 104, 110, 114
cost, 10, 17, 19, 21, 30, 39, 42, 44, 74, 96, 97, 101, 103, 142, 144, 145, 152, 155, 159, 189, 196
counsel, 83, 206
counseling, 25, 55, 63, 70, 94, 96, 105, 110, 119, 129, 138, 153, 167, 186, 189, 190, 197, 198, 202, 211, 214, 215

criminal statutes, 35, 70, 71
culture, 72, 121, 124
cure, 6, 21, 40, 131, 162, 212, 215
curricula, 65, 121, 193

D

data collection, 38, 66, 72, 74, 83, 190, 200, 211, 215
deaths, 31, 39, 190
deficiency, viii, 47, 141, 163, 202, 215
dental care, 102, 142
Department of Health and Human Services, viii, 43, 44, 47, 50, 118, 128, 141, 159, 161, 170, 179, 181, 183, 185, 215, 216
Department of Justice, 35, 47, 70, 71, 128, 203, 215
depression, 22, 27, 110, 137, 172
diabetes, 27, 109, 118, 123
disability, 27, 104, 166, 180
disclosure, 34, 71, 129
discrimination, 2, 3, 4, 5, 20, 22, 28, 29, 30, 33, 34, 35, 49, 51, 68, 71, 77, 105, 112, 114, 122, 124, 129, 130, 132, 167, 179
disease progression, 13, 32, 108, 110, 137
diseases, 27, 111, 153, 163, 180, 192
disorder, 67, 110
distribution, 53, 95, 96, 117, 145, 146, 149, 150, 154, 156, 165, 168
District of Columbia, 85, 88, 135, 148, 152, 157, 158, 162, 165, 209, 211, 214, 215
diversity, 4, 21, 23, 29, 62, 80, 99, 119, 121
doctors, 20, 105, 113, 129, 131, 185
DOJ, 47, 57, 64, 70, 71, 73, 75
DOL, 47, 66, 70, 71, 73, 75
Domestic Policy Council, vii, 7, 49, 79, 82
draft, 142, 185, 202
drug resistance, 98, 123, 204
drug treatment, 9, 17, 18, 57, 132, 142, 148, 153, 163, 171, 198
drugs, 9, 13, 24, 102, 110, 137, 139, 148, 150, 152, 163, 212, 215

E

economic downturn, 9, 62
education, 3, 16, 17, 20, 21, 45, 61, 82, 90, 91, 93, 98, 99, 103, 104, 107, 108, 112, 114, 121, 124, 125, 129, 132, 154, 197, 202

educational institutions, 1, 3, 7, 51
educators, 25, 70, 121
emergency, viii, 10, 60, 106, 130, 137, 138, 153, 161, 170, 171, 172, 185, 193, 194, 196, 198, 211, 214
employment, 28, 33, 70, 103, 104, 105, 129, 132, 203
enforcement, 34, 35, 68, 70, 77, 132
environment, 34, 36, 104, 129
epidemic, viii, 1, 2, 3, 5, 6, 7, 8, 9, 11, 13, 15, 16, 17, 18, 19, 29, 32, 33, 34, 36, 38, 39, 40, 48, 49, 50, 51, 53, 54, 56, 57, 60, 68, 72, 76, 77, 79, 80, 81, 82, 83, 89, 99, 114, 115, 117, 125, 129, 134, 148, 161, 162, 170, 190, 204
equipment, 18, 89, 99, 212
ethnic groups, 56, 123
ethnic minority, 65, 117
ethnicity, 2, 3, 15, 22, 43, 49, 77, 90, 99, 115, 121
evidence, 3, 7, 8, 9, 10, 13, 16, 17, 20, 24, 32, 34, 44, 49, 56, 57, 60, 61, 67, 75, 76, 93, 98, 133, 136, 171, 188, 213, 214
expertise, 25, 26, 37, 132
exposure, 18, 19, 44, 60, 96, 114, 153, 192, 214

F

Fair Housing Act, 34, 179
faith, 1, 2, 7, 8, 24, 50, 51, 70, 72, 82, 91, 112, 119, 152
families, viii, 5, 27, 40, 77, 82, 105, 141, 161, 162, 164, 213
family members, 166, 186, 203
family planning, 17, 26, 152, 192, 214
FDA, 37, 47, 59, 102, 136
fear, 4, 11, 33, 34, 95, 104
federal agency, 186, 211
federal funds, viii, 141, 142, 150, 151, 152, 164
Federal funds, 19, 38, 55, 59
Federal Government, 2, 5, 7, 23, 35, 36, 37, 38, 39, 48, 49, 50, 51, 52, 54, 62, 72, 74, 75, 77, 93, 96, 127, 128
Federal Register, 165, 180, 181
financial, viii, 26, 36, 96, 128, 131, 150, 161, 201, 211
financial resources, 36, 128
fiscal year 2009, 190, 192, 194, 200, 209, 211
flexibility, 36, 213
food, 28, 29, 51, 65, 67, 101
Food and Drug Administration, 37, 47

formula, 72, 74, 145, 146, 147, 148, 149, 150, 151, 154, 155, 156, 157, 158, 161, 164, 165, 167, 168, 169, 178, 181, 191, 209, 211
foundations, 8, 50, 131

G

GAO, 146, 147, 149, 151, 153, 154, 155, 157, 158, 159, 167, 168, 180, 183, 184, 185, 209, 211, 212, 213, 215
gay men, 12, 15, 16, 31, 41, 78, 121
gender identity, 2, 3, 49, 77
geography, 22, 121
Georgia, 42, 83, 88, 108, 135, 158, 174, 204, 205, 209, 212
gonorrhea, 18, 27, 111
governments, 1, 35, 36, 50, 51, 58, 63, 77
grant programs, 142, 164, 186
grants, viii, 26, 72, 74, 118, 132, 141, 145, 146, 147, 148, 149, 150, 151, 152, 153, 154, 156, 158, 159, 161, 164, 165, 169, 170, 178, 180, 184, 186, 190, 194, 198, 201, 205, 213, 215
growth, 113, 169
guidance, 57, 58, 63, 64, 65, 66, 105, 107, 165, 170, 186, 204, 206
guidelines, 23, 24, 25, 27, 36, 43, 44, 55, 60, 61, 63, 64, 65, 70, 94, 136, 147, 152, 190, 193, 206, 211, 216

H

HAART, 44, 46, 47, 89, 136, 137, 183, 188, 203, 212, 215
Health and Human Services, 37, 184
health care, vii, viii, 2, 4, 9, 22, 24, 25, 26, 27, 28, 29, 30, 33, 35, 45, 51, 62, 63, 64, 65, 66, 67, 70, 72, 85, 93, 94, 100, 102, 103, 104, 105, 107, 108, 112, 113, 115, 119, 120, 123, 124, 125, 129, 130, 132, 136, 137, 138, 139, 141, 142, 144, 145, 148, 153, 161, 170, 171, 184, 185, 186, 189, 190, 191, 192, 193, 194, 196, 197, 201, 203, 204, 206, 211, 212, 213, 214
health care costs, vii, viii, 2, 93, 141
health care professionals, 112, 184, 191, 192
health care system, 26, 29, 36, 100, 113, 132, 201
health condition, 4, 21, 23, 62, 109, 110
health education, 20, 61, 91
health information, 62, 122, 129, 130, 154

health insurance, 22, 80, 102, 104, 115, 142, 144, 145, 148, 162
health promotion, 56, 121
Health Resources and Services Administration (HRSA), viii, 37, 141, 170, 184, 186, 203
health services, 40, 110, 145, 202
health status, 4, 8, 22, 30, 123, 162, 204
heart disease, 22, 24, 27, 110, 118
hepatitis, 24, 27, 33, 60, 69, 97, 109, 110, 111, 138, 204, 205
herpes, 18, 27, 44, 111
HHS, viii, 25, 37, 39, 42, 44, 47, 50, 51, 55, 56, 57, 58, 60, 61, 63, 64, 65, 66, 67, 69, 70, 71, 73, 74, 75, 76, 78, 121, 139, 141, 142, 143, 147, 151, 152, 154, 155, 156, 157, 158, 159, 161, 170, 181, 183, 184, 185, 186, 192, 202, 213, 214
highly active antiretroviral therapy (HAART), 89, 188, 203
high-risk populations, 11, 16, 19, 26, 38, 59
Hispanics, 42, 119, 138
history, 6, 26, 99, 154, 194
homelessness, viii, 5, 22, 28, 33, 62, 123, 139, 161, 162, 163, 171, 172, 180
homes, 2, 27, 105, 129
hormone, 26, 102
hospice, 145, 171
House, 5, 7, 49, 85, 142, 147, 155, 157, 163, 168, 179, 181
housing, viii, 4, 5, 17, 21, 23, 25, 28, 33, 45, 51, 52, 62, 63, 64, 65, 67, 80, 84, 100, 101, 102, 103, 104, 105, 108, 115, 130, 132, 136, 161, 162, 163, 164, 165, 166, 167, 168, 169, 170, 171, 172, 179, 180, 181, 201, 202, 203, 206, 207, 213
Housing and Urban Development, 37, 47, 161, 164, 169, 178, 180, 181, 213
HUD, 21, 23, 37, 47, 52, 55, 57, 62, 63, 64, 67, 69, 71, 73, 74, 75, 161, 163, 164, 165, 166, 167, 168, 169, 170, 172, 178, 180, 181
human, vii, viii, 1, 2, 6, 34, 41, 42, 44, 45, 109, 135, 137, 138, 141, 161, 162, 171, 180, 183, 185, 202
human immunodeficiency virus, vii, viii, 1, 2, 6, 41, 42, 44, 45, 109, 135, 137, 138, 141, 161, 162, 180, 183, 185, 202

I

identification, 101, 114, 122, 142, 149, 206

immigrants, 99, 101, 106, 117
immigration, 80, 95, 124
immune system, vii, 2, 6, 111, 162, 172, 212
immunodeficiency, 137, 162, 180
improvements, 4, 22, 68, 162, 172
in transition, 103, 163
incarceration, 13, 64, 101, 104, 123, 130, 139, 202, 203, 204
incidence, 8, 10, 12, 14, 29, 30, 33, 39, 41, 42, 45, 53, 54, 55, 68, 74, 78, 82, 89, 91, 95, 99, 108, 110, 113, 123, 135, 156, 158, 162, 164, 180
income, viii, 4, 22, 46, 54, 70, 82, 103, 128, 141, 142, 144, 148, 162, 164, 166, 167, 180, 186, 201, 212
increased access, 96, 104, 108
Indians, 15, 43, 58, 138
industry, 24, 106
infants, 15, 141, 153, 192
infection, vii, 2, 3, 4, 5, 6, 8, 10, 11, 12, 13, 15, 16, 17, 18, 19, 20, 21, 24, 26, 27, 29, 30, 31, 32, 33, 38, 39, 41, 42, 43, 44, 45, 54, 56, 58, 61, 64, 68, 69, 74, 80, 82, 84, 91, 93, 94, 97, 98, 100, 108, 109, 111, 117, 121, 123, 129, 134, 137, 138, 162, 163, 166, 180, 190, 197, 211, 212, 214
informed consent, 186, 197, 211
infrastructure, 105, 113, 125, 130, 131, 213
initiation, 24, 32, 41, 44, 45, 114, 118
Injection Drug Use/User, 48
inmates, 202, 203, 204, 205
insecurity, 46, 54
institutions, 16, 24, 35, 51, 70, 91, 96, 98, 104
integration, 22, 25, 44, 57, 64, 69, 76, 83, 119
internist, 111
intervention, 44, 132, 137, 141, 145, 152, 191, 201, 202, 205, 213
investment, 5, 36, 40, 82, 123, 131, 132
investments, 3, 4, 5, 10, 19, 25, 36, 39, 49
Iowa, 88, 158, 174, 210, 212
issues, 4, 22, 23, 24, 25, 27, 28, 29, 33, 36, 38, 50, 54, 69, 72, 80, 83, 84, 90, 91, 95, 105, 107, 112, 114, 120, 126, 127, 128, 130, 137, 138, 159, 163, 184, 186, 187, 202

J

job training, 80, 101, 104, 115
jurisdiction, 16, 55, 167, 169, 187, 191, 194
justification, 156, 158, 159

L

languages, 91, 106, 119, 124
Latinos, 3, 13, 15, 22, 29, 30, 32, 33, 42, 53, 56, 57, 67, 68, 69, 84, 115, 117, 118, 119, 123, 138, 188
laws, 16, 34, 35, 56, 70, 71, 77, 93, 97, 149, 186, 187, 197
lead, 26, 29, 50, 51, 53, 67, 68, 102, 110, 111, 125, 192, 205
leadership, 1, 5, 35, 36, 39, 40, 51, 56, 68, 70, 77, 103, 112
learning, 4, 53, 94, 114
legislation, 102, 108, 142, 143, 168, 186, 196
life expectancy, 21, 114, 181
lifetime, 10, 42, 44, 93, 142, 144, 170
literacy, 26, 45
liver, 110, 111
local government, 2, 5, 7, 10, 19, 36, 48, 51, 59, 66, 72, 165, 211
Louisiana, 88, 109, 174, 205, 210, 212

M

magnitude, 5, 68
MAI, 141, 154, 159
majority, 6, 15, 31, 93, 97, 119, 131, 153, 167, 185, 198
man, 91, 94, 104, 106, 107, 110, 119, 120, 121, 123, 124, 128, 129, 131, 132
management, 26, 27, 28, 44, 45, 62, 65, 66, 80, 107, 108, 137, 145, 153, 172, 181, 192, 201, 202, 203, 206, 207, 213
marketing, 20, 57, 61, 89
Marshall Islands, 158, 211, 215
Maryland, 43, 88, 157, 175, 178, 210, 211
materials, 67, 96, 134, 202
matter, iv, 95, 119, 153, 205
media, 20, 35, 60, 70, 89, 93
median, 164, 166, 167, 180, 189
Medicaid, 4, 22, 37, 44, 47, 64, 105, 125, 142, 144, 148, 153, 156, 189, 196, 206, 212, 213, 214
medical history, 102, 130
Medicare, 22, 37, 47, 64, 102, 136, 142, 144, 148, 156, 189, 196, 212, 213, 214
medication, 9, 18, 23, 25, 32, 34, 45, 63, 64, 98, 102, 108, 110, 113, 123, 207
medicine, 112, 113, 114, 119, 131

mental health, 3, 17, 22, 24, 25, 26, 27, 28, 33, 34, 57, 62, 63, 65, 67, 102, 110, 120, 125, 128, 137, 138, 142, 145, 171, 202, 203
mental health professionals, 202
mental illness, 27, 110, 111, 139, 201
messages, 90, 91, 93, 95, 112, 119, 121, 124
messengers, 90, 91, 95
meta-analysis, 42, 45
metropolitan areas, viii, 42, 117, 127, 141, 142, 144, 145, 147, 151, 155, 156, 157, 166, 170, 190
Mexico, 82, 83, 84, 88, 89, 91, 93, 108, 113, 121, 124, 130, 176, 210, 212
Miami, 119, 174, 208
Minneapolis, 82, 83, 84, 93, 95, 117, 125, 175, 208
minorities, 7, 16, 24, 29, 56, 82, 93, 112, 115, 117, 118, 119, 124, 125, 130, 132, 154
misconceptions, 20, 89
Missouri, 88, 175, 210, 212, 215
models, 28, 33, 59, 72, 108, 121, 181, 186, 191
moderators, 83, 134
Montana, 88, 158, 210
morbidity, 27, 29, 30, 94, 109, 132
mortality, 5, 27, 29, 30, 31, 32, 94, 110, 132, 186
mortality rate, 29, 186

N

National Health Service, 25, 26
National HIV/AIDS Strategy, vii, 1, 2, 6, 7, 19, 36, 39, 42, 47, 48, 49, 50, 51, 52, 62, 72, 73, 75, 76, 77, 79, 82, 118, 132, 134, 171, 181
National Institutes of Health, 43, 44, 48, 159, 213
national strategy, 7, 49
National Survey, 14, 44, 45
Native Americans, 84, 99, 117, 119, 201
needy, 21, 22, 23, 52, 62
negotiating, 13, 96
New England, 106, 114, 135, 136, 137, 139
nurses, 20, 25, 26, 113, 114
nutrition, 27, 67, 103, 109, 145

O

Obama, 7, 34, 49, 81, 132, 142, 143, 155, 158
obstacles, 97, 100, 101
Office of National AIDS Policy (ONAP), vii, 5, 7, 49, 79, 134

officials, 7, 49, 73, 74, 91, 135, 184, 187, 188, 193, 194, 195, 196, 197, 198, 199, 200, 202, 203, 205, 206, 207, 212, 213, 214, 215
Oklahoma, 88, 158, 176, 180, 210, 212
operating costs, 166, 167
operations, 40, 136, 142, 155
opportunities, 9, 62, 64, 65, 80, 94, 104, 113, 114, 185, 192, 194
oral health, 108, 109, 145
outreach, 7, 49, 59, 70, 96, 99, 121, 145, 154, 201, 202

P

Pacific, 14, 16, 31, 43, 47, 58, 90, 91, 99, 106, 115, 117, 124, 148
Pacific Islanders, 14, 43, 58, 91, 99, 106, 115, 117
participants, 80, 84, 85, 89, 90, 91, 94, 95, 96, 97, 98, 99, 102, 104, 107, 108, 109, 111, 113, 114, 118, 121, 122, 123, 125, 127, 128, 129, 130, 131, 132, 172, 207
pathogens, 110, 192
penalties, 129, 151
PEP, 18, 60
perinatal, 41, 89, 93, 94, 136, 190
permit, 153, 199, 200
personal stories, 83, 134
persons with disabilities, 163, 166, 180
pharmaceutical, 8, 24, 131, 136, 145, 150
Philadelphia, 106, 177, 179, 205, 208
physicians, 25, 26, 27, 45, 66, 113
platform, 4, 22, 92
pneumonia, 88, 135
policy, 1, 7, 13, 14, 15, 17, 34, 36, 38, 40, 46, 55, 57, 62, 69, 72, 98, 102, 103, 118, 130, 131, 132, 163, 170, 181, 213
policy issues, 7, 17, 72
policy makers, 14, 15, 118, 131, 132
pools, 4, 22
population, 11, 12, 13, 14, 15, 16, 18, 19, 26, 30, 31, 40, 42, 53, 59, 80, 90, 93, 95, 97, 104, 106, 107, 109, 110, 111, 113, 115, 117, 118, 121, 122, 124, 144, 162, 186, 202, 212, 213
poverty, 4, 22, 33, 46, 100, 104, 109, 115, 123, 124, 163, 179
pregnancy, 9, 18, 89
President, v, vii, 1, 2, 5, 6, 38, 47, 48, 50, 72, 76, 79, 80, 81, 82, 83, 132, 141, 142, 155, 156, 157, 163, 164, 168, 169, 179

Presidential Advisory Council on HIV/AIDS, 48, 52, 71, 77, 134
presidential nominating conventions, 34
prisoners, 60, 187, 203, 204, 205, 206, 207
prisons, 64, 91, 96, 132, 137, 139, 202, 203, 205
probability, 17, 18, 89
professionals, 8, 20, 25, 26, 27, 81, 113, 114, 192, 202
progress reports, 39, 73, 213
project, 72, 106, 165, 166, 167, 193, 194, 198, 199, 201, 204, 205, 214
prophylaxis, 18, 19, 44, 60
protection, 34, 168
public education, 3, 11
public health, 3, 8, 10, 16, 34, 35, 39, 46, 54, 56, 65, 68, 70, 71, 74, 77, 83, 91, 95, 121, 128, 132, 139, 152, 153, 185, 192, 204
Public Health Service (PHS) Act, viii, 121, 141, 142, 212, 215
public investment, 19, 22, 130
public policy, 130, 131, 132
public resources, 127, 132
Puerto Rico, 3, 7, 12, 13, 14, 83, 88, 96, 108, 110, 117, 127, 130, 148, 152, 158, 165, 177, 210, 212, 215

Q

quality of life, 9, 26, 89

R

race, 2, 3, 15, 22, 43, 49, 77, 95, 99, 115, 121, 139
radio, 20, 60, 92
reality, 4, 89, 115
recommendations, 7, 26, 40, 49, 50, 52, 55, 56, 57, 58, 60, 66, 69, 71, 73, 74, 79, 80, 82, 83, 85, 86, 89, 94, 96, 98, 100, 101, 102, 108, 111, 113, 117, 121, 126, 130, 132, 134, 152, 163, 168, 179, 186, 189, 190, 193, 194, 196, 197, 211, 212, 214
reform, 22, 102, 108
regulations, 128, 151, 179, 180
Rehabilitation Act, 34, 129
reimburse, 196, 214
remediation, 75, 76
rent, 167, 169, 172
replication, 98, 110

requirements, 38, 72, 74, 102, 127, 128, 153, 158, 164, 200
researchers, 65, 162, 171, 172, 181
resource allocation, 38, 40, 51, 72
resources, viii, 3, 9, 10, 11, 12, 15, 16, 18, 22, 25, 28, 36, 38, 39, 40, 41, 42, 43, 44, 45, 46, 49, 51, 54, 56, 58, 63, 71, 72, 74, 78, 82, 92, 97, 105, 110, 117, 127, 128, 132, 135, 136, 137, 138, 161, 164, 165, 168, 179, 192, 216
response, vii, 1, 2, 6, 7, 8, 9, 11, 19, 24, 25, 29, 33, 36, 37, 39, 40, 48, 49, 50, 54, 74, 76, 77, 79, 90, 103, 118, 137, 153, 168, 170, 171
restrictions, 56, 148
risk factors, 20, 95, 120, 190, 214
risks, 16, 26, 28, 34, 56, 89, 90, 211
RNA, 45, 46
rules, 36, 38, 84, 165
rural areas, 22, 28, 44, 82, 105, 112, 124, 125, 127, 130, 131, 201

S

safety, 29, 62
scaling, 5, 38, 54, 60
school, 20, 33, 35, 61, 65, 70, 90, 91, 93, 96, 113, 121, 129, 131, 154
science, 2, 48, 91, 93, 95, 98, 192
scope, 80, 105, 113
security, 5, 28, 62
selective serotonin reuptake inhibitor, 110, 137
Senate, 142, 155, 157, 164, 185
sentencing, 71, 205
service organizations, 90, 171
service provider, 24, 28, 57, 132, 214
sex, 12, 13, 14, 17, 33, 41, 42, 43, 44, 45, 46, 56, 78, 80, 89, 91, 96, 97, 98, 99, 115, 121, 122, 130, 163
sexual activity, 17, 20, 34, 96, 98, 153
sexual behavior, 18, 42, 97
sexual health, 3, 20
sexual orientation, 2, 3, 49, 77, 80, 82, 93, 114, 124
sexuality, 36, 45, 93
sexually transmitted diseases, 17, 24, 33, 111, 204
sexually transmitted infections, 21, 26, 27, 61, 111
shelter, 29, 171, 201
shortage, 25, 81, 113, 125
small communities, 83

Social Security, 48, 102
social services, 17, 25, 63, 80, 101, 113, 115, 124, 131, 166, 172, 206, 207, 211
social support, 35, 206
social workers, 26, 28, 101
society, 2, 4, 7, 35, 104
software, 200, 215
South Dakota, 88, 159, 210, 212
specialists, 20, 26, 95, 96, 108, 110, 206
SSA, 48, 70, 73, 75
stability, 28, 53, 103
stakeholders, 2, 39, 48, 52, 79, 91, 118, 134
state, viii, 4, 5, 22, 36, 39, 46, 48, 53, 66, 73, 87, 117, 142, 144, 145, 149, 150, 151, 152, 158, 164, 165, 184, 186, 187, 188, 189, 190, 191, 192, 193, 194, 195, 196, 197, 198, 200, 201, 202, 203, 204, 205, 206, 207, 211, 212, 213, 214, 215
states, viii, 14, 34, 41, 43, 45, 57, 89, 127, 135, 136, 138, 141, 142, 145, 146, 148, 149, 150, 151, 152, 155, 157, 158, 161, 162, 164, 165, 170, 180, 181, 184, 185, 186, 188, 190, 191, 194, 196, 197, 200, 201, 202, 203, 204, 205, 206, 211, 212, 213, 214, 215
statistics, 92, 138, 145, 156, 158
statutes, 46, 71
statutory authority, viii, 36, 141
sterile, 18, 89
stigma, 2, 3, 4, 5, 20, 29, 30, 33, 34, 35, 46, 49, 51, 68, 77, 95, 96, 105, 109, 118, 120, 124, 125, 129, 130, 132, 137, 139, 201
stress, 107, 110, 137, 172
substance abuse, 3, 24, 25, 26, 27, 48, 57, 61, 62, 63, 65, 98, 102, 110, 128, 138, 142, 145, 159, 192, 194, 201, 202, 203, 204, 213, 214
substance use, 16, 17, 27, 33, 67, 69, 115, 120, 121, 123
support services, viii, 63, 82, 100, 105, 141, 142, 145, 148, 149, 170, 181, 203, 206, 213
suppression, 33, 46
surveillance, 15, 16, 18, 19, 38, 40, 41, 42, 43, 45, 46, 53, 56, 57, 58, 59, 62, 78, 80, 90, 99, 135, 138, 139, 179, 186, 187, 190, 198, 199, 211, 214, 215
survival, 30, 44, 89, 110, 114, 122, 212, 215
survival rate, 30, 89, 114, 212, 215
survivors, 109, 131, 132
symptoms, 26, 110, 203
syndrome, viii, 141, 162, 163, 180, 202, 215
syphilis, 18, 27, 42, 46, 111, 138

T

target, 16, 18, 25, 38, 55, 56, 76, 90, 98, 99, 120, 121, 128, 186
teachers, 91, 93
technical assistance, 69, 71, 76, 112, 166, 193, 197, 201
technical comments, 185, 202
technology, 62, 125, 130, 154
temporary housing, 170, 172
territorial, 5, 35, 36
territory, 50, 87, 88, 179
testing, viii, 6, 8, 24, 25, 33, 34, 53, 54, 55, 63, 68, 70, 94, 95, 96, 99, 128, 130, 136, 138, 143, 145, 148, 149, 152, 183, 184, 185, 186, 187, 188, 189, 190, 191, 193, 194, 195, 196, 197, 198, 202, 203, 205, 211, 212, 213, 214, 215, 216
TGA, 144, 145, 147, 156, 157
therapy, 9, 17, 18, 19, 21, 22, 23, 25, 28, 32, 33, 41, 43, 44, 45, 76, 89, 98, 110, 114, 118, 124, 137, 145, 171, 183, 188, 203, 213, 215
training, 24, 25, 26, 65, 66, 67, 95, 103, 104, 106, 112, 113, 114, 184, 186, 191, 192, 193, 197, 201, 213
training programs, 65, 114, 193, 213
transition period, 141, 146, 149, 151, 157, 158
translation, 84, 106, 202
transmission, viii, 2, 3, 5, 6, 8, 9, 11, 13, 15, 17, 18, 20, 26, 29, 32, 34, 35, 40, 41, 42, 43, 44, 45, 46, 52, 53, 57, 61, 70, 77, 78, 80, 89, 93, 94, 97, 98, 110, 135, 136, 154, 183, 185, 190
transportation, 22, 27, 28, 65, 67, 80, 84, 101, 105, 115, 130, 131, 145, 185, 201, 202
transportation infrastructure, 105
trauma, 110, 120, 137
treatment, vii, 2, 3, 4, 6, 9, 16, 18, 19, 21, 22, 23, 24, 25, 26, 27, 28, 30, 33, 34, 45, 54, 56, 57, 60, 61, 62, 63, 64, 65, 66, 67, 89, 92, 94, 97, 98, 100, 102, 103, 108, 109, 110, 111, 113, 114, 120, 123, 127, 128, 129, 130, 132, 135, 136, 137, 138, 142, 144, 145, 149, 154, 159, 168, 170, 171, 172, 181, 188, 189, 192, 194, 202, 203, 205, 206, 213
tuberculosis, 24, 110, 111, 204

U

uninsured, viii, 4, 9, 22, 112, 141, 142, 152, 186, 189
urban, 15, 42, 43, 44, 80, 103, 105, 106, 112, 119, 123, 124, 125, 141, 144, 170, 201
urban areas, 15, 103, 105, 106, 119, 124, 125, 141, 144, 170
USA, 41, 43, 136, 138, 212

V

violence, 13, 28, 120, 129
vision, 3, 49
vulnerability, 13, 32

W

waiver, 148, 150, 167
Washington, 1, 32, 83, 88, 96, 97, 103, 104, 105, 121, 131, 173, 177, 209, 210, 212, 213, 215, 216
wealth, 1, 6
wellness, 20, 115
White House, v, vii, 1, 5, 7, 49, 50, 79, 81, 82, 83, 84, 85, 159
Wisconsin, 88, 158, 178, 205, 210, 212
workers, 66, 70, 113, 120, 186
workforce, 25, 27, 62, 66, 104, 106, 112, 113, 128, 136, 138

Y

young adults, 7, 82
young people, 20, 91, 93, 136